AF333788

Assessment of Urinary Sediment by Electron Microscopy

Applications in Renal Disease

Assessment of Urinary Sediment by Electron Microscopy

Applications in Renal Disease

Anil K. Mandal, M.B.B.S., F.A.C.P.

Co-Chief of Nephrology
and Professor of Medicine
Wright State University
and Chief of Nephrology
Veterans Administration Medical Center
Dayton, Ohio

Plenum Medical Book Company
New York and London

Library of Congress Cataloging in Publication Data

Mandal, Anil K.
    Assessment of urinary sediment by electron microscopy.

    Includes bibliographies and index.
    1. Kidneys — Diseases — Diagnosis. 2. Urine — Examination. 3. Electron microscope,
Transmission. I. Mookerjee, Basab K. II. Title. [DNLM: 1. Kidney Diseases — diagnosis. 2.
Microscopy, Electron — methods. 3. Urine — analysis. QY 185 M271a]
RC904.M325   1987   616.6′107′58   87-14153
ISBN 0-306-42521-1

This book is dedicated to those friends whose benevolence and compassion have reinforced my perseverance in the pursuit of many ventures, especially

Sheldon C. Sommers, M.D., *New York, New York*
Carl M. Kjellstrand, M.D., *Stockholm, Sweden*
Vincent W. Dennis, M.D., *Durham, North Carolina*
J. Charles Jennette, M.D., *Chapel Hill, North Carolina*
William M. Bennett, M.D., *Portland, Oregon*
Richard D. Bell, Ph.D., *Chicago, Illinois*
Robert W. Schrier, M.D., *Denver, Colorado*
John D. Conger, M.D., *Denver, Colorado*
Kim Solez, M.D., *Edmonton, Canada*
James B. Hudson, M.D., *Augusta, Georgia*
Dinko Susic, M.D., *Belgrade, Yugoslavia*
and
Krishan K. Malhotra, M.D., *New Delhi, India*

Special thanks to H. Verdain Barnes, M.D., Professor and Chair, Department of Medicine, School of Medicine, Wright State University, and Mr. Alan Harper, Director, Veterans Administration Medical Center, Dayton, Ohio, for their support in my continuing ventures.

Foreword

Anil K. Mandal, M.D., is one of the trailblazers in the use of the transmission electron microscope in the study of the urinary sediment.

In this book, he reviews his extensive efforts to tie his vast clinical experience to his elegant basic research with the electron microscope. The pictures are comprehensive, and the clinical correlates are nicely outlined in tables and text.

It may astonish some readers that a book for fellows and clinical nephrologists has been written on the use of the transmission electron microscope in the study of urine. Some may view this as a sophisticated research instrument. I, however, applaud the effort. So many discoveries and advances in basic science lie unutilized because clinicians are not aware of the tools available or have little instruction in their use. Maybe that is the reason why so many tests have come and gone, have been found useless and dropped, or have simply been abandoned after being judged too complicated—some because they were, others because they were never applied and interpreted properly. The whole field of research seems to be pulling ahead and away from clinical medicine. Therefore, an effort like this one, which rapidly and clearly tries to introduce an advanced research examination technique into clinical medicine, is worthy of admiration and support.

The cells, fragments of cells, and their end products that are seen in the urine ought to reflect what goes on in the kidney. Depressingly, though, this prediction is not being borne out by analyses of urinary sediment by ordinary light microscopy. In the old days, when disease categorization was simpler, this technique was extensively used, but now it simply has not kept pace with the increasingly sophisticated classifications based on renal biopsy. Electron microscopy, which takes our observations down to the subcellular level, should be a more useful tool, and one's first impression upon studying Dr. Mandal's work is that it is. In any case, it is now available for independent investigation and clinical trials. The ultimate extent of its success and clinical utility cannot be known. Time will tell, but one wishes it well. We do need better noninvasive diagnostic methods to diagnose what goes on in the kidney and to follow changes in renal morphology.

Carl M. Kjellstrand, M.D.
Karolinska Hospital
Stockholm, Sweden

Preface

In my rounds, whether in general internal medicine or in nephrology, I frequently ask team members, "Have you looked at the urinary sediment?" The answer often is "No." It is a curious phenomenon that physicians promptly order and review chest X rays, abdominal films, or even CAT scans of the kidneys but frequently do not examine the urinary sediment. When it comes to urinalysis in the course of a patient work-up, most individuals only glance at the laboratory slip. This practice is of little consequence in a patient without renal disease; however, it could lead to a misdiagnosis in severe renal disease. Indeed, I have successfully treated a patient with rapidly progressive glomerulonephritis who was initially sent for urological evaluation because of a microscopic hematuria. The finding of only a red blood cell cast during careful examination of a urinary sediment in the presence of 3^+ proteinuria facilitated the correct diagnosis.

Urine examination dates from the fourteenth century; however, scientific examination of the urine began in the early years of the eighteenth century. Lorenzo Bellini (1643–1704) was apparently the first to discover the importance of urine examination. According to Bellini, urine was composed of water, salt, and tasteless earth or tartar.[1] This observation was followed by a better understanding of the characteristics of urine, such as its specific gravity and urea and glucose content. In 1801, Jarrold described a method of testing for albumin in the urine.[1]

The next epoch-making step in urinalysis was made by Prout, in 1820. He emphasized the scientific basis for the examination of urine and demonstrated its great value in the diagnosis of disease.[1] In the same era, Richard Bright, from Guy's Hospital in London, established for the first time the relationship between albuminuria and kidney disease. His name has in the past been associated with kidney diseases, usually various glomerulonephritides, that were often grouped under the name Bright's disease.

Although the English microscopist Robert Hooke had examined urinary sediment using a microscope as early as 1665,[2] the microscopic study of urinary sediment did not become really popular until the nineteenth century. Yet the practice of microscopic examination of the urine never attained the momentum of such other techniques as ultrasound of the kidneys. This may be attributed to two reasons: (1) The technique requires some skill in the preparation of specimens and the interpretation of the findings, and (2) the limited resolution of the light microscope, whether phase contrast or polarizing, does not clearly delineate the morphology of the sediment components. These hindrances tended to diminish the enthusiasm of the observer and were probably responsible for the decline in the technique's popularity.

For the last decade, urinary sediment has been studied by electron microscopy. Immunofluorescence techniques have been less frequently used in the study of urinary sediment, and therefore there is little information in this area. Among the electron microscopy studies, the scanning technique has been used mostly to investigate the formation and composition of urinary casts. Transmission electron microscopy (TEM) has been used mainly to examine amyloid fibrils in urinary sediment. From these limited observations, it has, in the past, been difficult to validate the general usefulness of this technique in urinary sediment studies.

This author has used TEM to examine urinary sediments from patients with a variety of renal diseases. The high resolution of TEM permits delineation of the composition of the casts, identifies different cell types (i.e., tubule cells versus urinary tract cells), and reveals the severity of changes in the tubule cells and the presence of structures of clinical significance, such as myeloid bodies, fibrin, and amyloid fibrils.

The use of TEM for the study of urinary sediment is an important technological advancement in the practice of medicine. Thus, TEM of urinary sediment can be valuable in diagnosing and managing patients with acute renal failure in whom renal biopsy is risky. Furthermore, a TEM laboratory with one experienced technician can handle a large volume of specimens (5–6 a day) at a reasonable cost ($50–$75 a specimen), making this test attractive for clinical purposes as well as for research. Therefore, it seems reasonable to hope that frequent use of TEM in urinary sediment analysis may point up the value of a complete examination of the urinary sediment and improve the position of urinalysis relative to other diagnostic tests for renal disease.

This book emphasizes the feasibility and practicality of TEM in the examination of urinary sediment. For the sake of familiarity, and to preserve tradition, the results of light microscopy of urinary sediment are presented, albeit sparsely. Although the value of urinary sediment studies is highlighted, other tests are described briefly in some chapters to help the reader synthesize the findings that support the final diagnosis of a renal disease. An outline of the management plan is presented at the end of a chapter, as required. It is hoped that this book will be useful to all involved in the care of patients with renal disease.

Anil K. Mandal

Dayton, Ohio

REFERENCES

1. Wellcome HS: *The evolution of urinalysis; an historical sketch of the clinical examination of urine.* London, Burroughs Wellcome & Company, 1911, pp 247–266.
2. Hatcher J: Quackery, fraud, and scientific method: The history of urine testing. *Nurs Mirror* 1976; 142:65–66.

Acknowledgments

This book is a product of studies at the Augusta Veterans Administration Medical Center Transmission Electron Microscopy Laboratory, which is partly supported by the Medical Research Service of the Veterans Administration. It is enhanced by the high-quality electron micrographs, which are products of the dedicated effort of the entire staff of the Medical Media Service of the Veterans Administration Medical Center, headed by Thomas W. Lanier. Since the book is a by-product of research on acute renal failure, it is my pleasure to convey heartfelt thanks to Mrs. Nancy Parks, Administrative Officer, and her staff at the Research Service of the Medical Center for their pleasant and stimulating attitudes. Finally, it has been a most enjoyable experience sharing the transmission electron microscopy unit with a charming personality, Dr. Nayereh Khankhanian, of the Department of Pathology.

I am grateful to my colleagues, Drs. P. Allen Bowen, II, and Allan H. Sklar, for their interest and efforts in providing me with urine samples. I gratefully acknowledge the assistance provided by George N. Mize of the Department of Pharmacy, Veterans Administration Medical Center, in the study of aminoglycoside nephrotoxicity. I am especially thankful to Mrs. Barbara B. Price for her keen and sincere secretarial help in preparing this book, and also to Miss Susan Trivelpiece and Miss Donna Tumm for their secretarial assistance. Despite her late appearance, my research assistant, Christiana E. Hall, B.S., was most helpful in the final organization of the manuscript, and I am grateful for her assistance. Finally, I must express my appreciation to Janice Stern of Plenum for encouraging me to write this book and for providing help in accomplishing the task.

A.K.M.

Contents

3   Acute Renal Failure

4   Aminoglycoside Nephrotoxicity

5   Bacteriuria and Pyuria

Basab K. Mookerjee, M.D., and Saleem Khan, M.D.

6 Renal Transplant Rejection

7 Hepatorenal Syndrome

8 Neoplasms and the Kidney

9 Glomerular Disease

10 Acute and Chronic Interstitial Nephritis

1

The Microscopy of Urine

The validity of routine microscopy of urinary sediments has been controversial, with many pathologists reporting that microscopy of the urine, the way it is performed, is practically useless except for the bacteriological work-up.[1] Valenstein and Koepke[2] have cautiously recommended that microscopy be reserved for urine specimens with abnormal physicochemical characteristics. By and large, it is true that urine microscopy adds little to the diagnosis when the results of the chemical examination, especially for protein and blood, are negative. Donauer[3] compared results by dipstick and by microscopy in 13,479 urine specimens. He found that 12% of the specimens with negative chemistry findings were positive microscopically, whereas 54.6% of the specimens with a positive test for albumin were positive microscopically. Though arguments against routine urine microscopy may be valid in terms of cost-effective analysis, it would be difficult to measure the price of one misdiagnosis for the lack of it. Furthermore, the usefulness of urine microscopy is enhanced by the proper collection of samples and by using suitable techniques to examine them.

In 1820, "Osborne had stated that much uncertainty and consequent mistrust of observations on the urine arose from the carelessness with which these observations were made. The physician one day examines urine which has been just passed, the next day, he examines urine which has lain in the laboratory for several hours. At one time, morning urine is examined, at another time, urine which has been produced after a drink, is examined."[4] Osborne was absolutely right in his statement. To ascertain whether urinary changes had been produced by a renal disease, rather than by diuresis, the urine should always be obtained and examined under the same circumstances.

Urine microscopy requires more interest, care, and skill than time and money. I have found that lack of interest in urine microscopy is largely the result

1

of the physician's inexperience. Most urinary sediment constituents, such as hyaline casts, finely granular casts, and red blood cells (RBC) or white blood cells (WBC) in unstained wet preparation, have the same optical density as water. Because of this low optical density, it is difficult to examine these structures by conventional light microscopy (LM) and to interpret findings correctly. Light micrographs of urinary sediment for the purpose of demonstration are even more difficult to interpret. Such difficulties are frustrating and lead physicians to believe that urinary sediment examination is not worth the time and that the examination should be done by technicians. Though this may be true, better LM technique can make the structures in the sediment easily visible and interpretable.

COLLECTION OF SAMPLES

Because night urine is concentrated, and thus more acid, first voided morning urine is always preferred for analysis. Formed elements are more likely to be found in a concentrated urine than in a dilute urine. Similarly, urinary casts are found more frequently in an acid urine than in an alkaline urine. The freshly voided specimen should be allowed to cool for a few minutes before it is centrifuged, since it has been shown that sediment forms better in a cool specimen than in a warm one. Also, sediment forms better in a nonturbid urine than in a turbid urine. Turbidity of urine may be the result of an alkaline pH or the presence of large amounts of phosphates and/or large numbers of pus cells or bacteria.

After a urine sample has been collected, its color, which can be quite informative, should be noted. The following list of colors may indicate the underlying condition:

Color of urine:	Condition:
Red	Hematuria (blood), hemoglobinuria (hemoglobin), beeturia (excessive consumption of beet), myoglobinuria (myoglobin)
Purple	Presence of porphyrin (upon standing)
Brown or yellow-brown	Presence of bilirubin, quinine, phenacetin
Orange or reddish orange	Presence of Gantrisin, rifampin, Pyridium, azulfidine
Black	Melanoma (presence of melanin), alcaptonuria (presence of homogentisic acid)
Blue	Methemoglobinemia (presence of methyline blue)
Cream	Filariasis (a tropical disease)

As mentioned earlier, urine should be examined within a few minutes of collection. If for some reason an immediate examination is not possible, the container should be capped and refrigerated to minimize bacterial overgrowth and the conversion of urea into ammonia, since ammonia (NH_3) will alkalinize the urine and dissolve formed elements.

If the urine on void is turbid and its pH is alkaline, a few drops of 10% acetic acid should be added to lower the pH. If the turbidity is the result of the presence of phosphates, the urine will clear upon acidification; if the turbidity is the result of the presence of WBC, the urine will become more turbid upon acidification.

PREPARATION FOR CENTRIFUGATION

Ten milliliters of urine is poured from the urine container into a conical clear plastic tube (15 ml), and its pH is checked by the dipstick method. If the pH is 6 or above, it is wise to acidify the urine with a few drops of acetic acid before centrifugation. In the case of dilute urine, it is preferable to centrifuge three or four tubes of 10 ml of urine each to ensure adequate sediment formation. The tubes are placed in a table top centrifuge and centrifuged at 1,500–3,000 revolutions per minute (rpm) for 10 min. While waiting for the sediment to precipitate, it is useful to determine the urine's chemical characteristics using a dipstick. In the absence of proteinuria, casts are unlikely to be found, irrespective of the method used. If the urine is positive for blood, the urine must be examined under the microscope to determine if RBC are present. After 10 min of centrifugation, the tubes are examined for sediment. If the sediment is inadequate, further centrifugation generally will not increase sediment volume. Two tubes containing adequate amounts of sediment are chosen; one is used for LM, the other for transmission electron microscopy (TEM).

FIXATION, STAINING, AND MICROSCOPY

Fixation

The supernatant is pipetted gently from each tube, leaving the sediment undisturbed. For LM, no fixation is necessary. For TEM, the sediment is resuspended in a 4% glutaraldehyde (pH 7.4) and 10% formalin (7:3) in a phosphate buffer and recentrifuged for uniform fixation (see the following section for details).

For light microscopy, the sediment is mixed with the remaining urine, a drop of the mixture is placed on a glass slide, cover slipped, and examined through a bright light microscope. To the remaining sediment, a drop of toluidine blue and basic fuchsin (epoxy tissue stain) (Electron Microscopy Sciences, Fort Washington, PA) is introduced and mixed thoroughly by pipette. The mixture is incubated for 5 min to ensure thorough staining of the material. A drop of the stained specimen is placed on a glass slide and cover slipped. The cover slip flattens the drop to a thin liquid film, which facilitates good optical resolution.

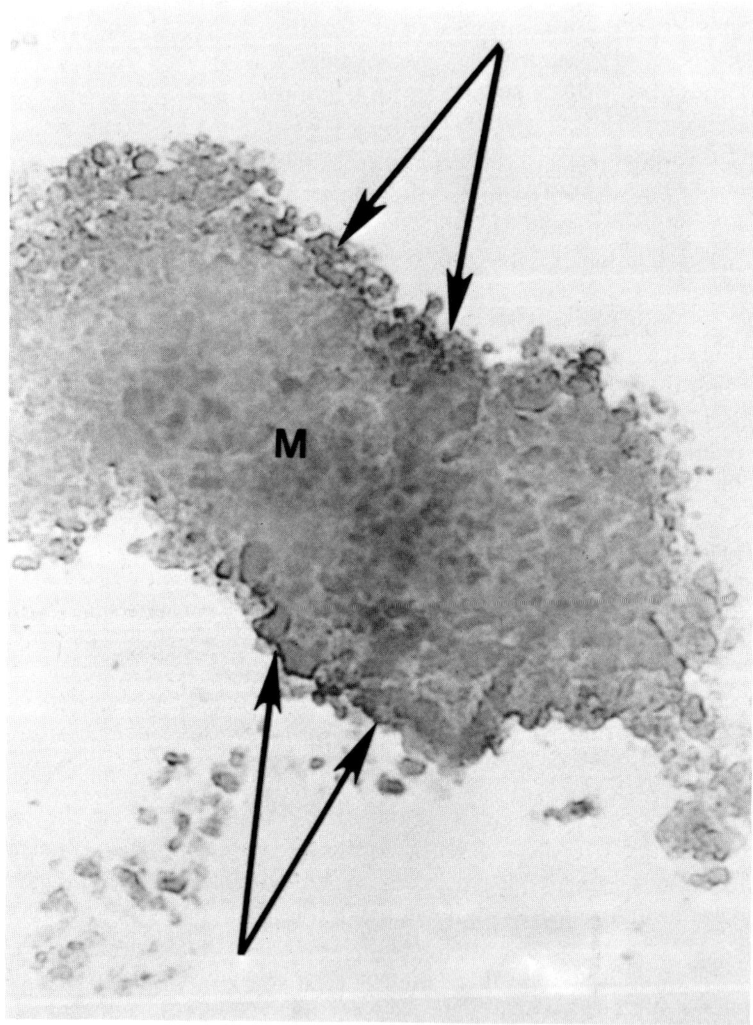

Figure 1-1.   A light micrograph of a red blood cell cast in an unstained wet preparation. The dark, clear areas are membrane-bound vesicles (double arrows), which adhere to the protein matrix (M) ($\times 400$).

As mentioned earlier, because of the low density of casts, and/or the presence of RBC or WBC, it is difficult to see these structures under bright light, but by partially closing the diaphragm, they can be seen.

Brody, Webster, and Kark[5] have shown that phase-contrast microscopy permits visualization of transparent objects without loss of definition. "Not only are the hyaline casts clearly visible, but maximum definition is not sacrificed and is available for other elements of the sediment. With the vastly improved definition by phase contrast, RBCs either free or in a cast are easily distinguished. Recognition of WBC is improved because their lobulated nucleus is usually visible and they can thus be more readily distinguished from the eccentrically placed, round nucleus of epithelial cells. If the urine is acidified this difference is even more striking. Bacteria appear much more dramatically."

Staining

Though phase-contrast microscopy is better than bright field microscopy, staining the sediment with epoxy tissue stain will obviate the need for it. This stain absorbs light and casts are easily seen (Figs. 1-1–1-3). It also stains epithelial

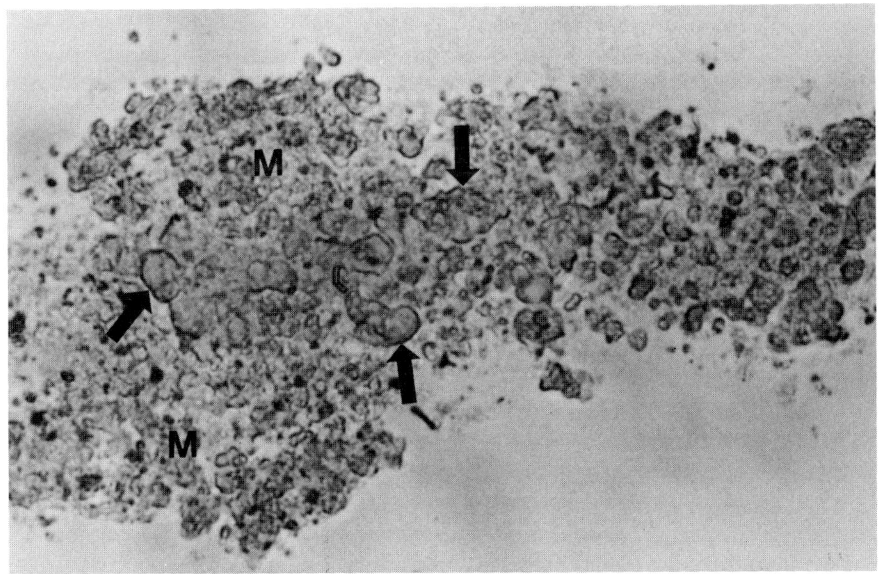

Figure 1-2. A light micrograph of the cast in Figure 1-1 as a stained wet preparation. Membrane-bound vesicles (arrows), which are remnants of RBC, and the matrix of the cast (M) are discernible (epoxy tissue stain, ×400).

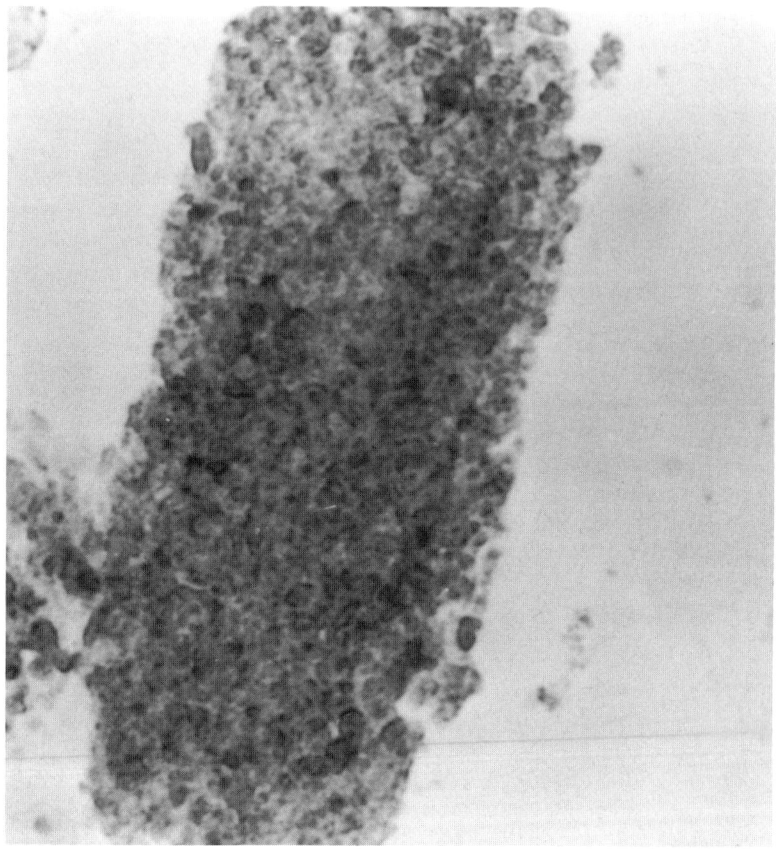

Figure 1-3. A light micrograph of a coarsely granular cast in a stained preparation. Small membrane-bound vesicles and the fibrillar network of the case are discernible (epoxy tissue stain, ×400).

cells (Fig. 1-4), but the cytoplasm does not stain well. The nuclei of WBC and RBC do not stain and are thereby distinguished from epithelial cells. As an alternative, 1% methylene blue can be used. Methylene blue stains the nuclei of WBC so they can be clearly distinguished from epithelial cells.

When the type of WBC is in doubt (neutrophil or eosinophil), a portion of the sediment in a third tube should be smeared on a glass slide and dried over a hot plate at low temperature. The slide can then be stained in a Hemastainer Automatic Slide Stainer (Smith, Kline Co., Wayne, PA, 19087), or manually. In manual staining, the slide is fixed in absolute methanol for a few seconds, stained with Wright stain for 2 min, and washed with phosphate buffer for 5

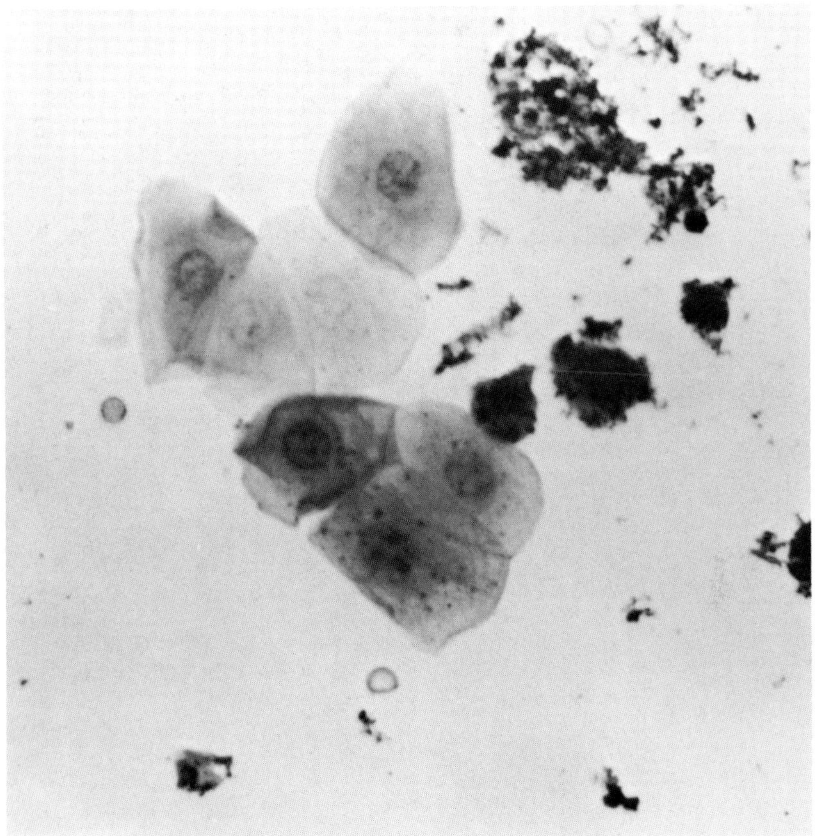

Figure 1-4.   A light micrograph shows clusters of epithelial cells, some of which stain better than others. Nuclei are clearly discernible, but cytoplasmic constituents cannot be identified (epoxy tissue stain, ×400).

min. After rinsing with deionized water, a differential count of the total number of WBC is made (Figs. 1-5 and 1-6).

Physicians often describe any epithelial cell seen under LM as a renal tubule epithelial cell. The author, who could not confirm this description, cautions that LM of urinary sediment, even after staining (Fig. 1-4), does not distinguish between types of epithelial cells, whether tubule epithelial cells or squamous (transitional) epithelial cells. Schumann has stated that bright field microscopy is useful for the early detection and preliminary evaluation of hematuria, leukocyturia, and urinary tract infections. However, the following urine sediment findings are difficult, if not "risky," to interpret using unstained bright field

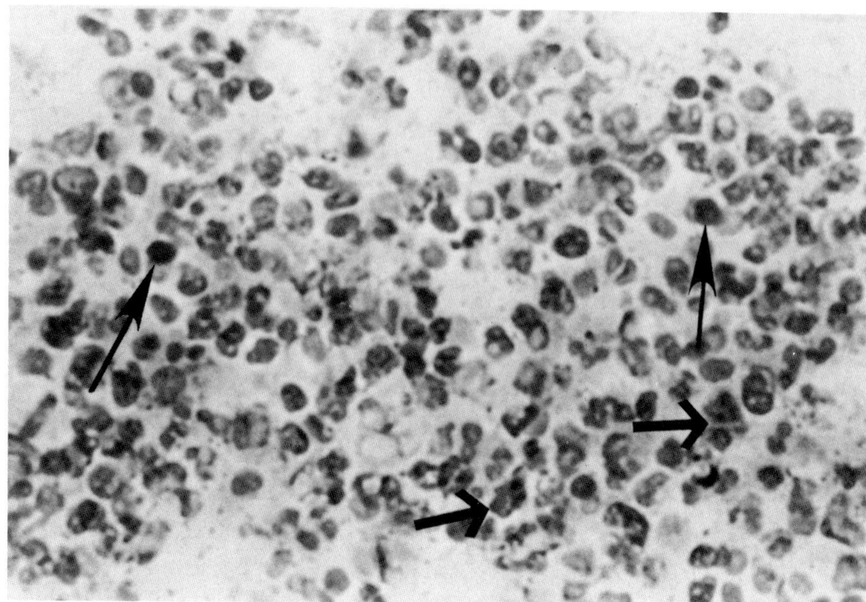

Figure 1-5. This urinary sediment shows numerous cells. These cells include neutrophilic leukocytes (thick arrows) and lymphocytes (thin arrows) (from a patient with anuric acute renal failure) (Wright stain, × 1,000).

microscopy. These include mononuclear cells (lymphocytes, plasma cells, eosinophils), renal tubular epithelial cells, and renal epithelial fragments.[6] As will be seen later, LM of thick (plastic) sections can readily distinguish tubule epithelial cells from transitional epithelial cells.

No matter how thorough or meticulous the LM technique, whether by phase-contrast or polarized light, the urinary sediment study is only complete by TEM.

Transmission Electron Microscopy

Most of the earlier electron microscopy studies were by scanning electron microscopy (SEM) (to be discussed later), but there were occasional reports of urinary sediments demonstrating amyloid fibrils[7] or myeloid bodies in Fabry's disease by TEM.[8] Since information on TEM study of urinary sediment was meager, the author had first to device a suitable technique. The idea of the study of urinary sediment by TEM developed from the problems in determining the morphological changes in the kidney in acute renal failure (ARF). In clinical practice, ARF is often equated with acute tubular necrosis (ATN), even when there is no histological evidence for the latter. Since most patients with ARF are very ill, renal biopsy is not feasible. It is, however, essential to obtain

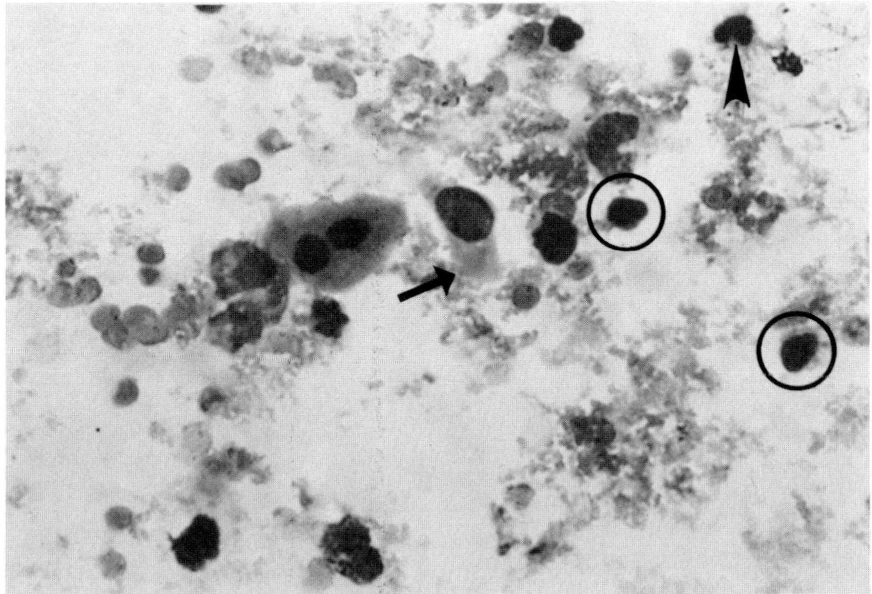

Figure 1-6. This urinary sediment shows a plasma cell (arrow), lymphocytes (circles), and a neutrophilic leukocyte (arrowhead). The prominent binucleated cell is either a uroepithelial cell or a plasma cell (from a patient with stage III myeloma, sepsis, and acute renal failure) (Wright stain, ×1,000).

information on the morphological changes in the kidneys, which can aid in the prognosis and guide the nephrologist in long-term management. It was conceived that TEM of urinary sediment might be a useful, yet noninvasive approach in demonstrating renal morphology in ARF.

Initially, specimens were fixed in 4% glutaraldehyde in phosphate buffer (pH 7.4). Pellets were obtained, but they were so friable that they broke during dehydration in alcohol and several specimens were thus lost. The use of a glutaraldehyde–formalin mixture* in sediment fixation has solved the problem. The use of glutaraldehyde-formalin has certain advantages over the use of glu-taraldehyde alone. These are pellet formation is improved and the pellet is less friable so that it does not break during processing.

After the sediment is formed in the 15-ml tube, the supernatant is pipetted out and discarded; 2–3 ml of glutaraldehyde–formalin mixture are poured into the tube, and the sediment is mixed with the fixative; and the tube containing the sediment and the fixative is centrifuged for 5 min to ensure uniform sediment fixation. The tube is then refrigerated overnight to promote good pellet formation

---

* Glutaraldehyde–formalin mixture: 4% glutaraldehyde and 10% formalin in a ratio of 7:3.

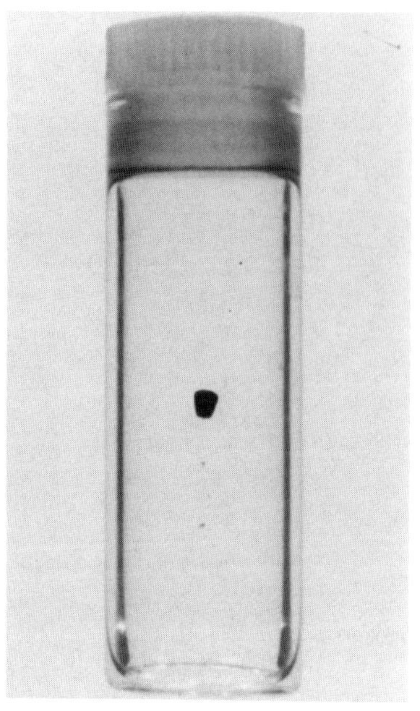

Figure 1-7.   A urinary sediment pellet in the center of the tube.

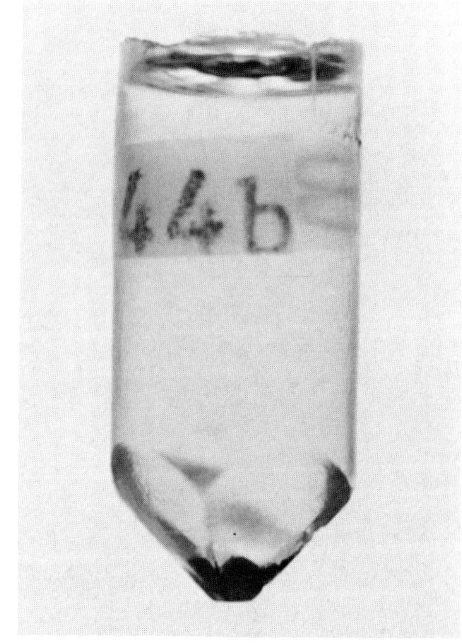

Figure 1-8.   Dark urinary sediment at the conical tip of the block.

(Fig. 1-7). The following morning, the pellet is rinsed and stored in 0.1 ml of cacodylate buffer until osmium fixation and dehydration. The sample is postfixed in 2% osmium in cacodylate buffer for 1 to 2 hr at 10° C. It is then rinsed with distilled water three times, 10 min each rinse, and dehydrated in 30, 50, 70, and 95% ethanol propylene oxide (10 min each). Fresh Spurr* (low-viscosity embedding media, Electron Microscopy Sciences, Fort Washington, PA) is added to the sample and allowed to penetrate overnight in a shaker. The following day, the sample is embedded in polyethylene capsules (size 00; Electron Microscopy Sciences) using fresh Spurr. The sample is then allowed to polymerize at 70°C in an oven for 16 hr. This processing is similar to that of tissue samples. The capsule with the urinary sediment embedded in Spurr is called a block (Fig. 1-8). Thick sections (0.5 μ) are cut from the blocks, using the Sorvall (Du-Pont) Ultramicrotome, and stained with epoxy tissue stain. This epoxy tissue stain (paragon 1301), as described by Spurlock, Skinner, and Kattine,[9] contains toluidine blue and basic fuchsin. The stain penetrates the plastic and stains the urinary sediment. The cellular details of the stained sediment can easily be

* For a description, see A.R. Spurr, *J. Ultrastruct. Res* 26:31–42, 1969.

observed; polychromatic staining can subsequently be obtained by flooding the thick plastic section with more paragon 1301. Thick sections are examined by LM to select areas for thin sectioning (Figs. 1-9–1-11). Thin sections (300Å) are cut with a Sorvall (Du-Pont) Ultramicrotome; they are then mounted on copper grids and stained with uranyl acetate (UA) in 50% ethanol and lead citrate (LC). These grids are examined using JEOL 100 cx electron microscope at 60 KV. After the sections are reviewed, important findings are searched for and photographed. From the negatives, 8 × 10-inch prints are made and the findings are analyzed in detail.

Transmission Electron Microscopy Study of Urinary Sediment

The contributions of TEM study of urinary sediments will be described in detail in later chapters. Briefly, they are as follows:

1. Transmission electron microscopy has unequivocally distinguished renal tubule epithelial cells from transitional epithelial cells or epithelial cells

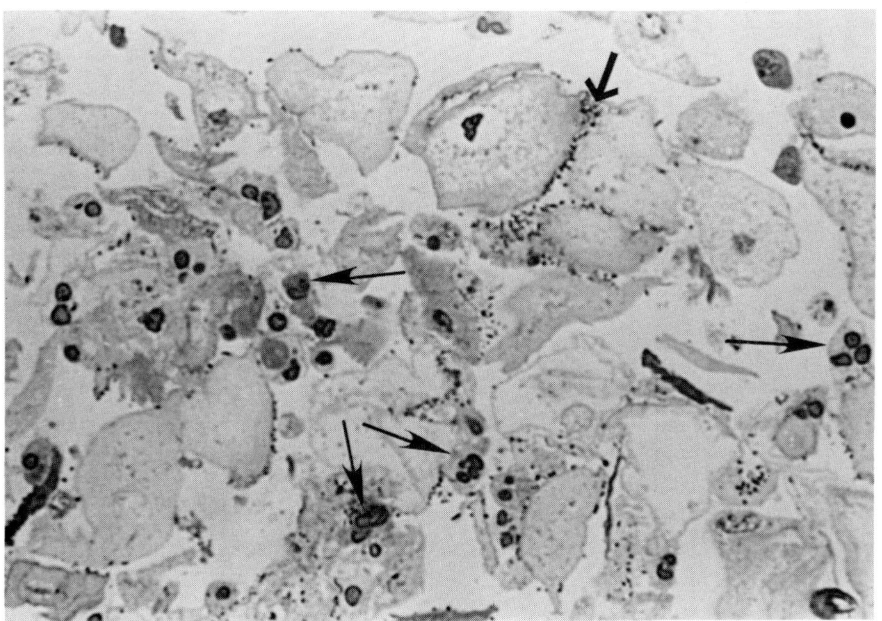

Figure 1-9. Transitional epithelial cells can be seen in this thick-section light micrograph. Note the interdigitating villi (thick arrow) between the cells; the small nuclei; and the pale cytoplasm, which contains few intracellular bodies. Several neutrophilic leukocytes (thin arrows) are clearly identifiable (this urinary sediment was obtained from a patient with a urinary tract infection) (epoxy tissue stain, ×400).

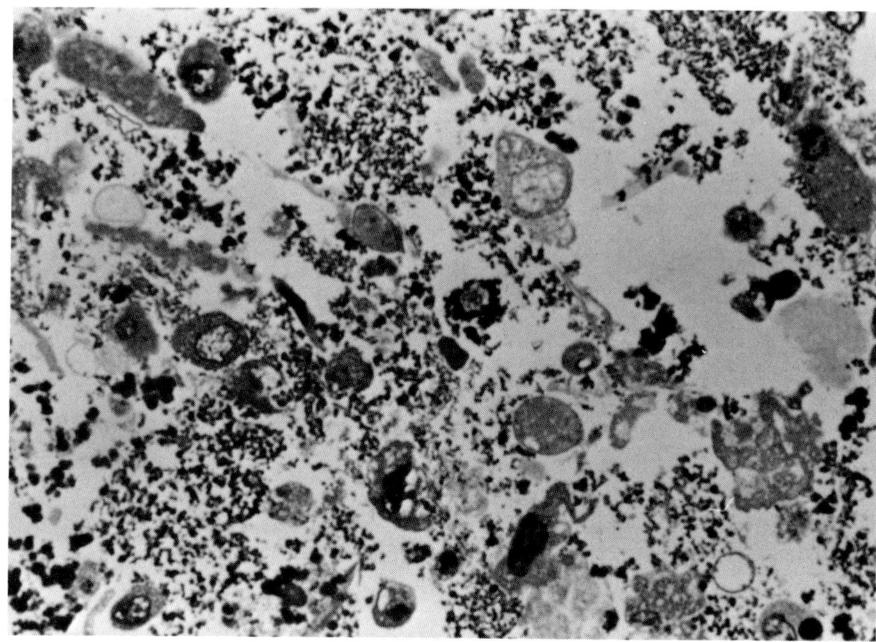

Figure 1-10.   In this thick-section light micrograph (0.5 μ), from the block of urinary sediment, are seen many cells that differ greatly from those seen in Fig. 1-9. The nuclei are large and the cytoplasm of the cell is dark; the cells appear rich in intracellular constituents. Among the cells, dark necrotic material is seen (this urinary sediment was obtained from a patient with ARF). The renal biopsy showed an atheroembolic disorder and focal cortical infarcts) (epoxy tissue stain, ×200).

of the urinary tract. Urinary cells are considered to be of renal tubule origin if they contain abundant cytoplasmic organelles, in particular, mitochondria, microvilli, and endoplasmic reticula (Fig. 1-12). These features are not characteristic of other cells that might be present in urinary sediment, i.e., RBC, bacteria, or transitional epithelial cells.[10,11] Well-preserved, renal tubule epithelial cells are almost indistinguishable from *in situ* tubule epithelial cells, and it is possible to identify the nephron segment(s) from which the cells under consideration have originated.

2. The predominant cell types found in the sediments of subjects without ATN were transitional epithelial cells, squamous epithelial cells, or cells of extraurinary tract origin (Figs. 1-13 and 1-14).

3. In LM studies, significant numbers of renal tubule cells in urinary specimens of healthy subjects were seen.[12] In TEM studies, only transitional epithelial cells were seen in urine obtained from healthy individuals (Fig.

1-15). Although these findings must be considered preliminary, it is suggested that earlier estimates of tubule cell desquamation rates in normal subjects should be reexamined.[13]

4. Transmission electron microscopy has demonstrated, in renal tubule cells, various serious changes that seems to correlate with the clinical course of ARF.[13]

5. This technique has demonstrated, unequivocally, the morphological characteristics of different types of casts, and the structure of myeloid bodies and fibrin. The latter finding has helped distinguish ATN from aminoglycoside nephrotoxicity and from transplant rejection.

Scanning Electron Microscopy

Lindner, Vacca, and Haber[14] and Haber and Lindner[15] have studied the composition and mechanism of the formation of various types of urinary casts by SEM. They found that the basic, fundamental structure of all the casts they studied is a mesh of fibrillar protein; hyaline casts are entirely complex proteinous material; cellular casts are blood or epithelial cells that closely adhere to the fibrillar cast matrix. These investigators showed, by SEM, that cells are

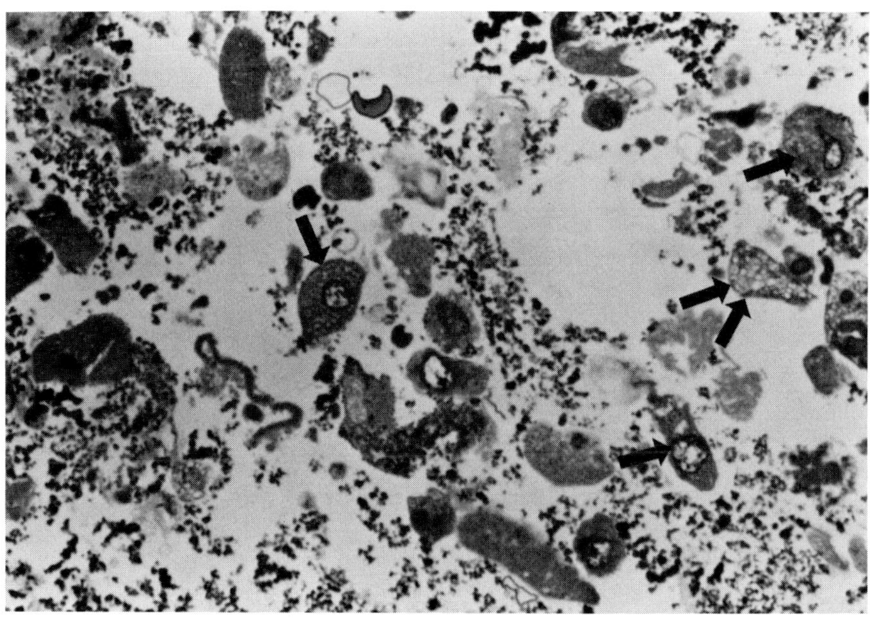

Figure 1-11.   In this light micrograph, from a thick section, as in Fig. 1-10, many cells are vacuolated (arrows). A lipid-laden cell (double arrows), similar to the oval fat bodies by conventional light microscopy, is shown (epoxy tissue stain, ×200).

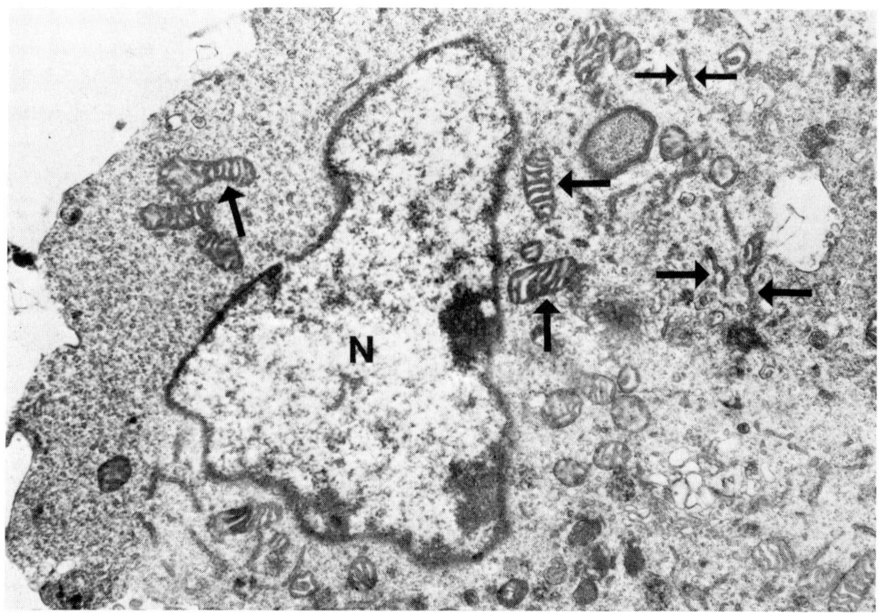

Figure 1-12.   In this normal-appearing distal tubule cell, the nucleus (N) and mitochondria (thick arrow) are intact. Many rough-surfaced endoplasmic reticula (between thin arrows) can be seen (UA + LC, ×4,800).

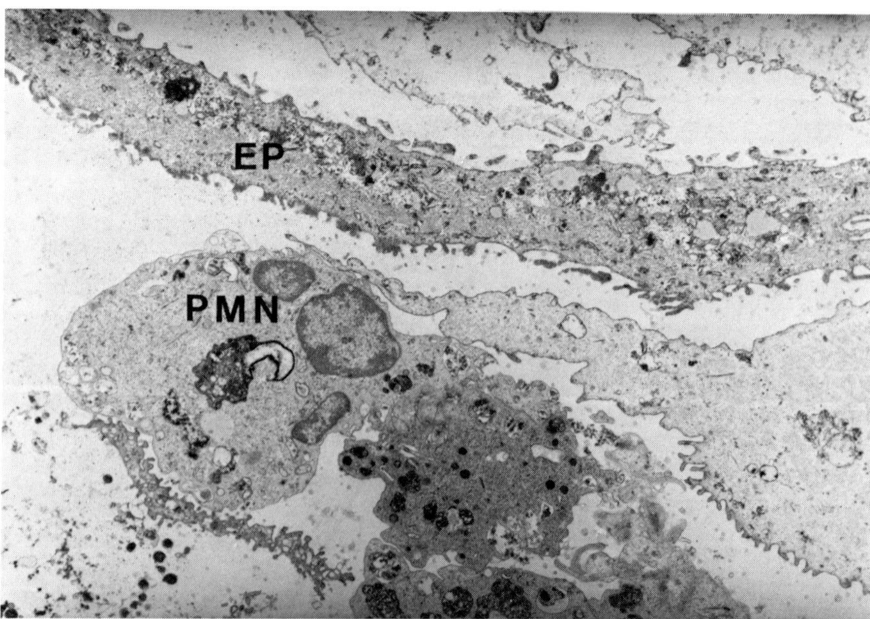

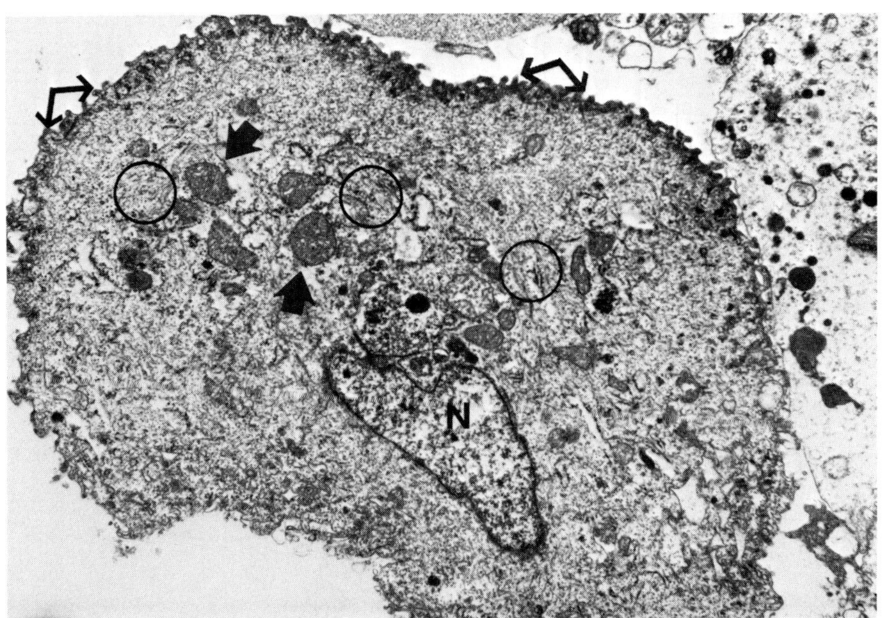

Figure 1-14. A squamous epithelial cell, characterized by a small nucleus (N), a few mitochondria (arrows), and small numbers of ribosomes, is seen. The cytoplasm contains numerous microfilaments (circles). As in transitional epithelial cells, these squamous epithelial cells show interdigitating villi at the cell periphery (double arrows) (UA + LC, ×5,000). From *Seminars in Nephrology,* Vol. 6, 1986, with permission.

attached to hyaline casts by encompassing fibrils, in contrast to the time-honored theory of their incorporation within the matrix during cast formation.

Though SEM provides a three-dimensional view that allows the examination of the surface of a structure, the low resolution (20 Å) of SEM, compared to that of TEM (2 Å), does not permit fine structure delineation. In using TEM, it was found that a granular cast contains cellular cytoplasm. The appearances of these casts observed by TEM are described in subsequent chapters.

Addendum: Recently, the fixative glutaraldehyde–formalin mixture has been modified in terms of pH and osmolality. Using 4% glutaraldehyde in phosphate buffer (pH 7.4), few or no casts were found in thick or thin sections,

Figure 1-13. This transmission electron micrograph of urinary sediment, from the urinary tract infection patient in Fig. 1-9, shows transitional epithelial cells (EP) and a polymorphonuclear neutrophil (PMN) (UA + LC, ×2,000).

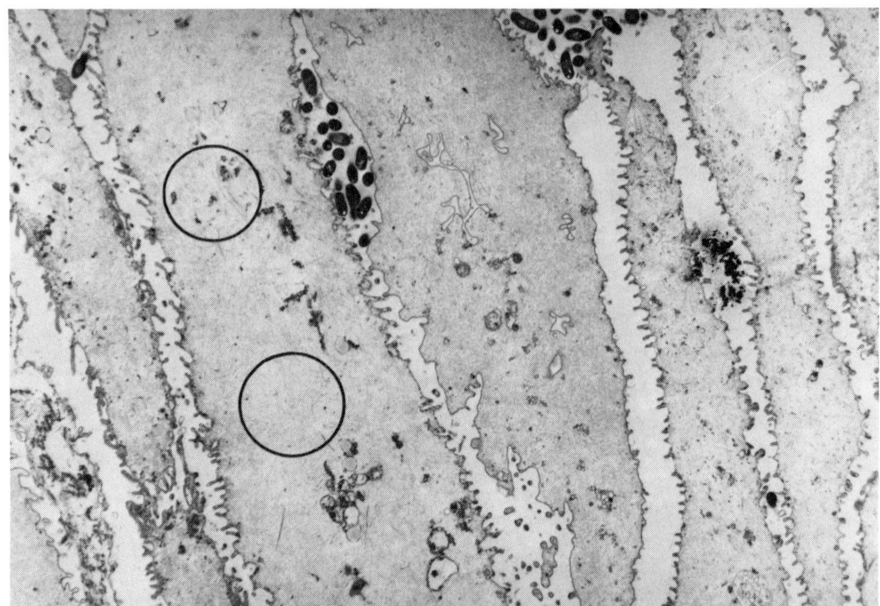

Figure 1-15. This transmission electron micrograph of urinary sediment pooled from urine samples collected by a group of doctors shows only transitional epithelial cells, which are characterized by interdigitating villi, and many filaments (circles). Note the conspicuous absence of mitochondria and endoplasmic reticulum (UA + LC, ×1,600).

although casts were found in wet preparations by conventional LM. Casts may dissolve in alkaline medium and thus disappear when the sediment is fixed in glutaraldehyde at an alkaline pH. In Chapter 2, it can be seen that casts are formed mostly in distal and collecting tubules where the urine is acid (pH 4.5–5) and has a high osmolality (900–1,300 mOsmole/kg). It was thus thought that if the urinary sediment were fixed in an *in vitro* environment resembling that of collecting tubules, the casts would be preserved. Indeed, with the glutaraldehyde–formalin mixture, at pH 5 and an osmolality of 900, many casts were found in both the thick and thin sections. In addition, structures are better preserved and the contrast is remarkably improved.

REFERENCES

1. Gyory AZ: Urine microscopy (Letter to the Editor). *Med J Aust* 1979; 2:369.
2. Valenstein PN, Koepke JA: Unnecessary microscopy in routine urinalysis. *Am J Clin Pathol* 1984; 82:444–448.

3. Donauer RM: The value of microscopic examination of urinary sediment (Letter to the Editor). *JAMA* 1978; 240:2044.

4. Osborne J: Method of examining the urine, in *A Sketch of the Physiology and Pathology of Urine*. London, Burgess and Hill Medical Booksellers, 1820.

5. Brody L, Webster M, Kark RM: Identification of elements of urinary sediment with phase-contrast microscopy. *JAMA* 1968; 206:1777–1781.

6. Schumann, GB: Cytodiagnostic urinalysis for the nephrology practice. *Sem Nephrol* 1986; 6:308–345.

7. Winer RL, Wuerker RB, Erickson JO, Cooper WL: Ultrastructural examination of urinary sediment: Value in renal amyloidosis. *Am J Clin Pathol* 1979; 7171:36–39.

8. Stachura I: Electron microscopy of urinary sediment in Fabry's disease (Letter to the Editor). *JAMA* 1977; 238:580.

9. Spurlock BO, Skinner MS, Kattine AA: A simple rapid method for staining epoxy-embedded specimens for light microscopy with the polychromatic stain paragon-1301. *Am J Clin Pathol* 1966; 46:252–258.

10. Mandal AK: *Electron Microscopy of the Kidney,* ed. 1. New York, Plenum Publishing Corp, 1979, pp 59–90.

11. Leeson TS, Leeson CR: *Histology,* ed. 2. Philadelphia, WB Saunders Co, 1970, pp 17–55.

12. Prescott LF: Th normal urinary excretion rates of renal tubular cells, leukocytes, and red blood cells. *Clin Sci* 1966; 31:425–435.

13. Mandal AK, Sklar AH, Hudson JB: Transmission electron microscopy of urinary sediment in human acute renal failure. *Kidney Int* 1985; 28:58–63.

14. Lindner LE, Vacca D, Haber MH: Identification and composition of types of granular urinary casts. *Am J Clin Pathol* 1983; 80:353–358.

15. Haber MH, Lindner LE: The surface ultrastructure of urinary casts. *AM J Clin Pathol* 1977; 68:547–552.

2

Proteinuria and Cylindriuria

Normal individuals excrete 100–150 mg (10 mg/dl) total protein in the urine in 24 hr. Electrophoresis of this urinary protein may reveal 40% albumin; 40% renal tissue proteins, consisting largely of Tamm–Horsfall (TH) protein; and 20% immunoglobulins. Such a small amount of protein in normal urine is not ordinarily detectable by the heat test or by the dipstick method, but these methods are quite sensitive and may detect protein in concentrated normal urine. Proteinuria that is so detected should be confirmed by a quantitative protein analysis of 24-hr urine; the types of proteins present can be determined by simple electrophoresis. If there is an electrophoretic monoclonal peak of globulin, immunoelectrophoresis of urine should be performed to determine the types of immunoglobulins present.

The formation of casts (cylinders) and the clinical significance of cylindriuria are discussed in this chapter. Since cast formation may be intricately related to protein excretion in the urine, it is important to acquaint the reader with the important aspects of proteinuria.

PROTEINURIA

Plasma protein is the major fraction of the proteins present in normal and abnormal urine. Normal glomeruli are barriers to protein, but glomerular capillary pores (70 Å) normally allow the passage of albumin (68 Å), most of which is reabsorbed by the proximal tubules. Only a small fraction (50–60 mg in 24 hr) appears in normal urine. In proteinuria, albumin filtration is increased, as is albumin reabsorption by the proximal tubules, but an excessive number of lysosomes (or "protein droplets") can be observed upon histological examination of the proximal tubules.

Small amounts of proteins that are antigenically similar to plasma globulins are also present in normal urine. These globulins are most likely to be free light chains. These light chains are lower in molecular weight (22,000–44,000 daltons) than is albumin (70,000 daltons) and are freely filtered by the glomeruli. Normally, minute amounts of light chains can be detected in the serum.[1] The amount of light chains filtered by the glomeruli is, therefore, small and almost completely reabsorbed by proximal tubules and catabolized there by lysosomal enzymes.[1] Normal urinary excretion of light chains (kappa and lambda) is 1–2 mg/day.

It is well established that a protein of nonplasma origin appears in normal urine. This protein, variously called uromucoid, mucoprotein, or TH protein, is produced by the tubules and is the main component of urinary casts. This subject will be discussed in detail later.

MEASUREMENT OF URINARY PROTEINS

Qualitative (Semiquantitative) Measurements

Qualitatively, the protein in the urine can be tested by (1) the heat test; (2) the sulfosalicylic acid test; and (3) the dipstick method.

The Heat Test

Heating urine to demonstrate the presence of protein is an old-fashioned method, which is still widely used in developing countries. Ten milliliters of urine is poured into a 15-ml glass test tube and the upper part of the tube is held in a bunsen burner. If a precipitate appears in the urine upon heating, a few drops of 10% acetic acid (not glacial acetic acid) is added. If the precipitate is the result of the phosphates present, it will dissolve and the urine will become clear; if the precipitate is the result of the proteins present, the urine will become turbid. In heavy proteinuria, the precipitate solidifies like the egg white of a hard-boiled egg. The degree of precipitate can be semiquantitated from 0 (no precipitate) to 4$^+$ (solid coagulum). The turbid coagulum formed in the upper layer of urine separates from the clear urine in the bottom of the test tube. The heat test is quite sensitive and can detect as little as 15–20 mg/dl of protein in the urine, but it is not as specific as the sulfosalicylic acid test or the dipstick method. Also, the heat test may be falsely positive in the presence of radiocontrast dyes, tolbutamide, or large amounts of such antibiotics as penicillin, nafcillin, or oxacillin. It should be remembered, however, that the heat test can be used to detect light-chain proteins (Bence Jones proteins).

The Sulfosalicylic Acid Test

Sulfosalicylic acid (5%) is added to a sample of urine and the degree of precipitate is noted, as in the heat test. This test is not as sensitive as the heat test, though it is more sensitive to albumin than to globulins. Light chains (Bence Jones proteins), however, are precipitated in this test.

The Dipstick Method

Here, a paper strip impregnated with the pH indicator dye tetrabromophenol and a buffer to maintain the pH in the paper at 3.0 is used to test for protein. Proteins change the color of the tetrabromophenol at a constant pH. The degree of color change is roughly proportional to the amount of protein present on a scale of 1^+ to 4^+, where $1^+ = 30$ mg/dl, $2^+ = 100$ mg/dl, $3^+ = 300$ mg/dl, and $4^+ \geq 2,000$ mg/dl. This quantitation is approximate. The correlation between quantitation based on color change and the quantitative analysis of protein in 24-hr urine is in the range of 60 to 70%.[2] This method does not give false positive results in the presence of radiocontrast dyes or antibiotics, but it is not as sensitive as the heat test or the sulfosalicylic acid test and therefore cannot detect a proteinuria of less than 30 mg/dl. In addition, this method does not detect Bence Jones proteins, as do the heat test and the sulfosalicylic acid test.

PROTEINURIA: QUANTITATIVE ANALYSIS

The above semiquantitative methods indicate the presence of proteinuria and roughly approximate its degree. To determine the severity of proteinuria, however, the total amount of protein excreted in 24 hr must be measured. The gel filtration biuret method has been adopted by the American Association for Clinical Chemistry as the "selected method" for urinary protein quantitation. Although accurate, the biuret method is cumbersome. The methods most widely used in the clinical laboratory are turbidimetric methods that employ trichloro-acetic acid or sulfosalicylic acid as precipitating agents. These methods are sensitive enough to quantify urinary protein directly, but they are not specific because the precipitating agents do not precipitate all protein classes uniformly nor do they precipitate all the proteins present, especially those at low concentrations. They are also susceptible to interference from drugs that precipitate protein in acidic solutions.[3] The 24-hr quantitative proteinuria is expressed as milligrams per liter. The total volume of urine excreted in 24 hr must be collected to calculate 24-hr proteinuria. This method does not distinguish the type of protein (albumin, globulin, or light chain); protein types are identified by electrophoresis and immunoelectrophoresis. Short of renal biopsy or selectivity study, electrophoresis of urine showing percentages of albumin and globulins excretion provide only estimate the degree of glomerular damage and the intactness of the barrier to protein filtration. A predominant globulin peak suggests either benign or malignant gammopathy.

Proteinuria is classified as (1) functional, (2) orthostatic, or (3) persistent.

Functional Proteinuria

In functional proteinuria, there are no demonstrable histopathological changes in the glomeruli and tubules. Urinary protein excretion increases two- to threefold following heavy exercise, febrile illness, congestive cardiac failure, emotional stress, norepinephrine infusion, and the prolonged assumption of the lordotic position; there is also increased formation of hyaline casts. This increase in proteinuria is attributable to a decrease in renal blood flow, with glomerular ischemia, and an increase in glomerular permeability to albumin. In functional proteinuria, both the proteinuria and the cylindriuria are transient, and tend to disappear in a few hours.

Similarly, increased urinary excretion of amylase in acute pancreatitis, of lysozyme in acute myelogenous leukemia, of myoglobin in rhabdomyolysis, and of hemoglobin in intravascular hemolysis occur without any discernible histopathological changes in the glomerular capillaries.

Orthostatic Proteinuria

Orthostatic proteinuria can be intermittent or fixed. Intermittent orthostatic proteinuria appears without any of the stimuli that induce functional proteinuria. This type of proteinuria occurs intermittently upon upright posture. The amount of 24-hr proteinuria is less than 1 g, and the renal biopsy study is normal or nondiagnostic. In fixed orthostatic proteinuria, the proteinuria almost always occurs when an upright position is assumed. Two 8-hr urine collections upon recumbency and upon upright posture should be analyzed to quantify proteins. In a typical orthostatic proteinuria, the recumbent sample should not contain more than 10 mg protein/dl, whereas the upright sample may contain 50 mg protein/dl or more. If the recumbent sample contains more than 15 mg protein/dl, and if the proteinuria is greatly increased in the upright sample, a diagnosis of orthostatic proteinuria is questionable. As in intermittent orthostatic proteinuria, the amount of 24-hr proteinuria is less than 1 g in fixed orthostatic proteinuria. Renal biopsy study is also noncontributory. In orthostatic proteinuria, the renal function is well preserved. In a 20-yr follow-up study of 43 patients with orthostatic proteinuria, a progressive decline in measurable qualitative proteinuria was documented. The quantitative 24-hr proteinuria was less than 150 mg and all patients had normal renal function.[4]

Persistent Proteinuria

In this condition, protein is detectable by the dipstick method, which is less sensitive than the heat test or the sulfosalicylic acid test, at all times and under all circumstances, although the sensitivity may vary. The amount of 24-hr proteinuria may vary from 2 g to 30–40 g. The persistent proteinuria may be the result of (1) glomerular disease (*glomerular proteinuria*), (2) tubular disease (*tubular proteinuria*), and (3) light chain proteinuria.

Glomerular Proteinuria

Glomerular proteinuria (>2 g in 24 hr) is often in the nephrotic range (>3.5 g/24 hr). It is generally associated with edema, hypertension, or renal insufficiency. Proteinuria of glomerular origin is corroborated by histopathological studies of renal tissue. Glomerular proteinuria results from an increase in glomerular capillary permeability to the passage of albumin and globulin. Because of the increased filtration of albumin, the tubules cannot reabsorb all the albumin and large amounts appear in the urine. The degree of damage of the glomerular basement membrane can be assessed by comparing the clearance of 1gG with that of albumin or transferrin (selectivity). A ratio of <0.1 (high selectivity) indicates minimal lesion disease (nil disease, foot process disease, or lipoid nephrosis). A ratio of >0.5 (poor selectivity) indicates membranous or membranoproliferative glomerulonephritis.

Tubular Proteinuria

Tubular proteinuria can be subdivided into proteins that are produced by the tubules and proteins that are normally reabsorbed by the proximal tubules.

Uromucoid or TH protein is produced by the tubules and a small amount normally appears in the urine (50 mg/day). This subject will be dealt with in more detail later. Such proteins as B_2 microglobulin, lysozyme, and light chains are normally reabsorbed almost completely by the proximal tubules. A small amount of these proteins will appear in normal urine. Though tubular proteinuria exists, the exact clinicopathological significance of tubular proteinuria, with the exception of B_2 microglobinuria and light chain proteinuria, is still unclear. Excessive amounts of B_2 microglobulin are found in the urine in acute and chronic proximal tubule dysfunction, such as aminoglycoside nephrotoxicity, in which B_2 microglobulinuria may be seen before renal failure becomes clinically evident.

Light Chain Proteinuria

Light chain proteinuria, which was once considered overproduction proteinuria, is now classified as a distinct clinicopathological entity. An excessive urinary excretion of light chain proteins, most commonly kappa, is associated with light chain nephropathy or light chain deposition disease.[1,5] This clinicopathological syndrome consists of proximal or distal renal tubular acidosis, proteinuria, and renal insufficiency. Histologically, nodular glomerulosclerosis resembling diabetic glomerulosclerosis, deposits of amyloid in the glomeruli, and positive immunofluorescence for kappa or lambda light chains or both in the glomeruli have been reported.[5,6] Excessive amounts of light chains in the urine may result, in part, from overproduction and, in part, from lack of tubular reabsorption. The concomitant presence of a large amount of albumin in the urine may be attributable to nodular glomerulosclerosis or amyloidosis or both.

FORMATION AND EXCRETION OF URINARY CASTS (CYLINDRIURIA)

There is unequivocal evidence that urinary mucoprotein, or TH protein, is the main component in urinary hyaline casts.[7–10] Casts previously designated granular casts and cellular casts are now considered hyaline casts that appear granular or that have cells embedded in their matrix.

Tamm and Horsfall, in 1950, reported the presence of a mucoprotein in normal human urine.[11] This mucoprotein was named for its discoverers. Thus far, all the evidence indicates that TH protein is produced by the kidney, specifically the ascending limb of Henle's loop, the distal tubule, the collecting tubule, and perhaps the proximal tubule. The TH protein will aggregate into gelatinous masses under certain conditions. These conditions include high concentrations of the mucoprotein, the acidity of the urine (pH <6), and the amount of sodium in the urine.[8,9,11] The daily excretion rate of TH protein is 0.05 mg/ml (50 mg total for a 24-hr urine volume of 1 liter). At concentrations over 50 mg/day, aggregation is likely to occur, particularly at low pH. The isoelectric point of TH protein (pH 4.8) is at or below the lower limit of urinary pH, so that the lower the pH of the urine, the more likely is the TH protein to aggregate. Thus, casts tend to persist longer in acid than alkaline urine.

Similarly, addition of 0.58 M sodium chloride to urine will precipitate most of the mucoprotein. Sodium, being the predominant cation in the urine, is considered to be the most important factor in aggregation of mucoprotein. Other cations, however, are equally effective, especially when there is less sodium in the urine, as in the nephrotic syndrome, congestive cardiac failure, or cirrhosis of the liver. Then, more potassium is excreted in the urine, and aggregation of TH protein can occur. Divalent cations, e.g., calcium, have an even greater effect on TH protein precipitation, but the concentration of calcium in the urine is not high enough to affect TH protein precipitation significantly. Urea is non-ionic and thus has a slight or no effect on TH protein aggregation.

It is clear that TH protein aggregation, or cast formation, occurs under conditions of low urine flow, acid urine, and high concentration of urinary sodium. Care must be taken, however, to restrict the term *cast* to structures that fit the following description. Casts must have formed within the lumen of the segments of the tubules that favor aggregation—the collecting tubules in which the urine is most concentrated, and lowest in pH. Hence, casts, by definition, are cylindrical structures of aggregated material that retain the shape of the tubule in the urine. Because of the cylindrical shape of casts, the presence of casts in the urine is frequently called *cylindriuria* (Fig. 2-1). Cells or necrotic material

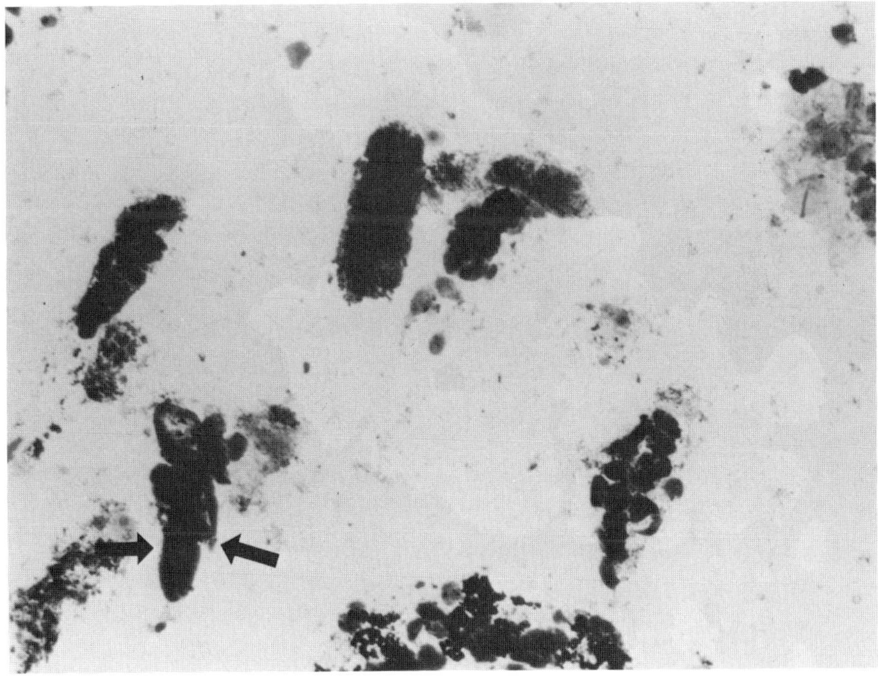

Figure 2-1. In this light micrograph of urinary sediment from a patient with severe hepatocellular disease and ARF, a wide variety of casts and desquamated epithelial cells (between arrows) are seen (epoxy tissue stain, ×100).

in the tubule lumen are embedded within the gelatinous matrix, like pieces of fruit in Jello, to form cellular (Fig. 2-2) or granular casts (Fig. 2-3); see also Fig. 1-3). In histological sections of the kidney, casts appear as collections of proteinous material within the tubule lumen (Fig. 2-4).

The composition and the physical characteristics of casts have been studied using immunofluorescence microscopy (IFM) and scanning electron microscopy (SEM). There is no mention of transmission electron microscopy (TEM) of casts in the literature. In an indirect immunofluorescence technique, antisera against TH protein, fibrinogen, albumin, $B1_c$ globulin, IgG, and IgM has been used to determine cast composition. The IFM technique showed strong positive reactions for TH protein in the matrix of all casts (Table 2-1). Positive reactions for other proteins were inconsistently found in casts associated with kidney disease. In addition, granules found in granular casts were positive for serum proteins, which

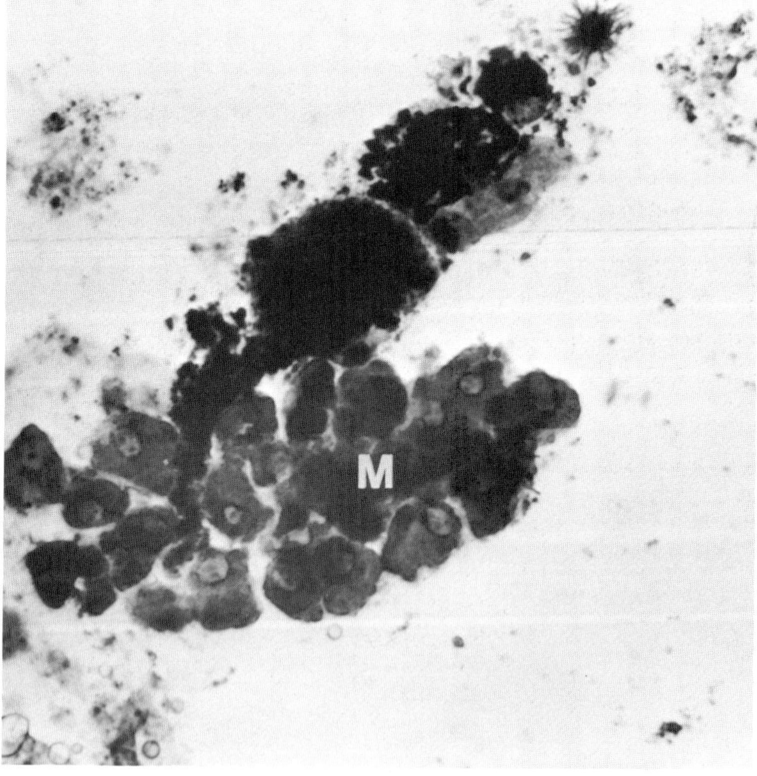

Figure 2-2.   Epithelial cells adhere to a homogeneous matrix (M) in this epithelial cell cast (epoxy tissue stain, ×400).

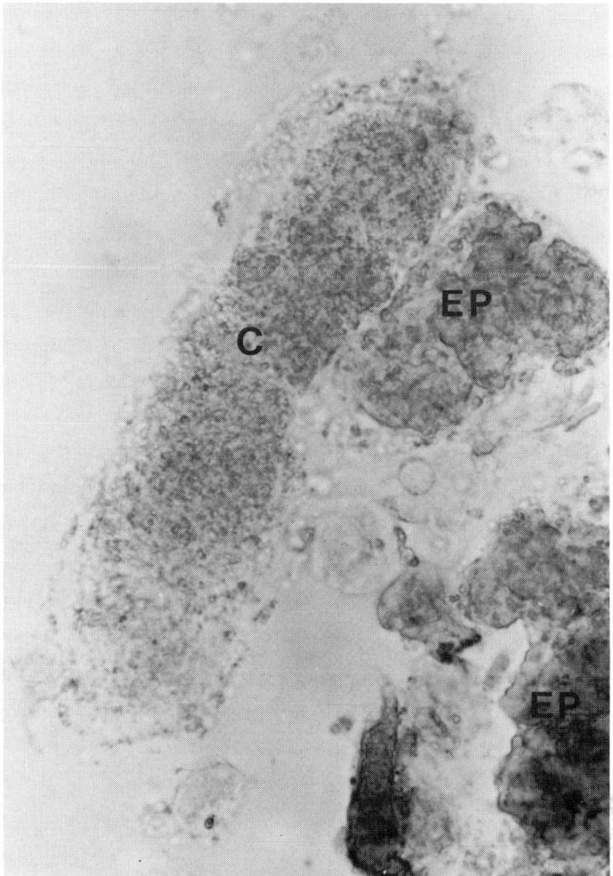

Figure 2-3. This is a light micrograph of a coarsely granular cast (C) from the patient in Fig. 1-2. Note the clusters of ill-defined epithelial cells (EP) (epoxy tissue stain, ×400).

suggests the incorporation of serum proteins in certain types of casts. The IFM technique also demonstrated that material reacting immunologically as TH protein is found in the cells of the ascending limb of the loop of Henle and the macula densa segment of the distal tubule, in particular.[12] Scanning electron microscopy has shown that the surface of hyaline casts can be smooth or, more frequently, fibrillar, with a wavy structure. In red blood cell casts, leukocyte casts, or epithelial casts, SEM has shown that blood cells or epithelial cells adhere closely to the fibrillar matrix of hyaline casts.[13] In many instances, blood cells or epithelial cells were found to be attached by encompassing fibrils.

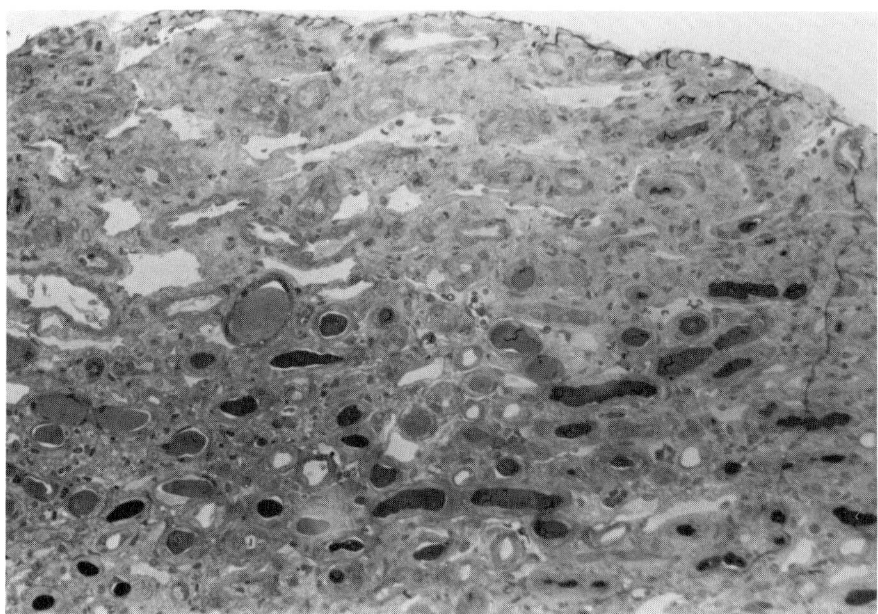

Figure 2-4. Thick sections (0.5 μ) from the renal biopsy of a patient with light chain nephropathy shows the kidney medulla. In the upper part of this light micrograph, there are a few tubules but mostly interstitial fibrosis; in the lower part, most of the tubules are dilated and filled with casts (epoxy tissue stain, ×400).

Table 2-1
Qualitative Composition of Urinary Casts of Various Origins

Antiserum	Ethacrynic acid; furosemide	Hydrochlorothiazide chlorthalidone after acidification	Football players	Patients with kidney disease
Antiuromucoid	+	+	+	+
Antifibrinogen	[(+)]	−	[(+)]	[(+)]
Antialbumin	−	−	−	(+)
Anti-B_{1C}/B_{1A}-globulin	−	−	−	(+)
Anti-γG-globulin	−	−	−	[(+)]
Anti-γM-globulin	−	−	−	[(+)]
Controls (normal rabbit serum)	−	−	−	−

Key: +, fluorescence in all samples and practically all casts; (+), fluorescence in all samples but not all casts; [(+)], fluorescence in some samples and some casts; −, no fluorescence in any sample.
Source: Adapted by kind permission from Imhof *et al.*[8]

Transmission electron microscopy of casts unequivocally identify structures in different types of casts, as follows:

Hyaline casts have a homogeneous electron-dense matrix, and the two-dimensional surface is coarse and pitted (Fig. 2-5). Granular casts consist of fine to coarsely granular and amorphous material that appears to be disintegrated cellular cytoplasm (Fig. 2-6). The many relatively intact cells adjacent to a granular cast indicate that this type of cast may be derived from an epithelial cell cast. Granular casts are most commonly found in association with acute tubular necrosis (ATN) and acute and chronic tubulointerstitial nephritis. In these conditions, tubule epithelial cells degenerate and desquamate; the degenerated epithelial cell products then are incorporated with TH protein to form granular casts as shown by TEM. By SEM study, however, there are indications that granular casts may be formed from degenerated granulocytes.[14] One argument against the latter theory is that the number of epithelial cells in ATN and acute tubulointerstitial nephritis far exceeds the number of granulocytes. Furthermore, TEM rarely shows neutrophilic leukocytes in urinary sediment that is predominantly necrotic tubule cells.

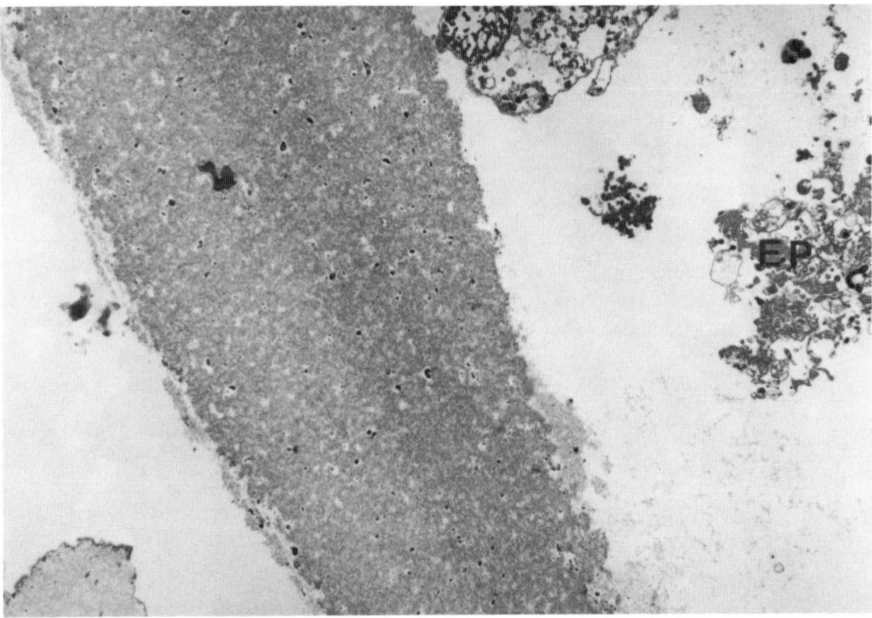

Figure 2-5. The ultrastructure of a hyaline cast from a patient with nephrotic syndrome. The cast, of homogeneous electron-dense material, has a coarse, pitted surface. Note the necrotic epithelial cells (EP) adjacent to the cast (UA + LC, ×2,000). From *Seminars in Nephrology,* Vol. 6, 1986, with permission.

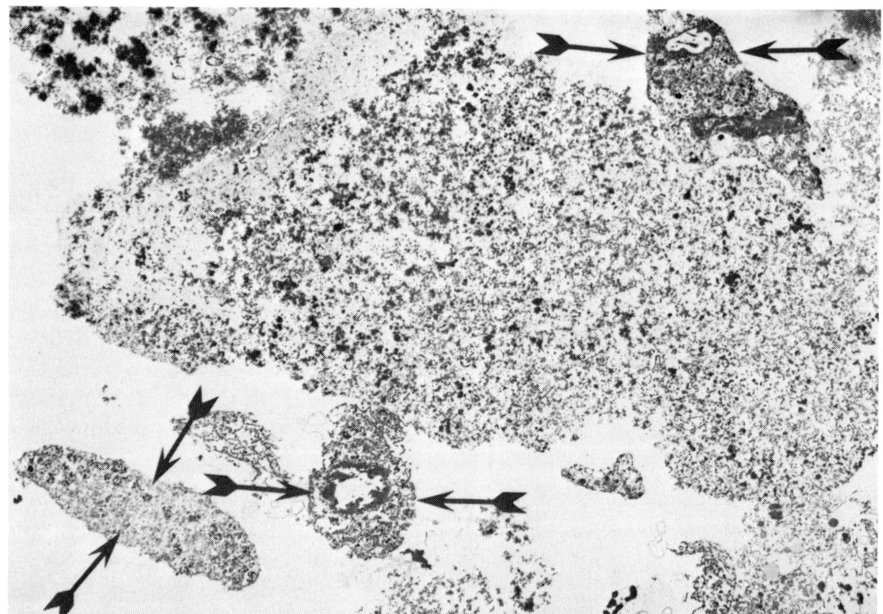

Figure 2-6.   A granular cast of finely granular to amorphous material. Adjacent to the cast are a number of relatively well-preserved tubule epithelial cells (between arrows) (UA + LC, ×1,000). From *Seminars in Nephrology,* Vol. 6, 1986, with permission.

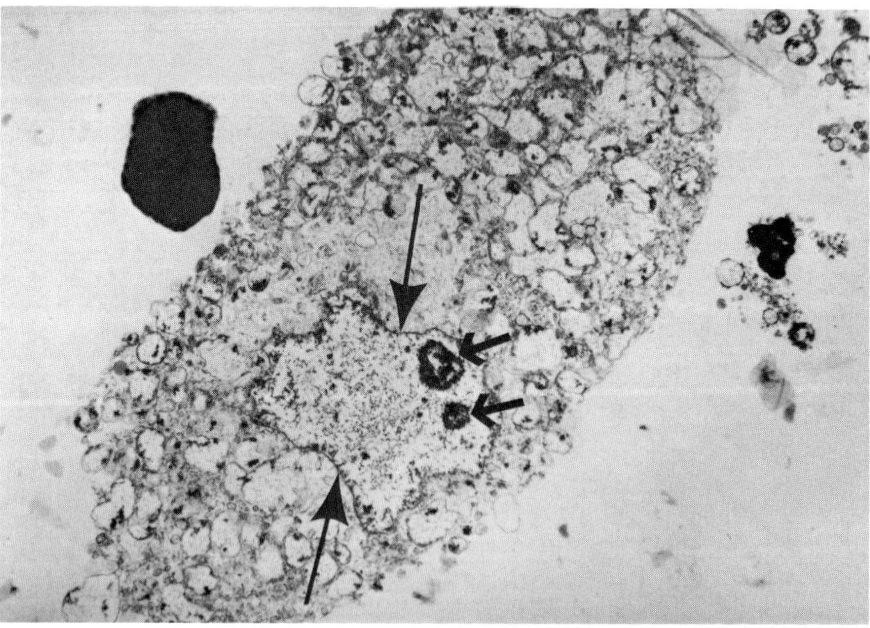

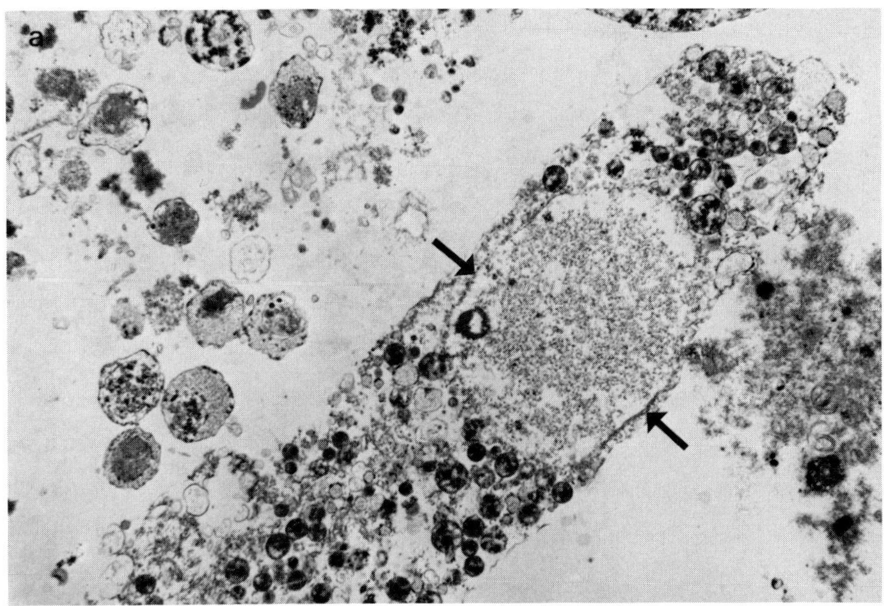

Figure 2-8a.   A cast from the patient shown in Fig. 2-2. Many severely damaged mitochondria are embedded within the cast matrix. The remnants of the membrane of a cell
that has undergone complete dissolution are shown (arrows), and cellular fragments sur-
round the cast. This transmission electron micrograph indirectly shows that such a granular
cast is a transitional form of a cellular cast (UA + LC, ×4,000).

Epithelial or epithelial cell casts consist of tubule but not transitional epithelial cells. In Fig. 2-7, an epithelial cast contains numerous swollen mitochondria, devoid of cristae but containing fine dark bodies, which is a sign of
ischemia; the nucleus with nucleoli is embedded within the matrix. The two
casts shown in Figs. 2-8a and 2-8b also appear to be epithelial casts, as indicated
by their abundant mitochondria.

Fatty casts are composed of fat granules (lipid droplets) embedded within
the homogeneous matrix (Fig. 2-9). These fat granules are not electron dense,
which suggests that these particular lipids are not osmiophilic and, therefore,
are likely to be saturated fatty acids[15] or cholesterol esters. These fat granules

Figure 2-7.   A transmission electron micrograph of urinary sediment from the patient shown
in Fig. 2-1 shows a cellular cast. Mitochondria are vacuolated and the nucleus shows dissolution, but the nuclear membrane is still intact (long arrows) and the nucleoli (short arrows)
are well preserved (UA + LC, ×4,000).

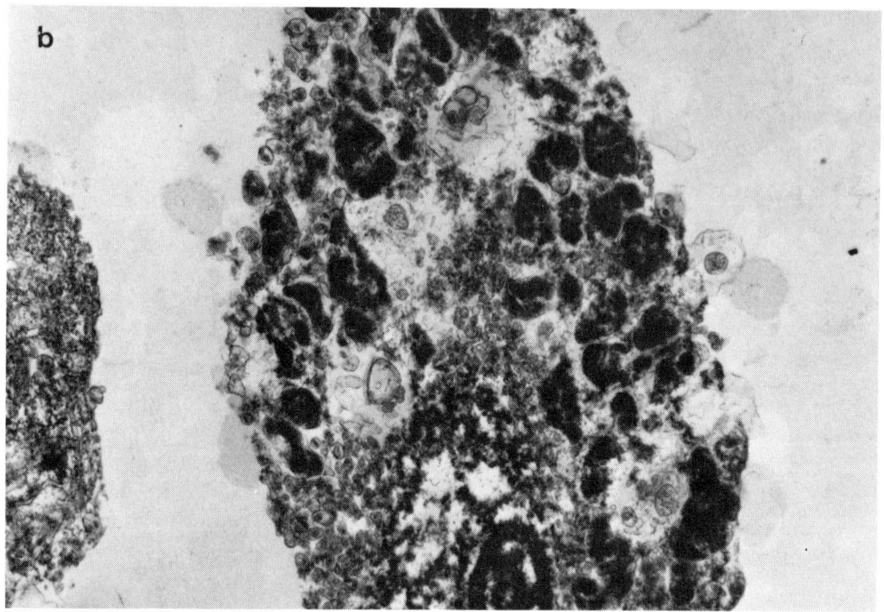

Figure 2-8b. In this transmission electron micrograph from the urinary sediment of the patient shown in Fig. 2-7, a cellular cast contains many mitochondria that are severely damaged, enlarged, and fused (UA + LC, ×13,000).

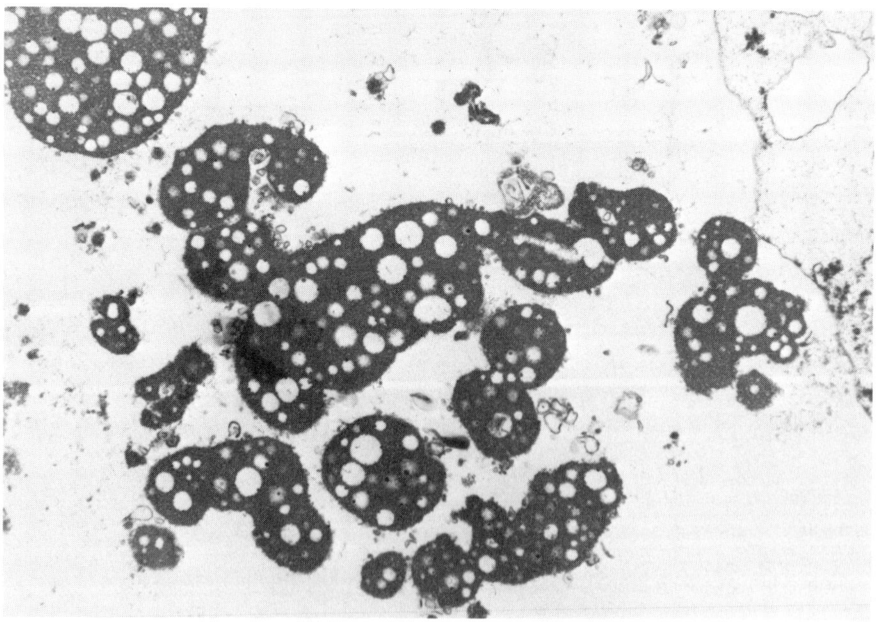

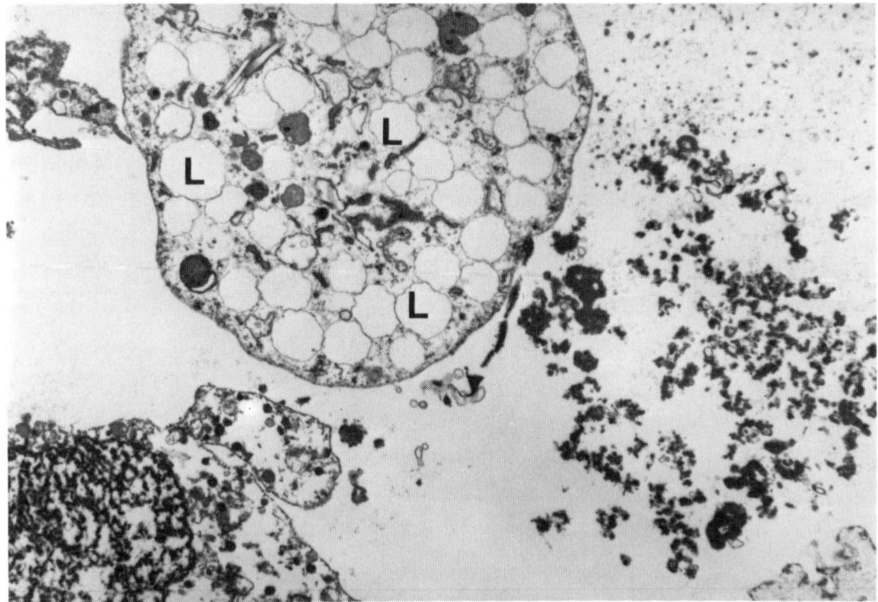

Figure 2-10. In this transmission electron micrograph, a swollen cell is studded with lipid droplets (L). In light microscopy, this is called an oval fat body. From the urinary sediment of the patient shown in Fig. 2-5 (UA + LC, ×2,600).

appear as doubly refractile bodies or shine brightly; they thus appear as maltese crosses under polarized light. In the lipiduria associated with proteinuria, the lipid droplets become embedded in the protein matrix to form either fatty casts (Fig. 2-9) or oval fat bodies (Fig. 2-10) by LM.

THE CLINICAL SIGNIFICANCE OF CYLINDRIURIA

Cylindriuria is clinically significant diagnostically and pathogenetically; it is also of importance in prognosis and management.

Figure 2-9. In these fatty casts, fat granules (lipid droplets) have been embedded in the cast matrix (UA + LC, ×5,000).

Diagnosis

Though a few hyaline casts in a urine sample may be considered normal, the presence of granular casts, epithelial casts, leukocyte casts, red blood cell casts, or fatty casts is almost always abnormal. Since TH protein aggregates rapidly when the urine flow is slow, when the pH is low, and when sodium concentrations are high, any condition that decreases the glomerular filtration and the urine flow rate will favor TH protein aggregation and cast formation. Thus, a physiological condition such as strenuous exercise could lead to excessive urinary cast formation and excretion. By and large, these casts will be hyaline casts and they will tend to diminish in number after 1–2 hr of exercise.[8] It has been reported that the cast excretion rate correlates directly with TH protein concentration in the urine ($p < 0.01$) and inversely with the urine flow rate; the cast excretion rate, however, does not correlate with TH protein excretion rate.[8] Serum protein excretion during exercise also increases and seems to accelerate cast formation, though this has not been demonstrated experimentally.[8] All in all, the presence of hyaline casts in the urine, however many are present, has little or no pathological significance.

Granular casts, red blood cell casts, leukocyte casts, epithelial casts, or fatty casts, however, are found in the urine of patients with acute or chronic renal parenchymal diseases. Though the presence of granular casts can imply a variety of renal parenchymal diseases, red blood cell casts indicate acute glomerular injury. Thus, red blood cell casts are found in acute endocapillary or extracapillary proliferative glomerulonephritis, glomerular infarction or necrosis, vasculitis, and malignant hypertension associated with glomerular infarction. Red blood cell casts are commonly found in association with acute glomerular injury, but this is not an exclusive finding for acute glomerular lesion. Red blood cell casts have also been found in ATN by this author (Fig. 2-11) and by other authors.[16] The presence of leukocyte casts characterizes acute or chronic pyelonephritis and such sterile pyuric conditions as membranous glomerulonephritis, renal vein thrombosis, or tuberculosis of the kidney. Epithelial casts are likely to be found in association with ATN of the ischemic or nephrotoxic type. In ATN, desquamated tubule epithelial cells become embedded in the gelantinous matrix of TH protein to form epithelial casts. A decrease in urine flow, or oliguria, and acid urine, which usually accompanies ATN, tends to enhance cylindriuria (Fig. 2-1). Similarly, epithelial casts may be found in acute tubulointerstitial nephritis, when ATN is a concomitant feature, and chronic tubulointerstitial nephritis, when desquamation of tubule epithelial cells occurs. In telescoped urinary sediment, all types of casts occur, with RBC and WBC. This type of urinary sediment, which was once considered pathognomonic for lupus nephritis, has been found to be nonspecific. Therefore, telescoped urinary sediment can be found in any type of acute diffuse proliferative glomerulonephritis or malignant

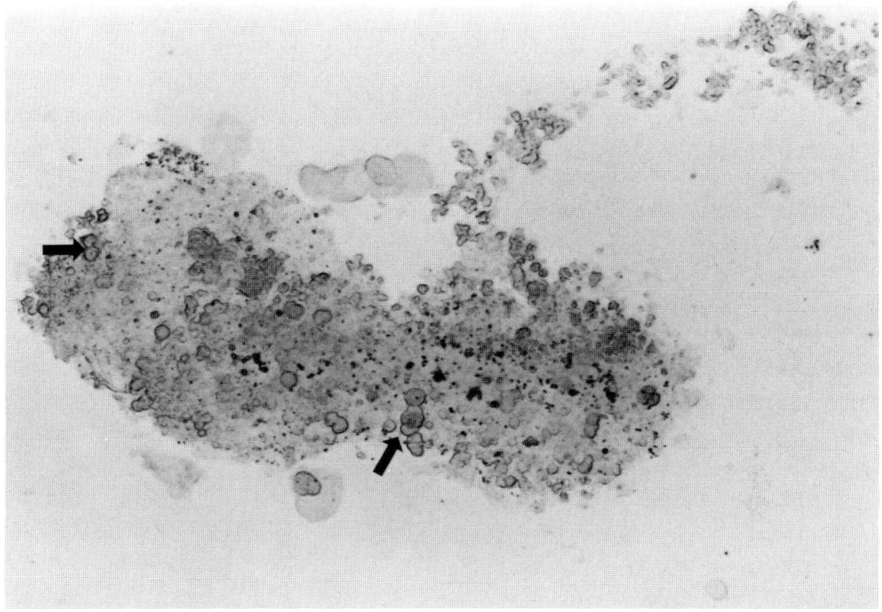

Figure 2-11. This light micrograph of urinary sediment from the patient shown in Fig. 2-1 is of a red blood cell cast. Red blood cells (arrows) are seen embedded in the matrix. The dark material may be hemosiderin pigments (epoxy tissue stain, ×400).

hypertension but is not considered diagnostic for a certain type of glomerulonephritis.

Fatty casts, waxy casts, and oval fat bodies are found in the urine of patients with nephrotic syndromes of diverse etiology. Heavy proteinuria (>3.5g/24 hr) is usually accompanied by lipiduria, which leads to the incorporation of lipid droplets into the cast matrix or epithelial cells.

Pathogenesis

Though casts are generally nonspecific with respect to the diagnosis of renal disease, some types of casts are more significant than others. For example, red blood cell casts generally indicate acute glomerular injury, whereas epithelial or granular casts point toward tubule epithelial cell injury. An important histological finding in acute renal failure (ARF) is the presence of large collections of proteinaceous material, especially in the collecting tubules of the renal papillae (Fig. 2-4). In ARF, a dilation of proximal and distal tubules, with flattening of the epithelium and filling of the lumen with large casts, is also a frequent finding.

Similarly, in myeloma, the tubules are frequently filled with large casts (to be described in Chapter 8). It has been proposed[17] that tubular obstruction by casts is one of the causes of oliguria in ARF. It has been demonstrated that furosemide increases urine flow without necessarily increasing the glomerular filtration rate, to convert oliguric to nonoliguric ARF, which may reflect the removal of intratubular obstruction by casts. Such relief of intratubular obstruction is possibly the result of an increase in urine flow and an alkalinization of the urine. Both tend to slow TH protein aggregation. Furthermore, it has been shown, in an elegant human study, that after administration of ethacrynic acid, the hourly excretion of TH protein remained within the normal range during the period of maximal diuresis. Thereafter, TH protein excretion decreased markedly. Though urinary cast excretion was at its maximum level during diuresis, the concentration and the hourly urinary excretion of TH protein were distinctly reduced.[8]

Prognosis and Management

It has been stated that TH protein is produced in large amounts in renal parenchymal diseases in which an excessive number of casts can often be demonstrated in the urine. Therefore, an excessive number of casts in the urine (cylindriuria) may have some relevance to the disease process. A few casts or the occasional cast in the urine, irrespective of type, may imply an inactive pathological process, whereas many casts suggest an active disease process. The appearance of red blood cell casts not previously noted along with other types of casts may signify an active glomerular lesion in addition to the existing renal lesions, which can lead to a rapidly progressive (crescentic) glomerulonephritis in association with membranous glomerulonephritis[18] or an acute diffuse proliferative glomerulonephritis superimposed on a diabetic nephropathy.[19] When the disease process is active, cylindriuria is of greater prognostic significance when it is accompanied by an increased proteinuria.

The urine of patients with renal parenchymal diseases should be monitored for protein by the dipstick method or the heat test and for casts by LM of the stained sediment to follow the course of the disease process and to determine the effect of treatment upon the pathological process. This is the simplest, most cost-effective test in the practice of nephrology. When there is no or slight proteinuria and occasional or no casts, the disease is inactive. There is no need for serum chemistry on every visit, but if the serum creatinine is elevated, even though the urine sediment is unconvincing, the pathological process may be smoldering, as in end-stage renal disease. It should be remembered that urine samples should be examined fresh, after checking the pH. Casts are unlikely to be found in alkaline urine, and lead to a false negative finding in the presence of active renal disease.

REFERENCES

1. Fang LST: Light chain nephropathy. *Kidney Int* 1985; 27:582–592.
2. Rennie IBD, Kee H: Evaluation of clinical methods for detecting proteinuria. *Lancet* 1967; 2:489–492.
3. Naccarato WF, Caffo AL: The performance characteristics of the urinary protein method for the Du Pont ACA Analyzer. *Du Pont Clinical Systems Technical Service Bulletin* 1982.
4. Springberg PD, Garrett LE, Thompson AL, *et al:* Fixed and reproducible orthostatic proteinuria: Results of a 20 year study. *Ann Intern Med* 1982; 97:516–519.
5. Ganeval D, Noel LH, Preud'Homme JL, *et al:* Light chain deposition disease: Its relation with AL-type amyloidosis. *Kidney Int* 1984; 26:1–9.
6. Alpers CE, Hopper J, Biava CG: Light chain glomerulopathy with amyloid-like deposits. *Hum Pathol* 1984; 15:444–448.
7. McQueen EG, McKenzie JK, Patel R, *et al:* Urinary mucoprotein and cast formation. *NZ Med J* 1969; 67:311–315.
8. Imhof PR, Hushak J, Schumann G, *et al:* Excretion of urinary casts after the administration of diuretics. *Br Med M* 1972; 2:199–202.
9. Rutecki GJ, Goldsmith C, Schreiner GE: Characterization of proteins in urinary casts. *N Engl J Med* 1971; 284:1049–1052.
10. McQueen EG: Composition of urinary casts. *Lancet* 1966; 1:397–398.
11. Tamm I, Horsfall FL: Characterization and separation of an inhibitor of viral hemagglutination present in urine. *Proc Soc Exp Biol* 1950; 74:108–114.
12. McKenzie JK, McQueen EG: Immunofluorescent localization of Tamm-Horsfall mucoprotein in human kidney. *J Clin Pathol* 1969; 22:334–339.
13. Haber MH, Lindner LE: The surface ultrastructure of urinary casts. *Am J Clin Pathol* 1977; 68:547–552.
14. Linder LE, Vacca D, Haber MH: Identification and composition of types of granular urinary casts. *Am J Clin Pathol* 1983; 80:353–358.
15. Mandal AK, Frohlich ED, Chrysant K, *et al:* A morphological study of the renal papillary granule: Analysis in the interstitial cell and in the interstitium. *J Lab Clin Med* 1975; 85:120–131.
16. Sweeney MJ, Forland M: *Methods of Diagnosing Renal Disease in Nephrology,* Stein JH (ed). New York, Grune & Stratton, 1980, pp 64–79.
17. Conger JD, Schrier RW: Renal hemodynamics in acute renal failure. *Ann Rev Physiol* 1980; 42:603–614.
18. Moorthy AV, Zimmerman SW, Burkholder PM, *et al:* Association of crescentic glomerulo-nephritis with membranous glomerulonephropathy, a report of 3 cases. *Clin Nephrol* 1976; 6:319–325.
19. Moonaham Y, Maxwell DR, Hamburger R, *et al:* Primary glomerulonephritis complicating diabetic nephropathy. *Hum Pathol* 1984; 15:921–927.

3

Acute Renal Failure

In adult inpatients, acute renal failure (ARF) commonly occurs in severe trauma, prolonged surgery, sepsis, cardiogenic shock, hypotension, or the use of aminoglycoside antibiotics.[1,2] This type of ARF is usually accompanied by acute tubular lesions or conventionally acute tubular necrosis (ATN) and, despite dialysis, the mortality rate of ARF, with the exception of ARF induced by drug or toxin, remains high.[3,4] Various mechanisms, including reduced renal blood flow, tubular obstruction, backleak of glomerular filtrate, increased catecholamine activity, and decreased prostaglandin production, have been proposed to explain ARF.[5] The results of experiments using pharmacological agents (vasodilator drugs) to increase renal blood flow and glomerular filtration rate, to wash out intratubular obstructions and increase urine flow, and to enhance cellular regeneration[6–9] have been encouraging, but no study has indicated the usefulness of these agents in human ARF, with one notable exception: In some patients furosemide may convert oliguric ARF to nonoliguric ARF. It has been shown that spontaneous nonoliguric ARF is associated with a significantly lower mortality rate than is oliguric ARF,[1] but there is no compelling evidence to date that the mortality rate of furosemide-induced nonoliguric ARF is significantly reduced.

CLINICAL SYNDROME

The clinical syndrome of ARF is well defined. Acute renal failure can occur after an ischemic or a nephrotoxic insult; within 48 to 72 hr a progressive azotemia, with or without oliguria, occurs. Clinically, ATN is suspected in most instances and is supported by the urinary sediment findings, increased urinary sodium and low urinary osmolality, and the high fractional excretion of sodium. Urinary sediment from patients with ARF has been examined by conventional light microscopy (LM) and variously described as containing "muddy-brown" casts, epithelial cell casts, coarse granular casts, red blood cell casts, renal tubule epithelial cells, red blood cells (RBC) and white blood cells (WBC). It should be mentioned, however, that in some patients with ARF, the urinary sediment may be excessive, whereas in other patients, the urinary sediment findings may be unconvincing. Findings of urinary sediment studies may be related to the severity of renal damage and, consequently, the ARF mortality rate. In one previous study, urinary sediments were examined in 97 episodes of ARF. Death occurred in 35% of the 47 episodes of ARF in which sediment abnormalities (as noted above) were present, compared to a significantly low ($p < 0.025$) mortality rate in 48 episodes of ARF in which there were no sediment abnormalities.[2]

This author has studied the urinary sediment using transmission electron microscopy (TEM) and found a significant correlation between sediment abnormalities, the severity of ATN, and the mortality rate of ARF.[10]

In this chapter, the value of TEM study of urinary sediment to elucidate the morphological changes of the kidneys in ARF are discussed, followed by a review of how this information might help in making a prognosis and planning the management of ARF.

Before clinicopathological correlations are discussed, clinical profiles and urinary sediment studies from several patients will be presented to illustrate how TEM studies of urinary sediments contribute to assessment of ARF.

URINARY SEDIMENT STUDIES

Urine specimens from 48 patients were analyzed using TEM. Thirty-one of these 48 patients had ARF secondary to ATN and were evaluated during an 18-month period ending July 1984. These patients were considered to have ATN on the basis of the following criteria: (1) an abrupt decline in renal function (increased serum creatinine concentration, ≥ 0.5 mg/dl per day) following a known ischemic or nephrotoxic insult; (2) the progression of azotemia after correction of any hemodynamic abnormality; (3) the absence of pyelocaliectasis, as shown by ultrasonography; (4) a fractional excretion of sodium ($\geq 2\%$); and (5) the presence of numerous epithelial cells (≥ 1 per HPF) in the urinary sediment by LM. For the purpose of comparison, urinary sediment shown to contain few or no epithelial cells by LM were obtained for TEM evaluation from 17 patients with diagnoses other than ATN.

Each patient with ATN was followed for at least 3 mos after the onset of ARF to assess the functional severity of acute renal illness and to determine the final clinical outcome. Functional severity was evaluated by the volume of urine

Table 3-1
Clinical Profiles of Patients with Acute Renal Failure[a]

Sediment type	No.	Age (years)	Sex	Etiology	Onset ARF to urine collection (days)	base	peak	Urine output	Dialysis intervention	Renal recovery	Duration of ARF[b] (days)
I	1	60	M	Arteriography	<1	1.4	6.4	O	Yes	No	84[c]
	2	61	M	AAA resection	72	2.0	16.8	A	Yes	No	92[c]
	3	58	M	Septic shock	<1	1.3	3.1	O	No	No	2[c]
	4	54	M	Sepsis	63	NA	12.5	A	Yes	No	87
	5	69	M	Unknown	3	NA	12.0	A	Yes	No	90
	6	68	M	Arteriography	1	1.7	6.2	O	Yes	No	8[c]
	7	70	M	Hypotension	2	1.4	5.8	O	No	No	4[c]
	8	72	M	Sepsis	1	1.0	1.8	O	No	No	2[c]
	9	63	M	Septic shock	20	2.6	7.2	O	Yes	No	24[c]
	10	53	M	Sepsis	2	1.5	2.1	O	No	No	2[c]
	11	21	M	Septic shock	2	1.0	2.0	O	Yes	No	2[c]
II	12	64	M	Contrast, cardiac surgery	4	1.7	3.2	NO	No	Yes	14
	13	55	M	Hypovolemia	38	1.7	3.5	NO	No	Yes	66
	14	71	F	Contrast	<2	1.5	3.5	O	No	Yes	7
	15	28	F	Aminoglycosides	2	0.7	1.5	NO	No	Yes	14
	16	23	F	Aminoglycosides	5	1.0	2.7	NO	No	Yes	28
	17	48	M	Aminoglycosides	1	2.0	4.8	NO	No	Yes	33
	18	65	M	Myocardial infarction	2	1.6	2.4	NO	No	Yes	9(13[c])[d]
	19	66	M	Rhabdomyolysis	24	1.0	10.2	NO	Yes	Yes	<180
III	20	74	M	Sepsis	2	NA	10.6	A	Yes	No	74†
	21	53	M	Arteriography	7	1.3	9.9	NO	Yes	No	68
	22	71	M	Rhabdomyolysis	<1	NA	11.7	A	Yes	Yes	<14

(continued)

Table 3-1
(*Continued*)

Sediment type	No.	Age (years)	Sex	Etiology	Onset ARF to urine collection (days)	Serum creatinine (mg/dl) base	Serum creatinine (mg/dl) peak	Urine output	Dialysis intervention	Renal recovery	Duration of ARF[b] (days)
	23	43	M	Rhabdomyolysis	27	1.3	15.7	NO	Yes	Yes	64
	24	66	M	Arteriography	3	1.5	7.5	O	Yes	Yes	42
	25	64	M	Hemorrhagic shock	3	1.1	5.5	O	No	Yes	14[c]
	26	87	M	Hypovolemia	<1	2.2	5.4	O	No	Yes	7[c]
	27	61	F	Sepsis	10	2.0	>6.5	NO	Yes	No	20[c]
	28	48	M	Aminoglycosides	3	0.5	1.7	NO	No	No	15[c]
	29	58	M	Aminoglycosides	3	1.4	2.9	NO	No	Yes	14
	30	72	M	Hypovolemia	7	0.5	2.3	O	No	Yes	18[c]
	31	63	F	Sepsis	3	1.8	7.8	NO	No	Yes	17

[a] Key: ARF, acute renal failure; M, male patient; F, female patient; AAA, abdominal aortic aneurysm; NA, not assessed; A, anuria (<100 ml/day); O, oliguria (100 to 400 ml/day); NO, nonoliguria (>400 ml/day).

[b] In patients who did not regain renal function, the number of days represents the time interval between either the end of the observation period or death (†).

[c] Day patient died.

[d] Patient No. 18 regained renal function on day 9, but died from recurrent myocardial infarction on day 13.

Source: Adapted from Mandal, Sklar, and Hudson[10] by the kind permission of the editor of *Kidney International*.

output in the early phase of renal injury (patients with outputs > 400 ml in a 24-hr period, whether spontaneously or produced by a diuretic, were considered to have nonoliguric ATN), and in need of dialysis. Patients who died within 48 hr of the onset of ARF and who were not already on dialysis were excluded from the study. Clinical outcome was determined by recovery of renal function and patient survival. Patients who regained more than 50% of their lost renal function, as assessed by serum creatinine levels, were considered to have recovered their renal function. Patients who died within 14 days of the onset of ARF were considered not to have recovered renal function. Patients who lived for at least 2 months following the onset of ARF, were considered to have survived their acute renal illness.[10] The clinical profiles of 31 patients with ARF are presented in Table 3-1.

RENAL HISTOPATHOLOGY

Renal tissue specimens were obtained at autopsy from 4 subjects, by wedge biopsy during surgery in 1 patient, and by percutaneous needle biopsy in 1 patient. Specimens were studied by LM and TEM in all except one instance where examination was solely by LM.

The clinical profiles of the individual patients and their urinary sediment studies follow.

Patient No. 1, P. C., a 53-year-old white male was admitted to the Veterans Administration Medical Center, Augusta, Georgia on May 25, 1983, with a history suggestive of transient ischemic attacks. Multiple radiological studies using contrast material were done to evaluate the patency of his carotid and coronary arteries. There was evidence of a bilateral carotid artery involvement with total occlusion of the left internal carotid artery, and multiple occlusions in the coronary arteries. His admission serum urea nitrogen and serum creatinine concentrations were 20 mg/dl and 1.3 mg/dl, respectively. Shortly after the radiological studies were completed, serum urea nitrogen and serum creatinine levels increased to 58 mg/dl and 9.9 mg/dl, respectively, while urine output remained normal or high. On the basis of the onset of ARF after radiocontrast studies and the absence of oliguria, dye-induced ATN was suspected; but the possibility of an atheroembolic disorder of the kidney as the result of the catheterization of the atheromatous arteries could not be excluded. The patient was temporarily dialyzed (hemodialysis) to prepare him for carotid artery surgery. Following discontinuation of hemodialysis, his serum urea nitrogen and serum creatinine progressively increased to 100 mg/dl and 12 mg/dl, respectively. An arteriovenous fistula was created and long-term hemodialysis was undertaken three times a week.

A urine sample was collected 7 days after onset of ARF and fixed for TEM analysis. The findings of TEM study of urinary sediment are shown in Figs. 3-1–3-6. The sediment contained many cells. In Fig. 3-1, the urinary sediment included necrotic tubule epithelial cells, RBC, a WBC (monocyte), and a cast consistent with ATN. Though the anatomy

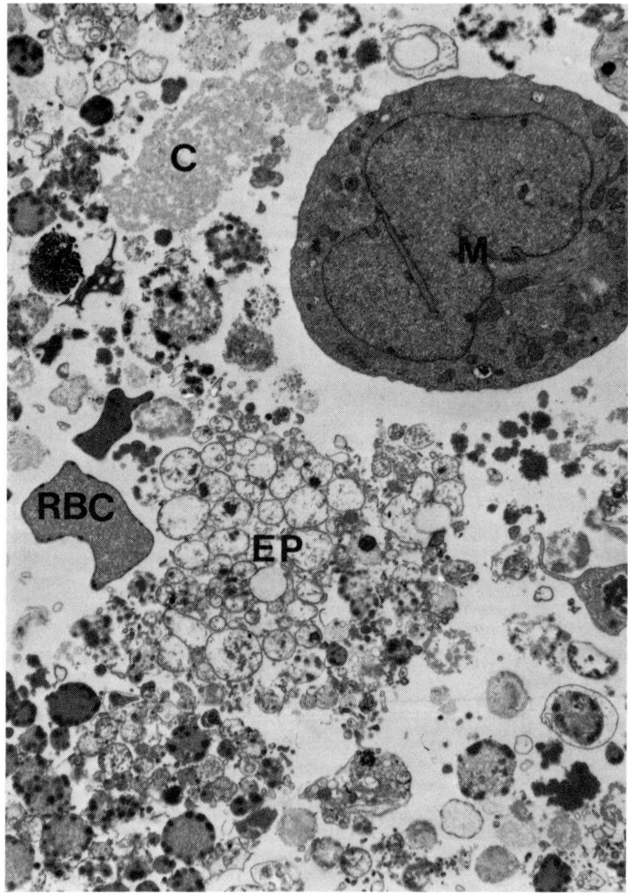

Figure 3-1.   This transmission electron micrograph shows a sediment consisting of a necrotic renal tubule epithelial cell (EP), a monocyte (M), a red blood cell (RBC), and a hyaline cast (C), which are commonly found in ATN (UA + LC, ×3,300). From *Seminars in Nephrology,* Vol. 6, 1986, with permission.

of the nephron segment of every cell observed could not be identified, many of the cells appeared to be of proximal tubule origin (Figs. 3-2 and 3-3). All the cells were rich in mitochondria, some of which were intact, whereas other mitochondria showed swelling with loss of cristae and still others contained dark bodies (a sign of ischemic change) (Fig. 3-4). Some of the mitochondria with ischemic changes were fused. In some cellular casts, the cellular membranes and constituents appeared intact (Fig. 3-5). Red blood cells (Fig. 3-1), neutrophilic leukocytes, lymphocytes, or monocytes (Fig. 3-1) had infiltrated

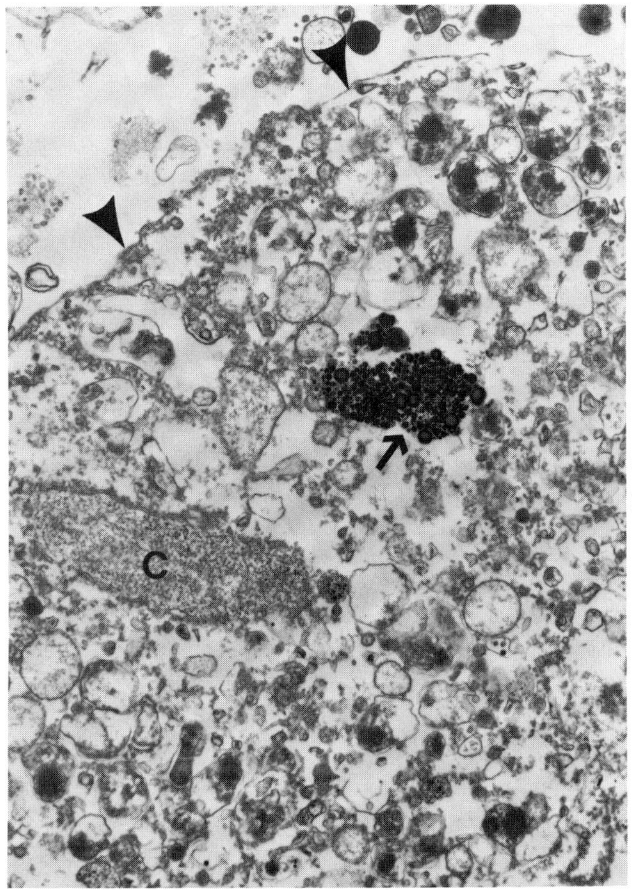

Figure 3-2.   A prominent luminal membrane (arrowheads) and many mitochondria suggest that this cell is of proximal tubule origin. A lysosome is shown (arrow). A granular cast (C) may be superimposed upon the cell (UA + LC, ×6,600).

the tubule cells, but no eosinophils were seen. Lysosomes were scattered throughout the sediment (Fig. 3-6).

Comments: The sediment findings were interpreted as consistent with ATN or acute tubulointerstitial nephritis. Because of the marked swelling of many mitochondria (Figs. 3-2 and 3-3), and ischemic changes in the mitochondria (Fig. 3-4) in many cells, the renal pathology was considered severe. Conversely, because of the presence of intact mitochondria in a few cells

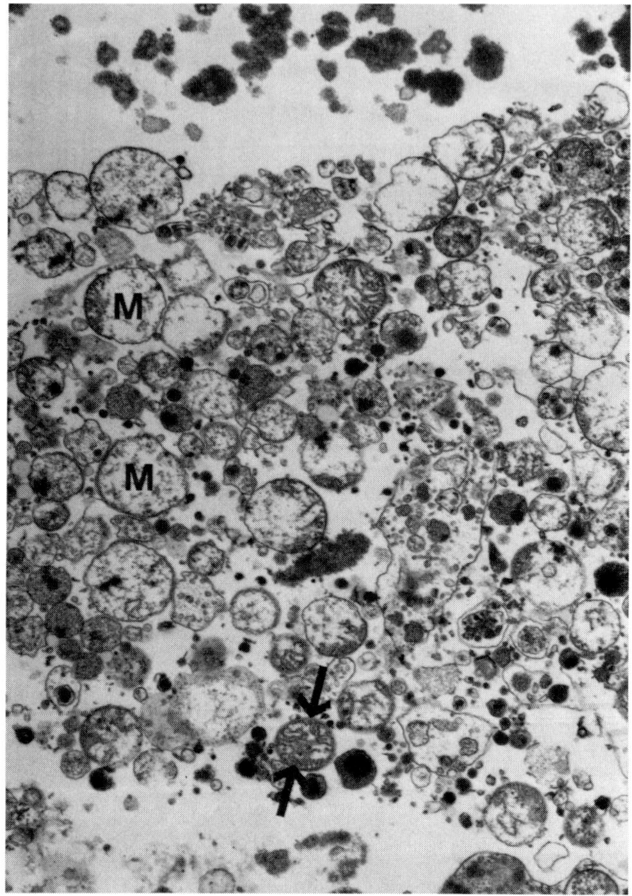

Figure 3-3.   In this tubule cell, apparently of proximal tubule origin, most of the mitochondria (M) are swollen and devoid of cristae, though a few (between arrows) appear intact (UA + LC, ×5,000).

(Fig. 3-5) and abundant lysosomes (Fig. 3-6), the possibility of a reversible process remained. Because of the results of the urinary sediment study, the prospect of a good recovery of renal function was considered unlikely for this patient.

Patient No. 2, H. K., a 61-year-old white male, was admitted to the Veterans Administration Medical Center, Augusta, Georgia on February 15, 1983, for the repair

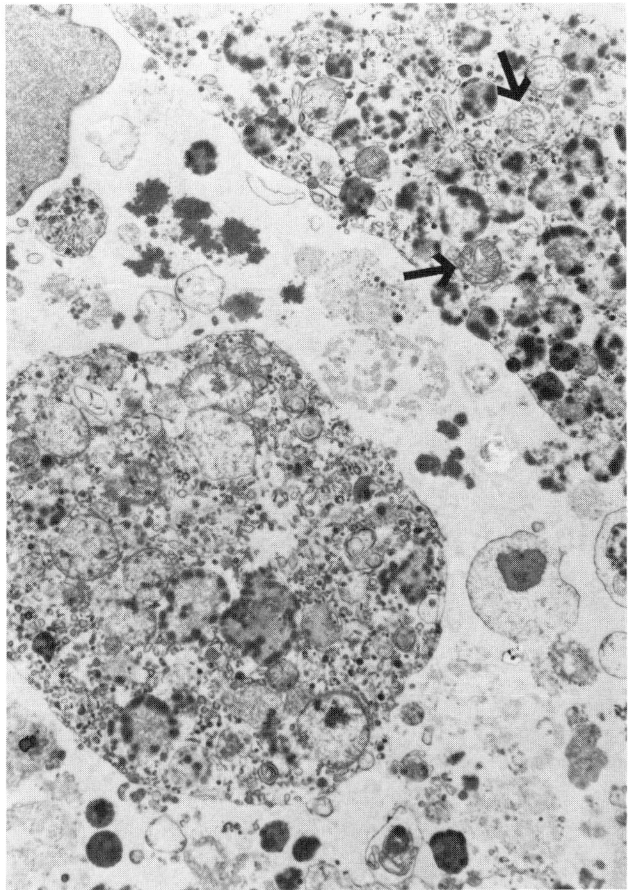

Figure 3-4.   In these tubule cells, which appear to have come from Henle's loops, many mitochondria reveal amorphous dark bodies (a sign of ischemia); few mitochondria (arrows) appear intact (UA + LC, ×3,300).

of an abdominal aortic aneurysm. At surgery, the aneurysm was found to be inoperable because of the multiple areas of extremely thin aortic walls, the large size of the aneurysm, and the extensive involvement of the aortic branches. The aortic aneurysm was treated by a wrapping procedure. Immediately following this surgical procedure, anuric acute renal failure developed. The patient's serum creatinine increased from the baseline level of 2 mg/dl to 16.8 mg/dl. His 24-hr urine output was less than 100 ml, and subsequently dropped to 0. Initially, an arteriovenous shunt and, later, an arteriovenous fistula were created to provide hemodialysis three times a week. The patient's severe hypertension

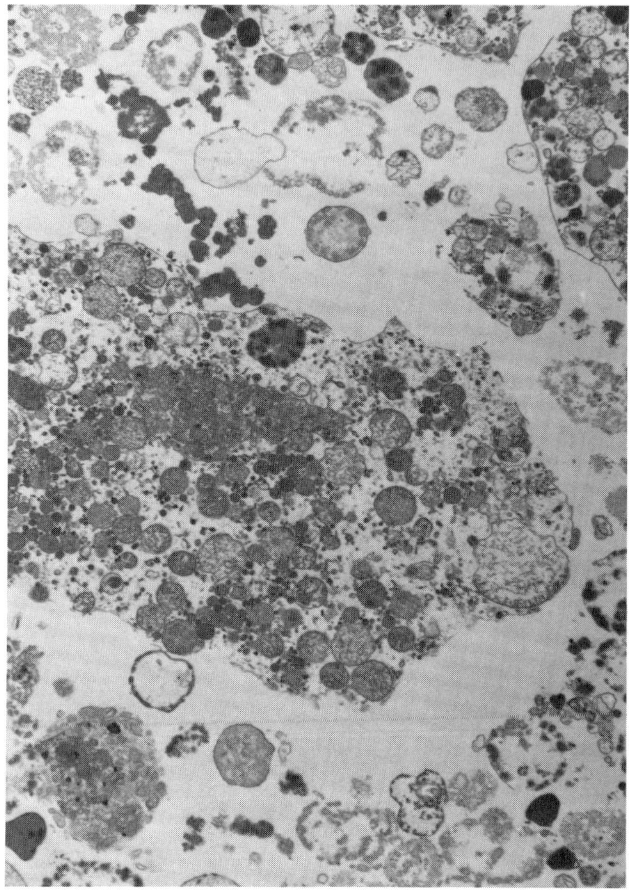

Figure 3-5.   In this renal tubule epithelial cell cast, most of the mitochondria appear intact (UA + LC, ×3,300).

required medication with minoxidil, propranolol, and captopril. He also developed a *Staphylococcus aureus* septicemia from the arteriovenous shunt, which was, however, successfully treated. A urine sample was collected 72 days after the onset of ARF and fixed for TEM analysis. The patient died suddenly at home, possibly from a ruptured abdominal aortic aneurysm.

The TEM study of urinary sediment showed severely necrotic tubule cells. No more than one mitochondrium could be seen in any cell, but plasma membrane infolds separating tubule cells were found (Fig. 3-7), as was a fragment of a necrotic glomerular capillary loop (Fig. 3-8).

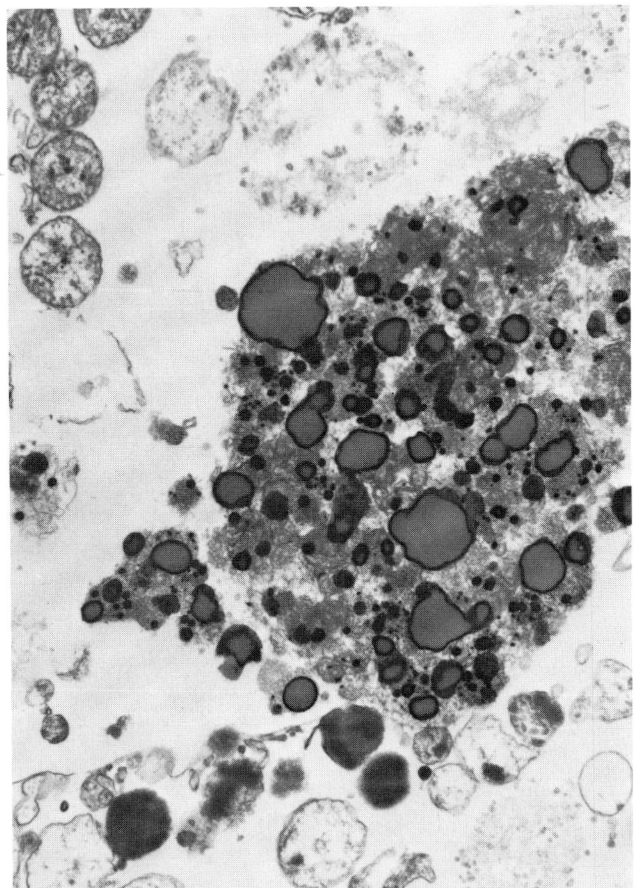

Figure 3-6. Many giant lysosomes, shown here, are seen, suggesting repair activity by renal tubule cells (UA + LC, ×6,600).

Comments: The findings of the urinary study showed little or no chance of renal recovery in this patient. His history revealed that he had anuric ARF from which he never recovered.

Patient No. 3, H. M., a 60-year-old white male, was admitted to the Veterans Administration Medical Center, Augusta, Georgia on June 8, 1983, for the repair of an abdominal aortic aneurysm. On January 26, 1983, he had been seen in the clinic with a history of chest pain radiating to the back and abdomen. An abdominal bruit was heard

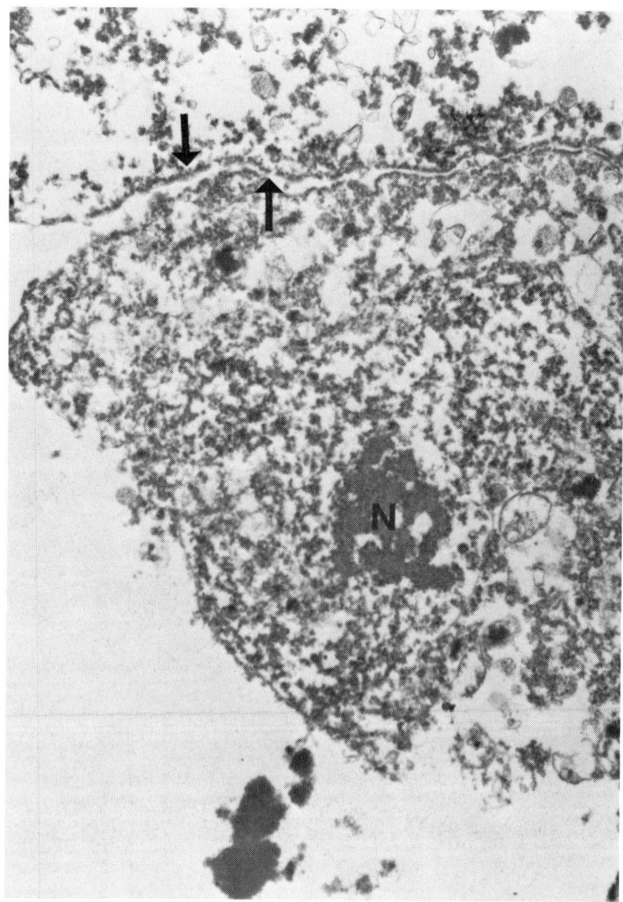

Figure 3-7. The urinary sediment from patient No. 2 shows severe necrosis of tubule cells, the nephron segment of which could not be identified. The cell nucleus (N) is condensed into a mushroom shape. The plasma membrane separating the cells can be identified, however (arrows) (UA + LC, ×13,500).

and a 4-cm fusiform abdominal aortic aneurysm was documented by an abdominal sonogram. A repeat sonogram of the abdomen on June 6, 1983 showed that the aneurysm had enlarged to 5.5 cm. A baseline 24-hr creatinine clearance (Ccr) in June of 1983 was 39 ml/min. On July 7, 1983, he underwent surgery with aneurysmectomy and placement of a Y-graft. For 12 hr prior to surgery, during surgery, and after surgery furosemide was infused at the rate of 20 mg/hr. The postoperative course is shown in Fig. 3-9. As seen in this figure, two days after surgery, his Ccr decreased to less than 10% of base line, but urine output remained unchanged and high. It was thought that he had nonoliguric ARF possibly the result of tubular ischemia. The finding of a markedly low fractional sodium excretion in the face of high urine output was intriguing. Five days after surgery, his urine output dramatically decreased from 3 liters to 600 ml in 24 hr and his Ccr decreased to 1 ml/min, despite continuous furosemide infusion. He became febrile and rectal bleeding was observed. A diagnosis of ischemic colitis was made. The precipitous drop in urine output led to the consideration of ATN or, because of the accompanying ischemic colitis, an antheroembolic disorder involving both the kidneys and the large bowel. A second operation was scheduled, but before this second surgery, a sample of urine was collected for TEM analysis. A left hemicolectomy with a low anterior resection and a transverse colostomy with a feeding catheter jejunostomy were performed. During surgery, the bilateral renal blood flow was believed to be normal, and a wedge biopsy was taken from the left kidney. The renal tissue was fixed for conventional LM and TEM studies. Following surgery, the patient became oligoanuric and progressively azotemic. Daily hemodialysis was initiated. He developed repeated episodes of septicemia. A third surgery required the ligation of the right inferior epigastric artery to control intestinal bleeding. His renal function did not appreciably improve, despite frequent hemodialysis. He died on October 7, 1983.

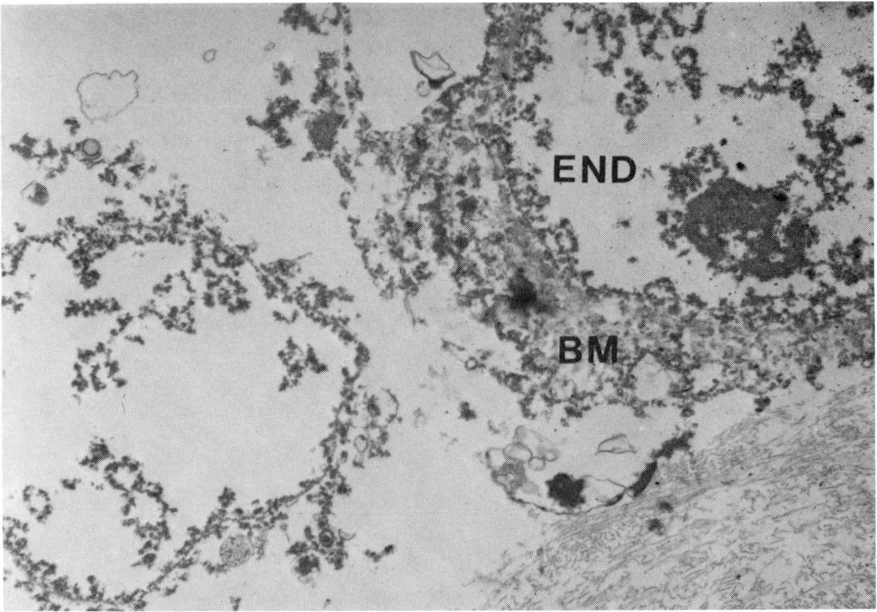

Figure 3-8. This transmission electron micrograph from patient No. 2 shows a segment that appears to be from a glomerular capillary loop. The disrupted basement membrane (BM) and a necrotic endothelial cell (END) are discernible (UA + LC, ×13,500).

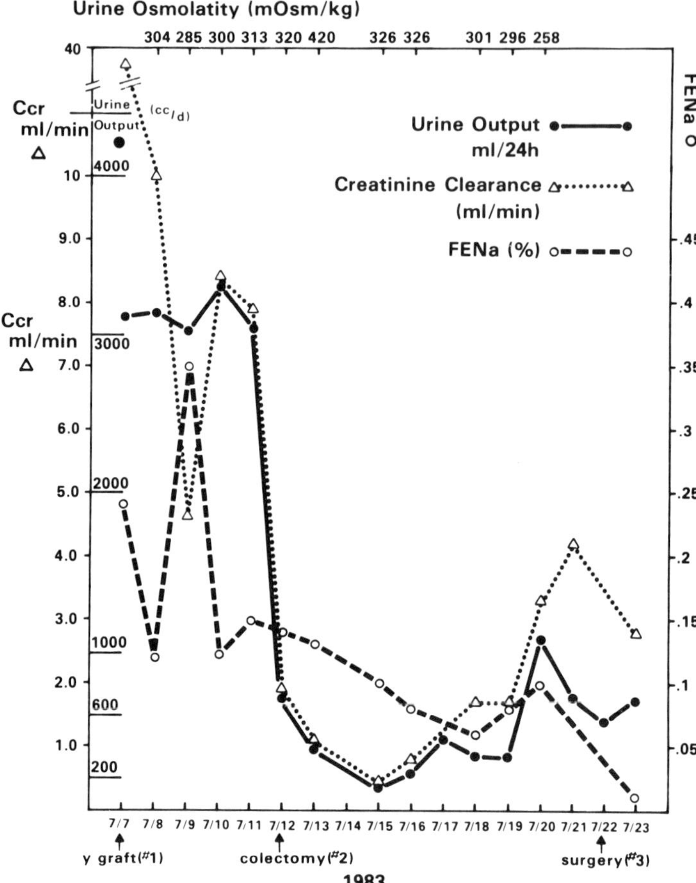

Figure 3-9. The interoperative and postoperative courses in patient No. 3. See the text for details. From *Seminars in Nephrology,* Vol. 6, 1986, with permission.

The TEM study of the urinary sediment showed severely necrotic tubule cells with total disorganization of the cell contents and barely recognizable mitochondria (Fig. 3-10). Many cells were so distorted that the nephron segments from which these cells originated were difficult to identify. Some cells had plentiful mitochondria and appeared to be of proximal tubule origin. These cells also sustained severe injury in that the mitochondria were either markedly swollen with complete loss of cristae (Fig. 3-11) or studded with amorphous dark bodies (Fig. 3-12).

Thick sections taken from the plastic blocks before thin sectioning revealed a needle-shaped cleft within a large arteriole (Fig. 3-13). This finding, reminiscent of cholesterol

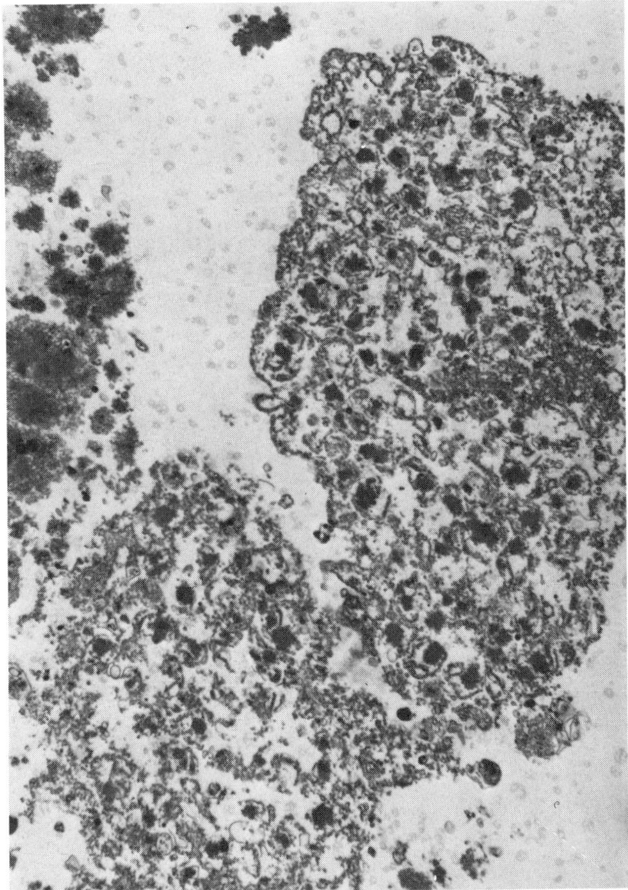

Figure 3-10. In this urinary sediment from patient No. 3, the necrotic tubule cells are barely recognizable. The cells lack mitochondria and much of the cytoplasm has been replaced by fluid (UA + LC, ×5,000).

emboli, established a diagnosis of an atheroembolic disorder of the kidney. Though glomerular sclerosis and interstitial fibrosis were seen, the tubules were essentially intact. The TEM study of thin sections revealed fairly intact tubules (Fig. 3-14). The findings (Figs. 3-13 and 3-14) were inconsistent with the necrotic appearance of the tubule cells in the urinary sediment shown in Figs. 3-10–3-12. Therefore, in an attempt to discover why the tubule epithelial cells were necrotic, sections were cut from the paraffin blocks for conventional LM and what, if any, pathology might have been missed. Conventional LM of paraffin-embedded sections revealed ATN (Fig. 3-15) and areas of infarct (Fig.

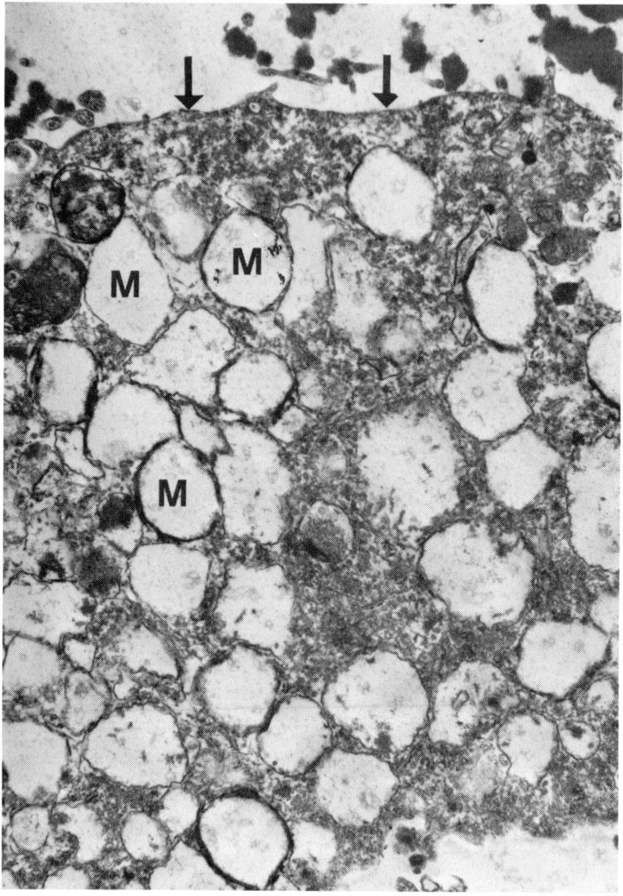

Figure 3-11. The urinary sediment again, from patient No. 3, shows a cell that appears to be a proximal tubule cell. The inner membrane (arrows) is still intact, but all the mitochondria (M) are markedly swollen and devoid of cristae (UA + LC, ×6,600).

Figure 3-13. This thick (plastic) section light micrograph shows needle-shaped clefts within the lumen of a large arteriole (between arrows). Not shown here is the transmission electron micrograph of the same arteriole, in which the cleft passes through and divides the endothelial layer. Close inspection of this micrograph shows that the cleft on the left has encroached on the endothelial layer, whereas the cleft on the right is separated from the endothelial layer by a chink in the lumen. Tubules (T) are few and far, separated by a prominent interstitial fibrosis (I) (epoxy tissue stain, ×400). From *Seminars in Nephrology,* Vol. 6, 1986, with permission.

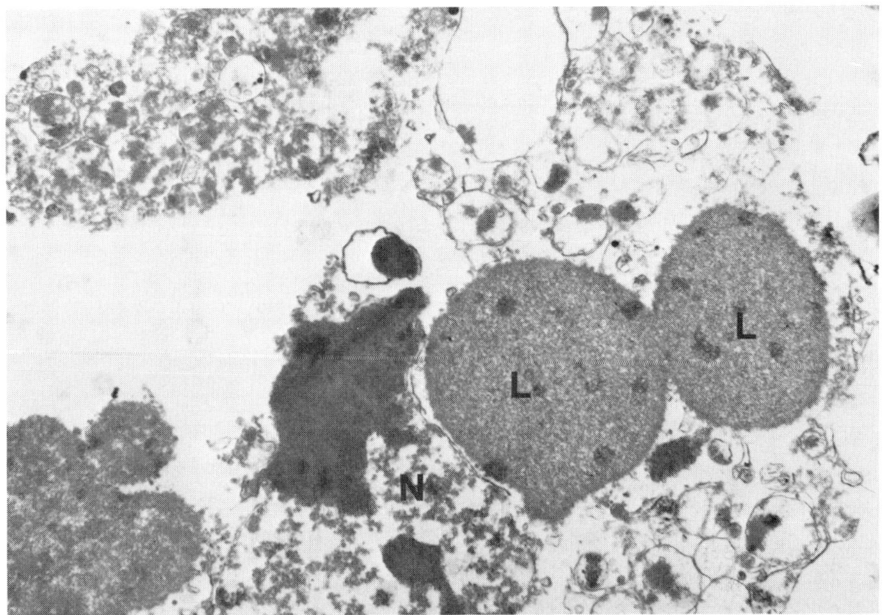

Figure 3-12. In this urinary sediment from patient No. 3 (see Figs. 3-10 and 3-11), a necrotic cell with dissolution of the nucleus (N) and many mitochondria with amorphous dark bodies can be seen. The large electron-dense granules appear to be lipid droplets (L) (UA + LC, ×6,600).

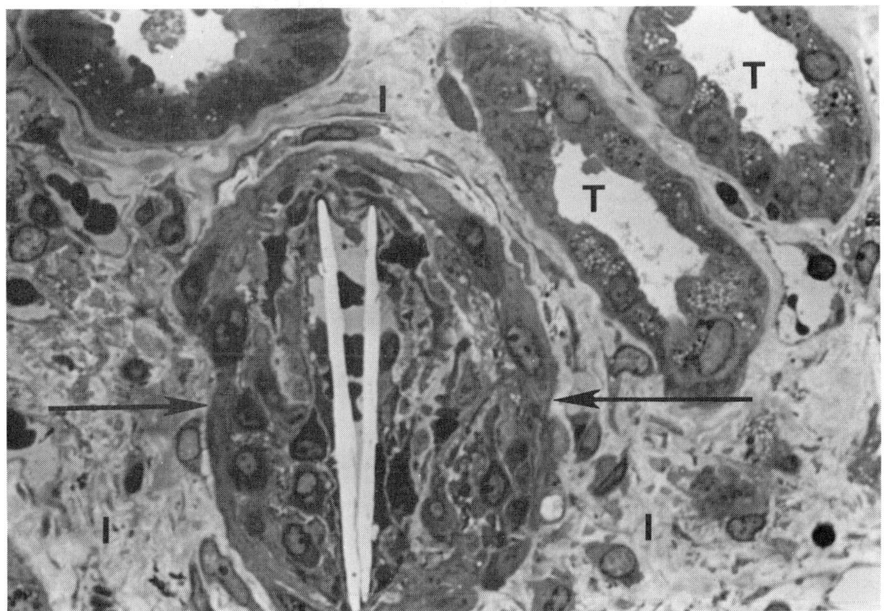

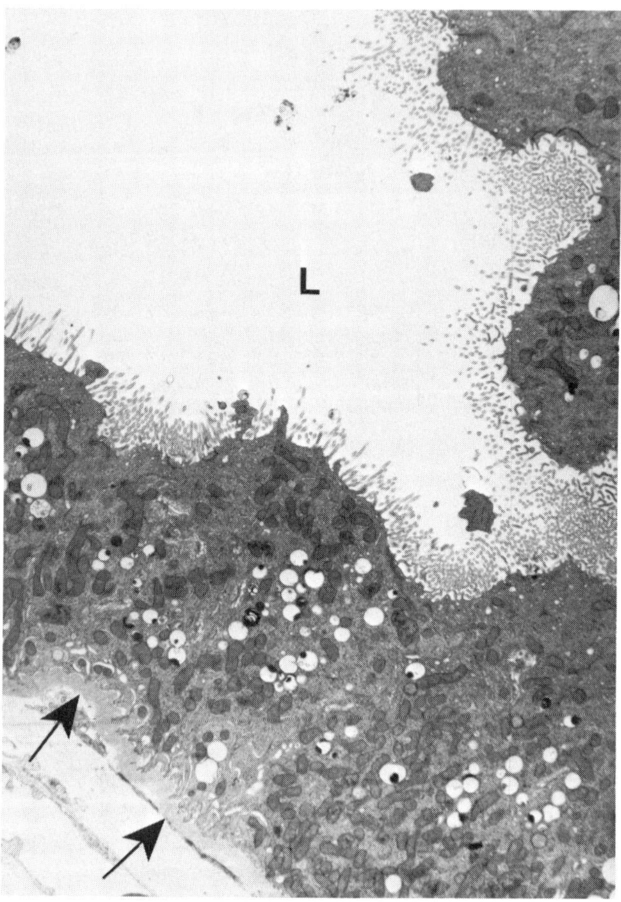

Figure 3-14. This transmission electron micrograph of a proximal tubule shows some disruption of the microvilli; also, fewer microvilli than normal are seen. Except for vacuoles, the proximal tubule cells appear to be intact. The basement membrane (arrows) and lumen of the tubule (L) are shown (UA + LC, ×2,000).

Figure 3-16. In this light micrograph, necrosis and thrombosis of a glomerulus (G) and widespread necrosis of the tubules (T) can be seen. Most of the tubules are empty, which might reflect shedding of the necrotic epithelium into the urine (H & E, ×200).

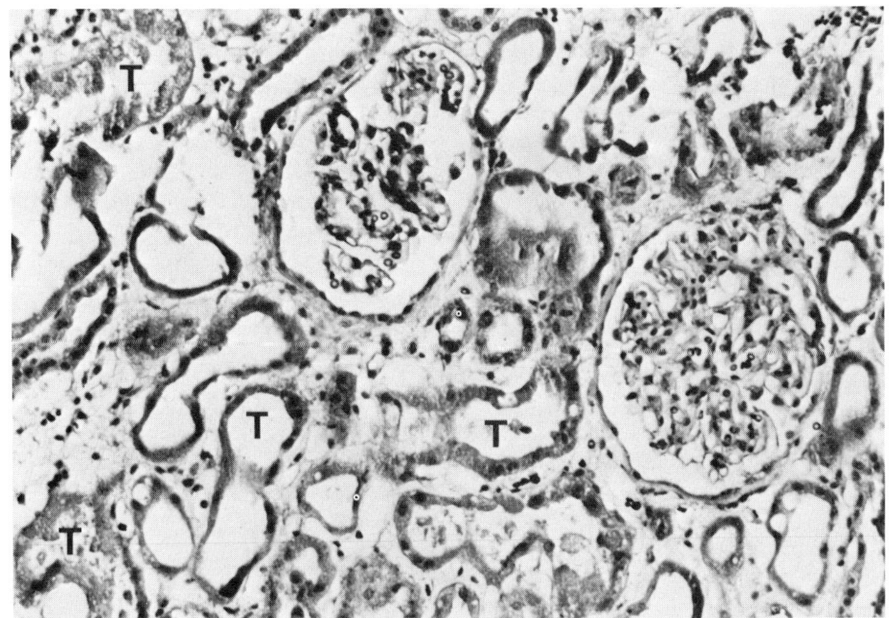

Figure 3-15.   In this light micrograph, the glomeruli appear essentially normal. Most of the tubules are dilated, with flattened (atrophic) epithelium and a few scattered tubules (T) show an epithelial necrosis (H & E, ×200).

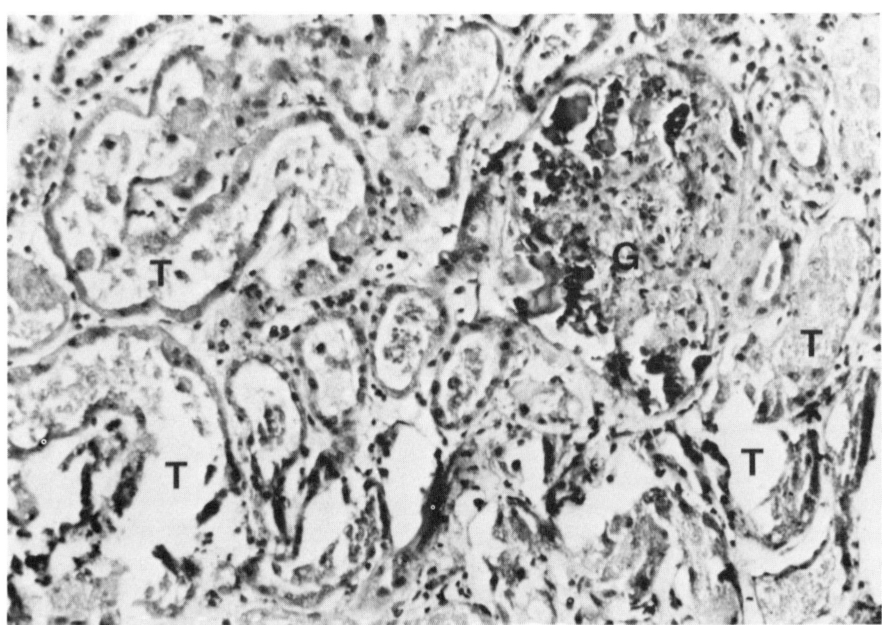

3-16). Thin sections from the remaining plastic blocks, however, revealed well-preserved distal and collecting tubules but necrotic tubule cells in the lumen of many of these intact tubules (Fig. 3-17). Apparently a necrosis of tubules occurred somewhere proximally and cells had been shed through the lumen of intact distal tubules only to appear in the urine. The necrotic tubule cells seen inside the lumen of a collecting tubule shown in Fig. 3-17 were similar to those in the urinary sediment in Fig. 3-12.

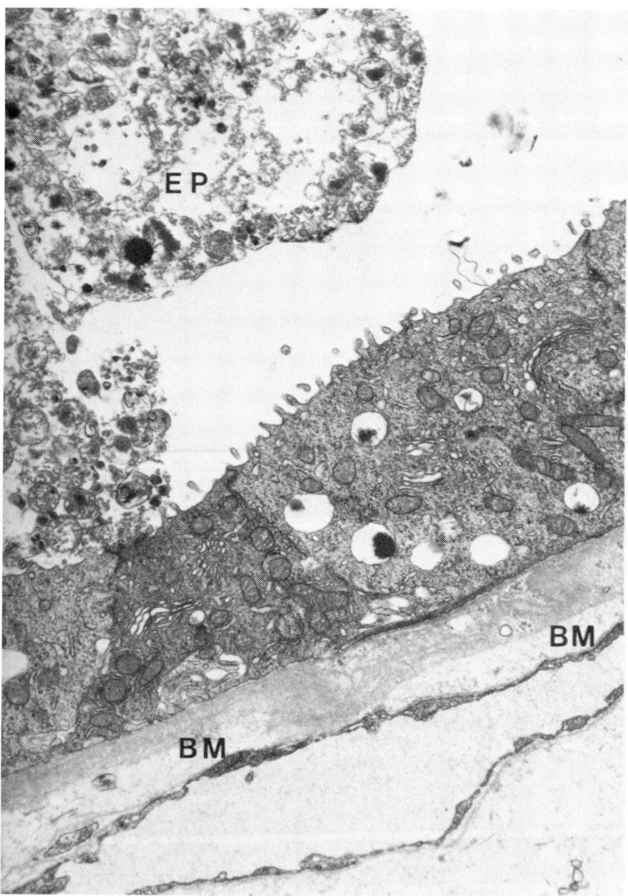

Figure 3-17. In subsequent TEM studies of the renal biopsy from patient No. 3, the collecting tubule cells appeared normal. The basement membrane (BM) of the collecting tubule, however, is thickened. Within the lumen, masses of necrotic tubule epithelial cells rich in mitochondria (EP) are seen. Because of excessive numbers of mitochondria, the necrotic cells are probably of proximal tubule origin (UA + LC, ×3,300). From *Seminars in Nephrology,* Vol. 6, 1986, with permission.

Comments: The results of a urinary sediment study indicated the presence of a severe necrotic renal lesion, which was subsequently found. Focal cortical infarcts and ATN were confirmed histologically. Fragments of necrotic tubule cells similar to those in the urinary sediment were found in the lumen of intact distal tubules, suggesting a proximal tubular necrosis.

Patient No. 4, B. F., a 71-year-old white male pharmacist, was admitted to the Veterans Administration Medical Center, Augusta, Georgia on August 25, 1983, with a history that he had stopped urinating for one week before admission. He stated that the

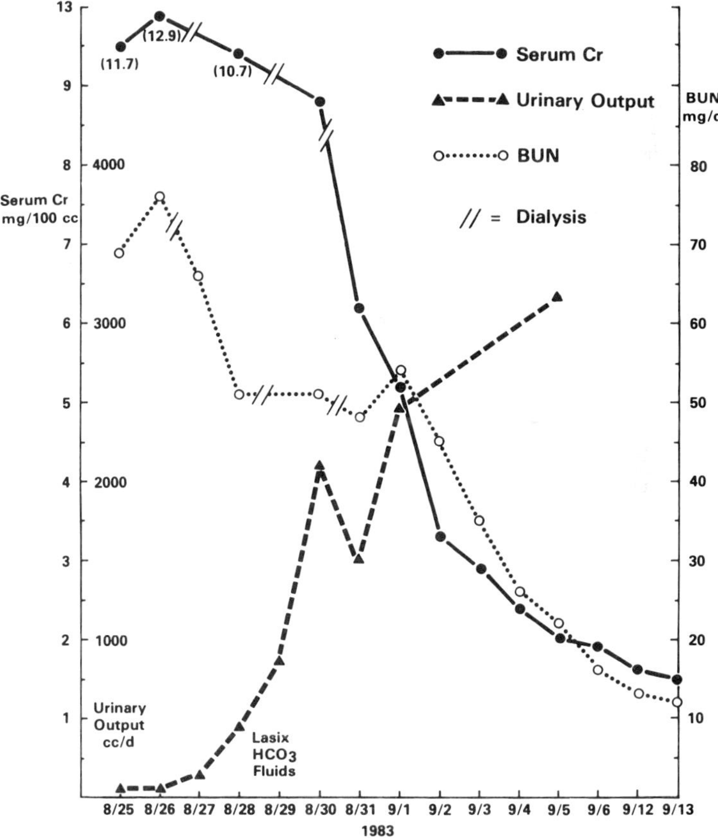

Figure 3-18. The hospital course of patient No. 4 is shown. Initially anuric, his urine output slightly increased after two hemodialysis treatments and markedly increased after rechallenge with fluids, bicarbonate, and furosemide. See the text for a full description. From *Seminars in Nephrology,* Vol. 6, 1986, with permission.

problem started after an episode that he described as gout. He went to his local physician who gave him an injection of Lasix® with no improvement of the condition. Three days before admission, he had nausea and vomiting and lost his appetite. He had a long history of recurrent gout and a long history of alcohol abuse. Since he was a pharmacist he had, on his own, started taking allopurinol (100 mg daily) from the time he stopped urinating. The admission physical examination revealed that he was poorly responsive, agitated, and anuric. Laboratory studies on admission showed a serum urea nitrogen of 69 mg/dl, a serum creatinine of 11.7 mg/dl, and a serum uric acid of 13.0 mg/dl. His renal function status before admission was unknown. Other serum chemistries on admission revealed a sodium of 142 mEq/liter; potassium, 4.2 mEq/liter; chloride, 96 mEq/liter; CO_2, 17.7 mEq/liter; phosphate, 9.92 mg/dl; and calcium, 7.0 mg/dl. A diagnosis of acute uric acid nephropathy was made; the possibility of rhabdomyolysis on the basis of a history of alcohol abuse and hyperuricemia, hyperphosphatemia, and hypocalcemia could not be excluded, however, an attempt to induce diuresis by intravenous fluid and furosemide met with slight or no success. The patient was also found to be anemic: A complete blood count showed WBC, 7.8×10^3; RBC, 3.14×10^6; hemoglobin, 10.1 g/dl; and hematocrit, 31.3%. The red blood cell indices were within normal limits. His general condition continued to deteriorate and, on August 26, 1983, his serum urea nitrogen and serum creatinine were 76 mg/dl and 12.9 mg/dl, respectively, and his serum uric acid had increased to 15.6 mg/dl. On August 26, 1983, hemodialysis was initiated. The hospital course is shown in Fig. 3-18. After two hemodialysis treatments, his serum chemistries showed urea nitrogen 51 mg/dl; creatinine, 10.7 mg/dl; and uric acid, 9.1 mg/dl. He was again challenged with normal saline containing bicarbonate and intravenous furosemide, after which his urine output increased dramatically and reached 3 liters in 24 hr. At the same time, his serum urea nitrogen and serum creatinine rapidly decreased. As shown in Fig. 3-18, in a period of 15 days his serum urea nitrogen and serum creatinine returned to normal levels.

First and second urine samples were collected for TEM analysis upon admission, and when urine output increased after the second furosemide challenge, a third sample was collected before his discharge from the hospital September 14, 1983. Two months after discharge from the hospital, he was seen in the renal clinic. He renal function was normal. A fourth sample of urine was collected for TEM analysis. The TEM study of urinary samples are presented in Figs. 3-19–3-24. In this patient, the urinary sediment was unique because the presence of many papillary (medullary) interstitial cells during both the oligoanuric and the recovery phase. During the oligoanuric phase, the cells showed severe changes, though the cellular anatomy was identifiable (Fig. 3-23). In human kidneys, the amount of papillary interstitial cell granularity is less than that in the rat kidney.[11] During the recovery phase, the sediment consisted mainly of interstitial cells (Fig. 3-24), though a few tubule cells (Fig. 3-22) were found. The cells during the recovery phase were better preserved than those during the oligoanuric phase. During the recovery phase, tight bundles of fibers, interpreted as uric acid crystals, were found in the urinary sediment.

Comments: The appearance of many papillary interstitial cells in the urinary sediment suggested that the renal medulla and papilla had sustained the brunt of the lesion. The latter portions of the kidney, however, were vulnerable to

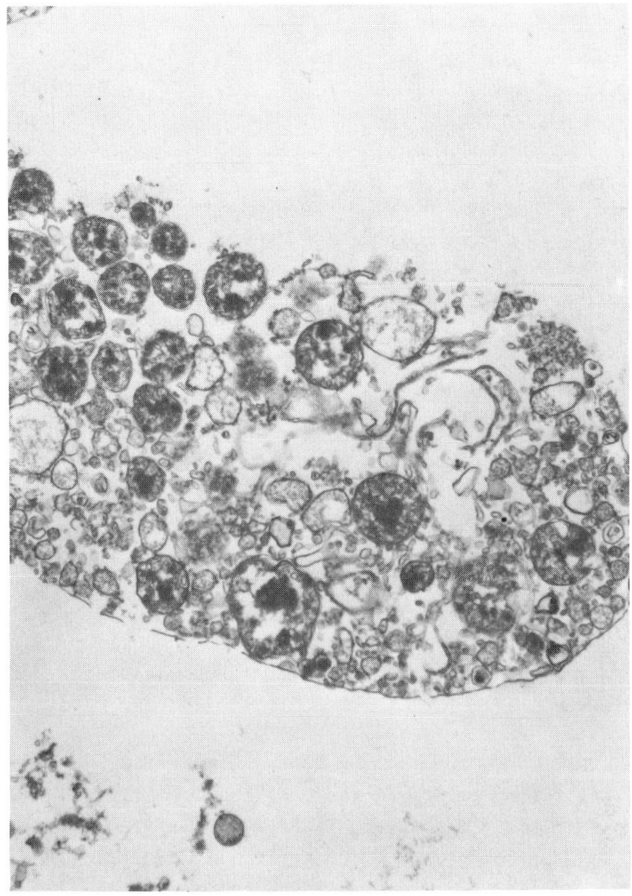

Figure 3-19. This transmission electron micrograph of patient No. 4 shows an epithelial cell cast in the oliguric phase of acute renal failure. The anatomy of the nephron segment cannot be identified from this cell, though all the mitochondria show ischemic changes. Few ribosomes and other cellular constituents are seen (UA + LC, ×6,600).

damage by uric acid deposits. The medullary interstitium was severely affected by this metabolic product, possibly through injury of the tubule basement membrane. The findings of the urinary sediment study indicated a uric acid nephropathy and a prospect for good renal recovery, which was confirmed clinically by the complete reversal of ARF in this patient.

Patient No. 5, R. B., a 74-year-old white male, was admitted to the Veterans Administration Medical Center, Augusta, Georgia on June 16, 1983, with a history of

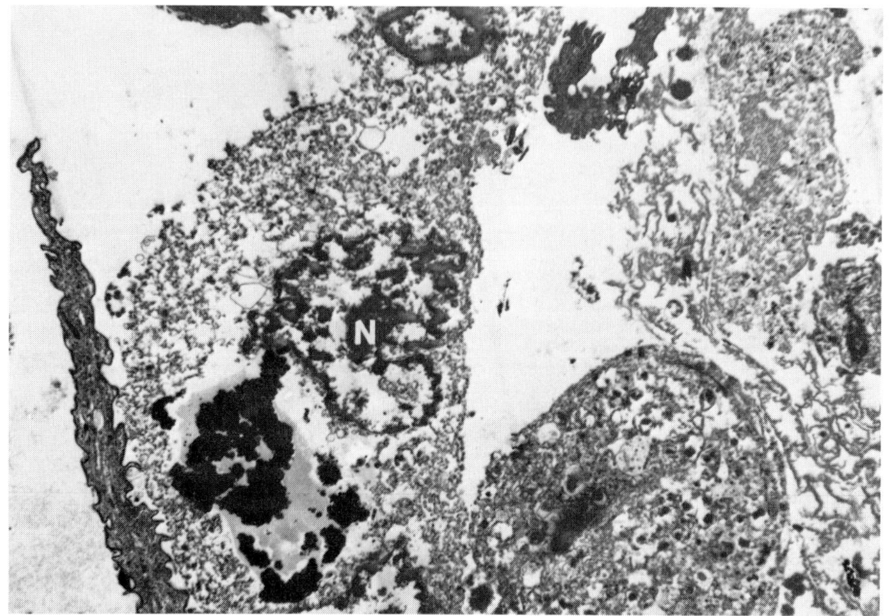

Figure 3-20.   During the oliguric phase of ARF (patient No. 4), many damaged tubule epithelial cells were found. Because cell nuclei (N) can be found, there is the potential for recovery of the nephron segments from which these cells originated (UA + LC, ×6,000).

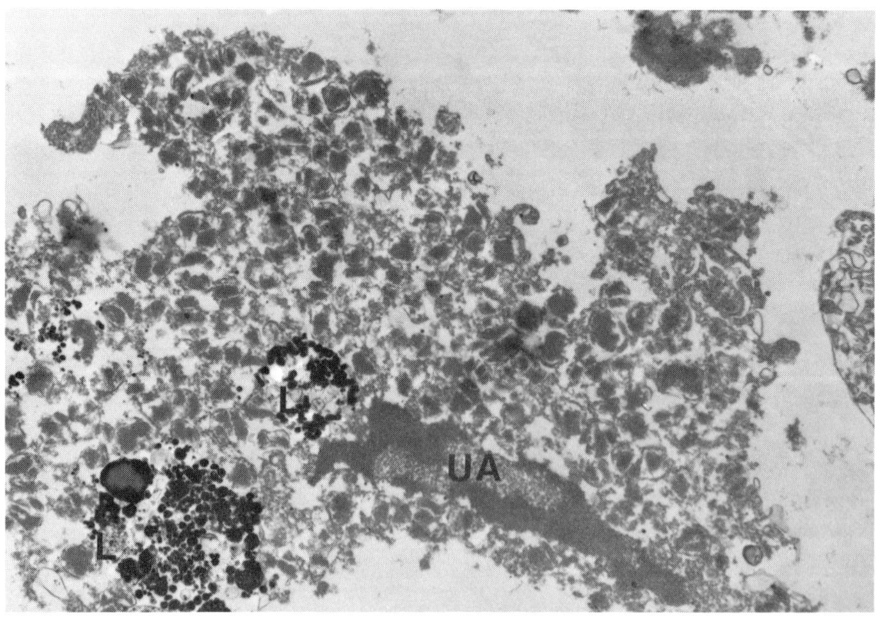

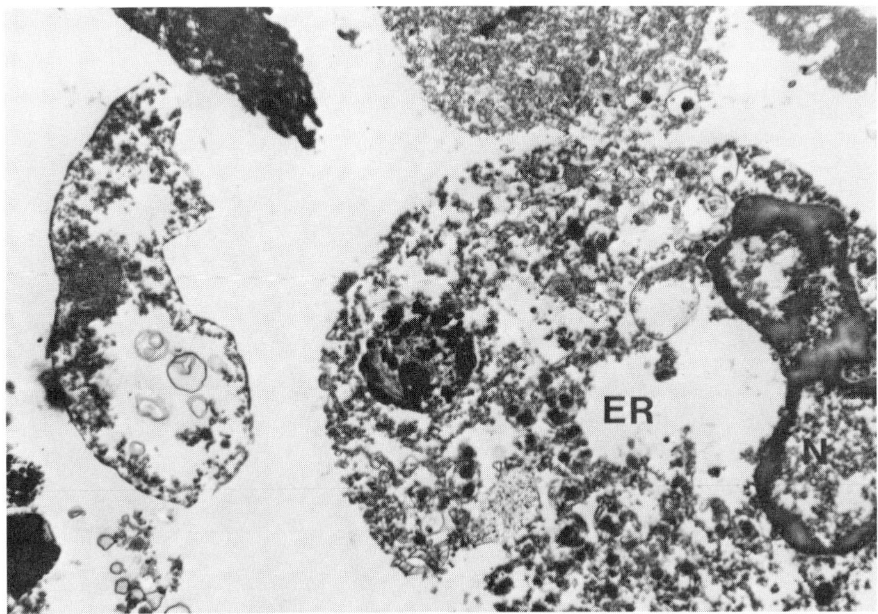

Figure 3-22.   This transmission electron micrograph shows a renal medullary interstitial cell during the polyuric phase (patient No. 4). Note the few dilated endoplasmic reticulum (ER). The nucleus (N) shows dissolution (UA + LC, ×5,000).

inability to pass urine and obtundation for 24 hr before admission. The patient had fractured his right femur one week before admission. Admission serum chemistry showed urea nitrogen, 145 mg/dl; creatinine, 15 mg/dl; potassium, 6.2 mEq/liter; calcium, 7.6 mg/dl; and phosphate 14 mg/dl. There was no previous history of renal disease. Nalfon, a nonsteroidal antiinflammatory agent had been prescribed before admission. Upon admission, a straight bladder catheter was inserted and a small (unmeasured) amount of urine was obtained and sent for urinalysis and culture. Urinalysis showed a specific gravity of 1.013; WBC, 25–30, along with clumps of WBC; RBC, 10–12; and epithelial cells, 8–10 in a high power fields. At the time of admission, the patient was afebrile, a peripheral WBC count was normal; 6 hr after bladder catheterization, however, he had a temperature of 101° F. A diagnosis of sepsis was made and blood samples were sent for culture. Both blood and urine cultures revealed the growth of *Proteus mirabilis*. Meanwhile, a sonogram of the kidneys revealed no evidence of urinary tract obstruction, but a thin cortex was

---

Figure 3-21.   A severely necrotic tubule epithelial cell during the oliguric phase (patient No. 4) is shown; two large lysosomes (L) are seen. The elliptical structure may be a uric acid (UA) crystal (UA + LC, ×6,600). From *Seminars in Nephrology,* Vol. 6, 1986, with permission.

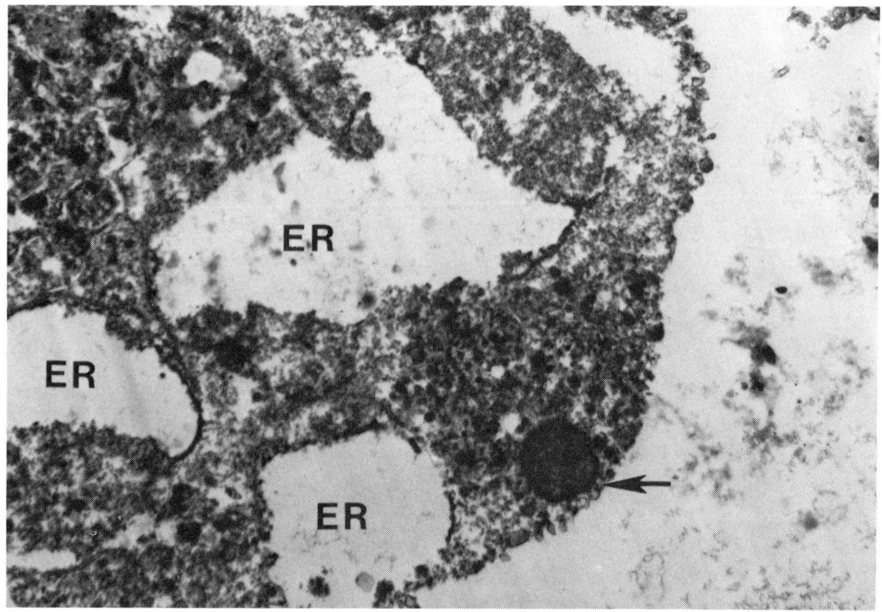

Figure 3-23.   A renal papillary interstitial cell during the polyuric phase is shown. This cell is characterized by many markedly dilated endoplasmic reticula (ER), many ribosomes, and an electron-dense granule (arrow) (UA + LC, ×5,000). From *Seminars in Nephrology*, Vol. 6, 1986, with permission.

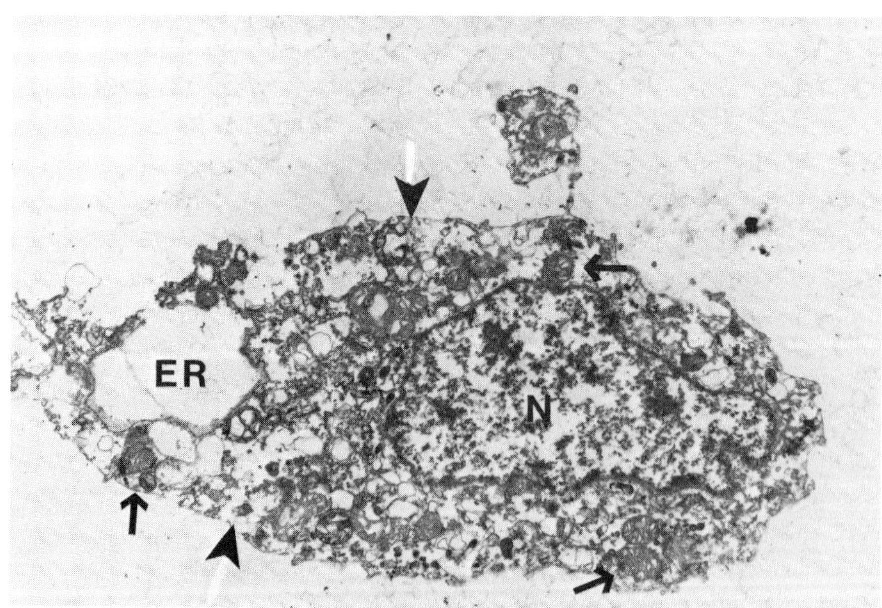

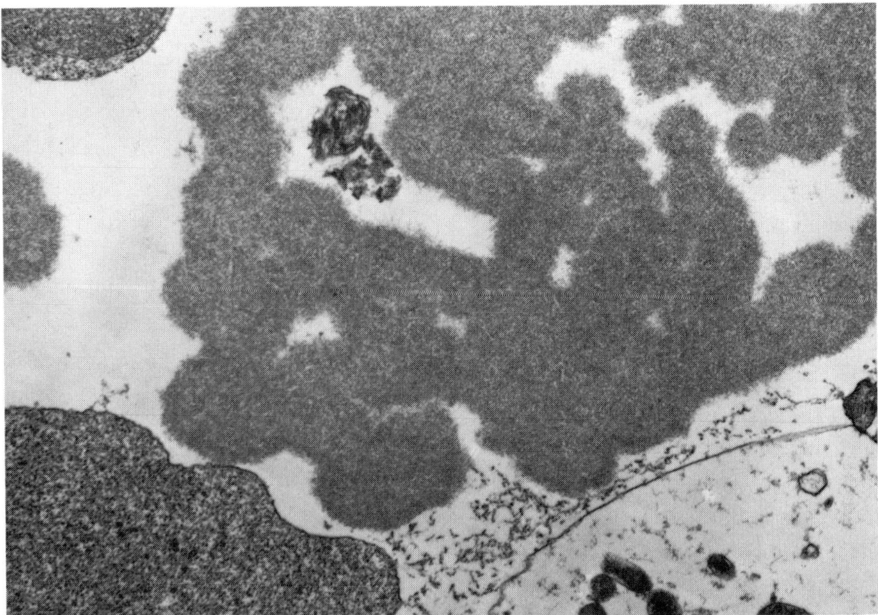

Figure 3-25. This transmission electron micrograph (patient No. 5) shows fibrin masses inside the lumen of a tubule cell (UA + LC, ×6,600).

described bilaterally. Daily hemodialysis was instituted and he was treated with gentamicin for sepsis. He recovered from sepsis, but his renal function did not improve. He remained oliguric to anuric and required hemodialysis three times a week.

Administration of fluids accompanied by diuretics failed to induce diuresis. Because of marked hyperphosphatemia and hypocalcemia, an initial diagnosis of rhabdomyolysis was made.

A urine sample was collected for TEM analysis 7 days after admission to the hospital. The TEM study of urine sediment revealed such thrombotic features as fibrin masses (Fig. 3-25) in the tubules. In addition, free clots and RBC showing evidence of hemolysis (Fig. 3-26) were found,[12] as were a few more tubule epithelial cells with necrotic changes. A more exact diagnosis of microangiopathic hemolytic anemia is suggested by these findings. An excessive number of lysosomes (Fig. 3-27) and occasional myeloid bodies in the tubule epithelial cells might represent an aminoglycoside effect, whereas the urinary sediment study showing features of renal thrombosis suggested a diagnosis of disseminated

◄────────────────────────────────

Figure 3-24. Several renal papillary interstitial cells, similar to the one shown here, were found in the urine sediment two months after patient No. 4 recovered from ARF. This reasonably well-preserved cell shows an intact nucleus (N) with nucleoli, many intact mitochondria (arrows), and dilated endoplasmic reticula (ER), a characteristic feature of this cell. The cellular membrane (arrowheads) is also intact (UA + LC, ×3,300).

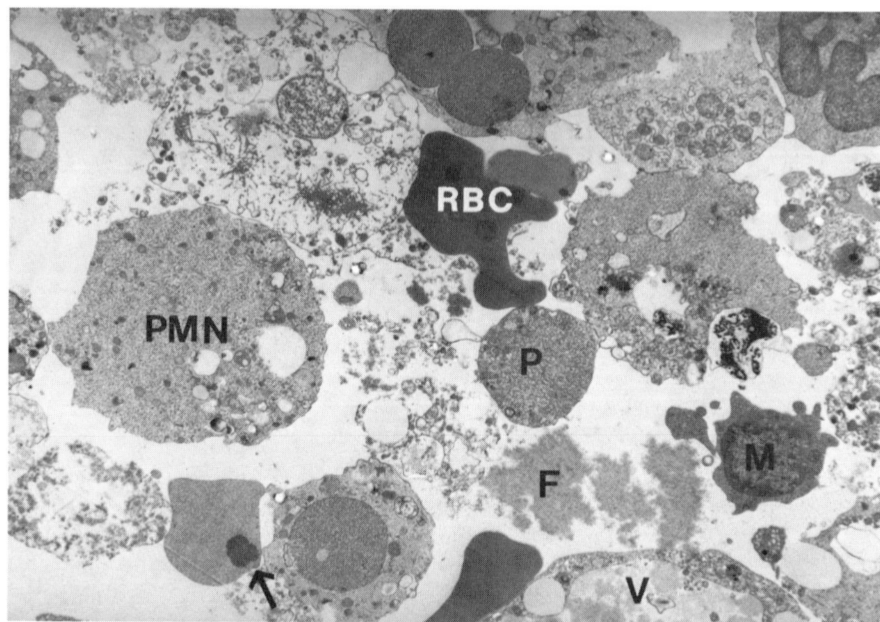

Figure 3-26. Fragments of a clot characterized by a degenerated polymorphonuclear neutrophil (PMN), a platelet (P), a monocyte (M), and red blood cells (RBC) are shown. The RBC shows bodies (arrow) such as are found in hemolytic anemia. An RBC is seen adhering to the wall of a necrotic segment of a vessel (V), and a fibrin mass (F) is seen along the vessel wall (patient No. 5) (UA + LC, ×2,600).

intravascular coagulation (DIC). The patient died on November 4, 1983. An autopsy showed evidence of kidney and liver thrombosis (Figs. 3-28 and 3-29), and renal tubule necrosis.

Comments: The urinary sediment study prompted the diagnosis of DIC in this patient. It remained unclear whether the DIC caused the ARF or whether the DIC was superimposed upon the rhabdomyolysis and induced the ARF.

Patient No. 6, J. J., a 67-year-old white male, was admitted to the Veterans Administration Medical Center, Augusta, Georgia on December 30, 1983, with a 2-day history

Figure 3-28. This light micrograph of a paraffin-embedded section of an autopsied kidney from patient No. 5 shows thrombosis in glomerular arterioles (A) and in capillaries of the glomerular hilum (H). The glomerulus appears somewhat bloodless, and the tubules (T) are necrotic (H & E, ×200).

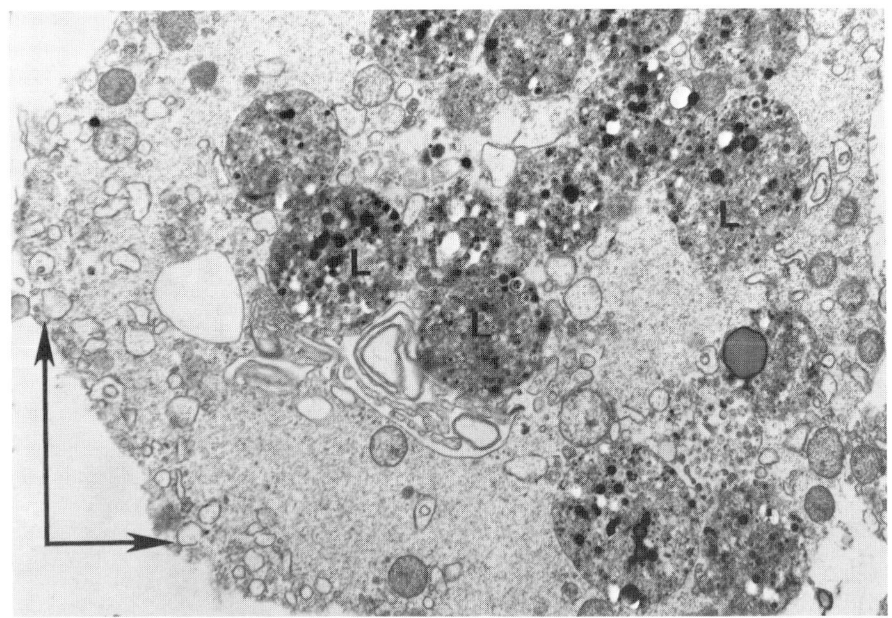

Figure 3-27. A proximal tubule cell shows apical pits (arrows) and a damaged luminal membrane. The many giant lysosomes (L) may be the result of the aminoglycoside effect (patient No. 5) (UA + LC, ×5,500).

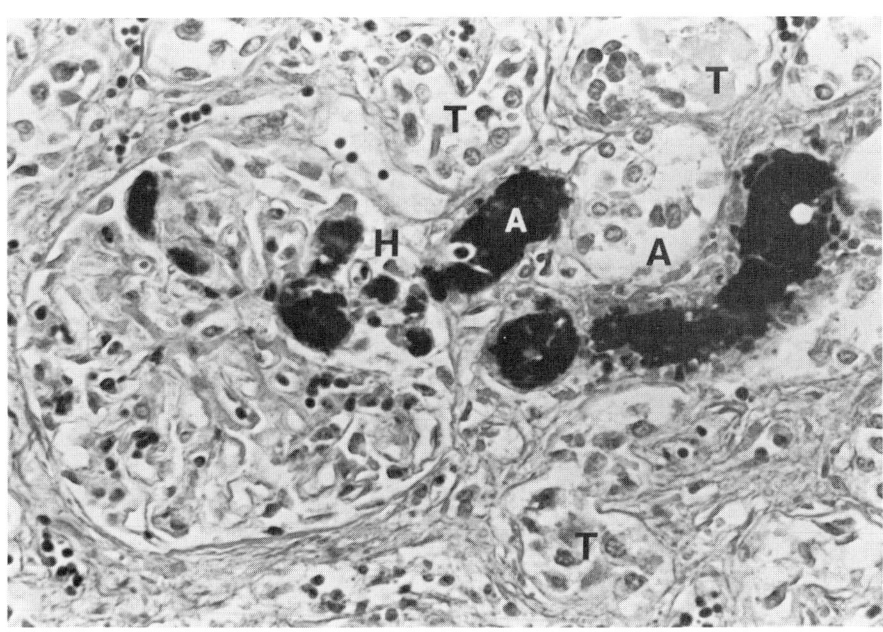

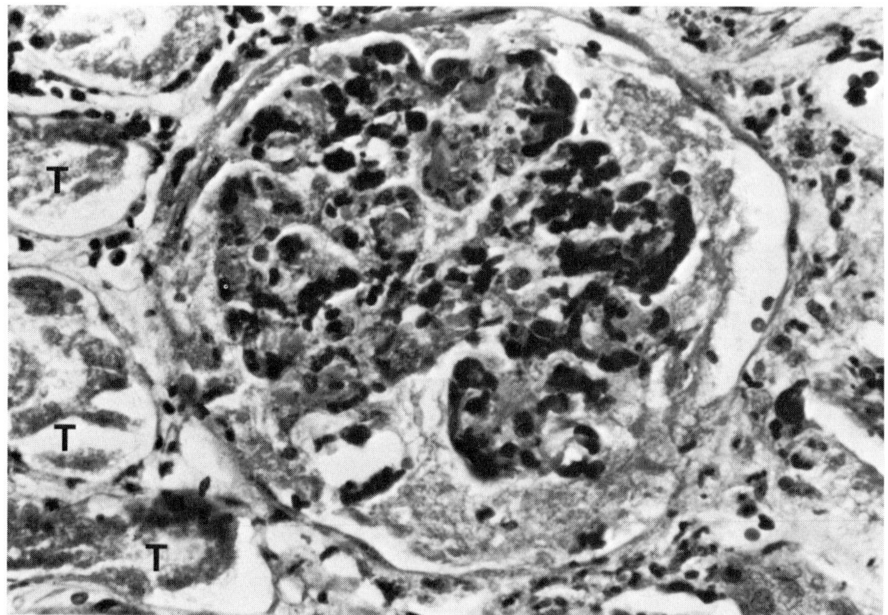

Figure 3-29. This section from patient No. 5 shows the glomerulus to be thrombotic and necrotic. Tubules (T) show a complete necrosis of cells and a separation of the epithelia from the basement membranes (H & E, ×200).

of chest pain, which had responded to four sublingual nitroglycerin tablets. On the day of admission, he had recurrence of chest pain, which was not relieved by nitroglycerin; he was, therefore, admitted for possible myocardial infarction. On his second hospital day, he suddenly complained of pain in both legs and developed mottling of the abdomen and legs. Both lower extremities felt cold and no pulse was palpable below the groin. The femoral pulses, however, were bounding. The patient passed Coca Cola-colored urine, the color of which was thought to be the result of myoglobinuria. An emergency abdominal aortogram revealed a decrease in blood flow below both femoral arteries. Streptokinase therapy was initiated. His serum chemistry on January 2, 1984, revealed a urea nitrogen of 42 mg/dl; creatinine, 2.1 mg/dl, and normal electrolytes. Before admission, his serum creatinine (Sr) had been 1.5 mg/dl. His condition, however, deteriorated rapidly; he became oliguric, and his serum urea nitrogen (SUN) and Scr continued to rise. Serum creatinine phosphokinase (CPK) on January 4, 1984 was 16,520 IU/L (normal, 24–195 IU/L). The patient was thought to have arterial thrombosis of both legs, which was not be reversed by streptokinase. On January 5, 1984, he underwent bilateral, above-the-knee amputation. From the morning of January 6, 1984, he became anuric and his Scr increased to 5.1 mg/dl. The subsequent course is illustrated in Fig. 3-30. Hemodialysis was initiated, but because of the patient's cardiovascular instability, ultrafiltration, combined with brief periods of hemodialysis, was begun. Intravenous

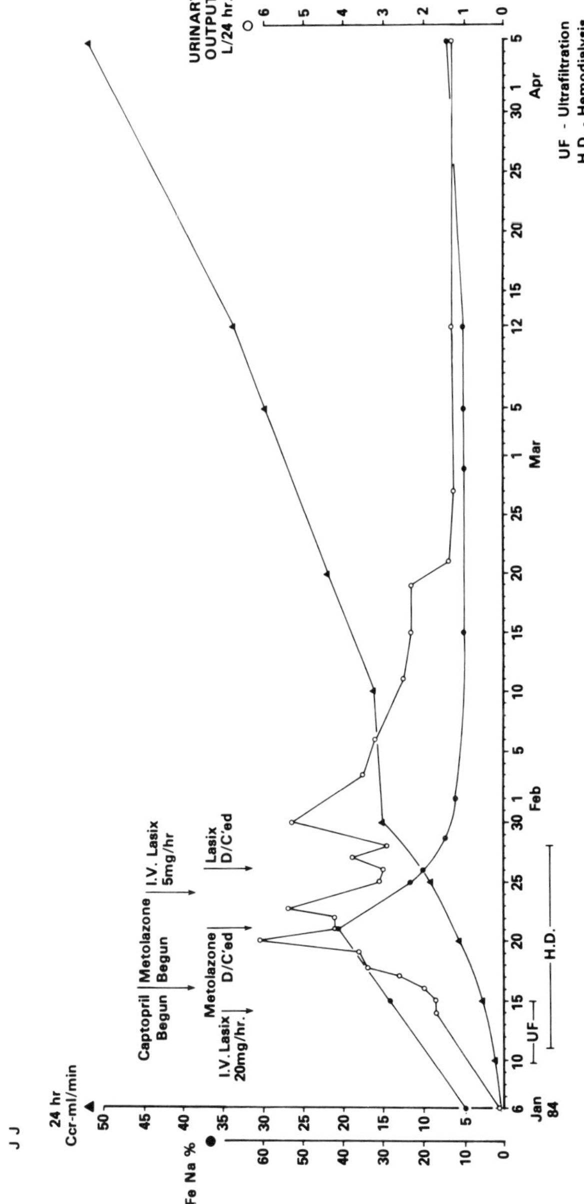

Figure 3-30. The course of the ARF in patient No. 6 is shown. See the text for details.

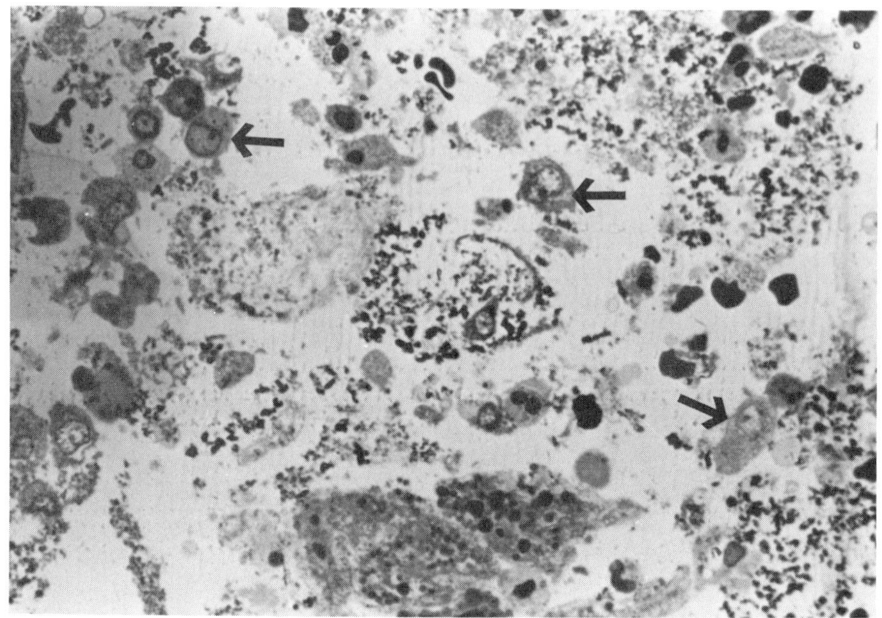

Figure 3-31.   This light micrograph shows many tubule epithelial cells characterized by large nuclei (arrows) (patient No. 6) (epoxy tissue stain, ×200).

infusion of furosemide (Lasix®) 20 mg/hr was initiated. Captopril was added to the regimen with the idea that the renin–angiotensin system is activated in ARF. His urine output promptly increased and remained in the range of 4–5 liters/day and then gradually decreased to normal. Simultaneously, the fractional excretion of sodium increased and decreased at the same rate as urine output. His 24-hr creatinine clearance showed a slow but progressive rise. After discharge from the hospital on March 9, 1984, he was followed frequently in the renal clinic and his renal function was monitored at each clinic visit. A 24-hr creatinine clearance, as of May 2, 1985, was 42.5 ml/min. On August 1, 1985, his SUN and Scr were 22 mg/dl and 1.4 mg/dl, respectively. The latest Scr level is better than the baseline level before his admission. A urine sample was collected for TEM analysis 3 days after the onset of anuric ARF.

The thick section stained with epoxy tissue stain (LM) showed many tubule cells (Fig. 3-31). The TEM study of urinary sediment showed proximal tubule cell necrosis (Fig. 3-32) and many WBC and white blood cell casts. An interesting finding was the presence of a segment of an arteriole with a cleft in the endothelial cell, suggesting cholesterol emboli (Fig. 3-33), which is a characteristic feature of an atheroembolic disorder of the kidney. The TEM study of a second urinary sediment during recovery from ARF and 42 days after the onset of ARF showed only squamous epithelial cells and a few bacteria (Fig. 3-34).[18]

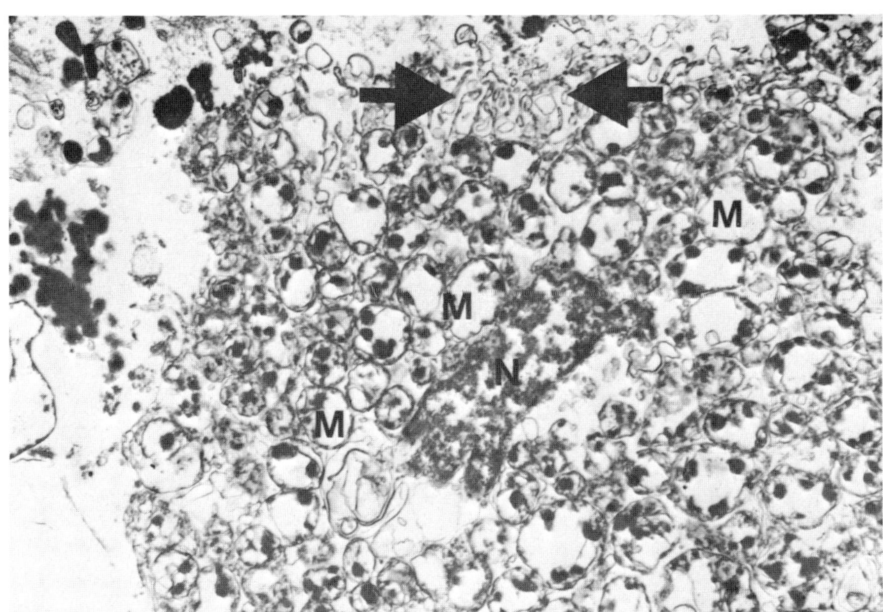

Figure 3-32.   This transmission electron micrograph shows a proximal tubule characterized by microvilli (between arrows) and numerous mitochondria (M). The mitochondria are swollen and devoid of cristae; their membranes, however, are intact. The nucleus (N) is atrophic (patient No. 6) (UA + LC, ×5,000). From *Seminars in Nephrology,* Vol. 6, 1986, with permission.

Comments: Severe ischemia of the lower extremities, passage of Coca Cola-colored urine, a marked elevation of CPK, hypocalcemia, and hyperuricemia suggested a diagnosis of rhabdomyolysis. The patient, however, had only a mildly elevated serum phosphate. His history of ischemic heart disease, livedo reticularis, and gangrene of the lower extremities suggested atheroembolic disease. The aortography surely had predisposed to the atheroembolic disorder of the kidneys and ARF. The finding of a cholesterol cleft in the segment of a vessel is supportive evidence of an atheroembolic disorder. The rhabdomyolysis was secondary to ischemia of the lower extremities and perhaps contributed to the development of ARF.

Patient No. 7, A. H., a 21-year-old black male, was admitted to the Medical College of Georgia Hospital on August 28, 1984, for evaluation of leukemia. He was in his usual state of health until 10 days before admission, when he developed a flu-like syndrome with chills, bleeding gums, and a stomach ache. He had noted easy bruising for some

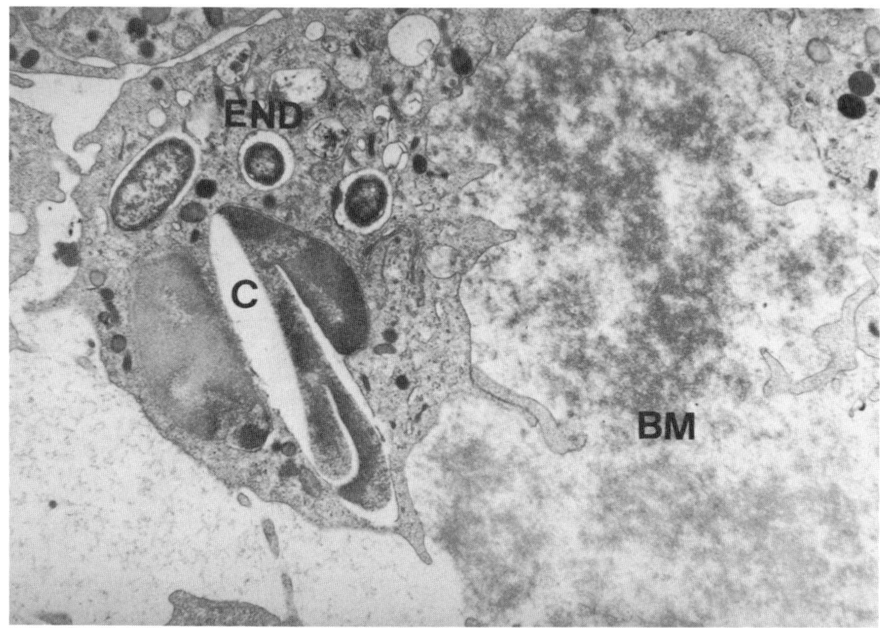

Figure 3-33.   A segment of an arterial vessel shows a thickened basement membrane (BM) and an endothelial cell (END). A cleft (C) can be seen in the endothelial cell (patient No. 6) (UA + LC, ×5,000).

time before admission. Physical examination revealed numerous hemorrhages in the retina and gums and a diffuse posterior cervical lymphadenopathy. His liver was enlarged, with a total span of 13 cm, but the spleen was not palpable. Stool occult blood was 4$^+$. Admission laboratory studies revealed WBC, 150,000/mm^3, with a differential of 80% blast cells. Serum chemistries revealed a urea nitrogen of 15 mg/dl; creatinine, 1.0 mg/dl; CO_2, 24 mEq/liter; potassium, 3.2 mEq/liter; uric acid, 5.3 mg/dl; and phosphate, 1.4 mg/dl.

A diagnosis of myelomonocytic leukemia was made and he was begun on chemotherapy on the second hospital day. On the fourth hospital day, he developed a tumor lysis syndrome, characterized by hyperphosphatemia (serum phosphate, 7.0 mg/dl) and marked acidosis, with a decrease in serum CO_2 to 7 mEq/liter. His serum urea nitrogen increased to 53 mg/dl, and his serum lactic acid level was 20 mEq/liter (normal, 0.5–2.2

Figure 3-35.   This tubule cell in which the nephron segment of origin cannot be identified is studded with large vacuoles (V). All the mitochondria (M) are swollen, and some contain amorphous dark bodies. Lipid droplets (L) are seen in necrotic cells, and the tubule basement membrane (BM) is fragmented (patient No. 7) (UA + LC, ×5,000).

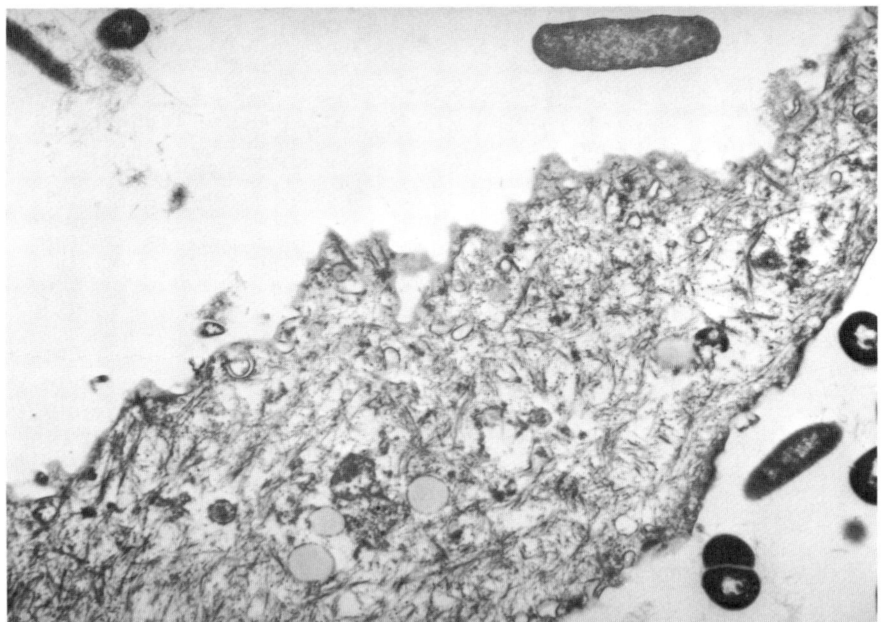

Figure 3-34.   This transmission electron micrograph shows a squamous epithelial cell characterized by many fibrils, scanty ribosomes, and few or no mitochondria (patient No. 6)
(UA + LC, ×5,000).

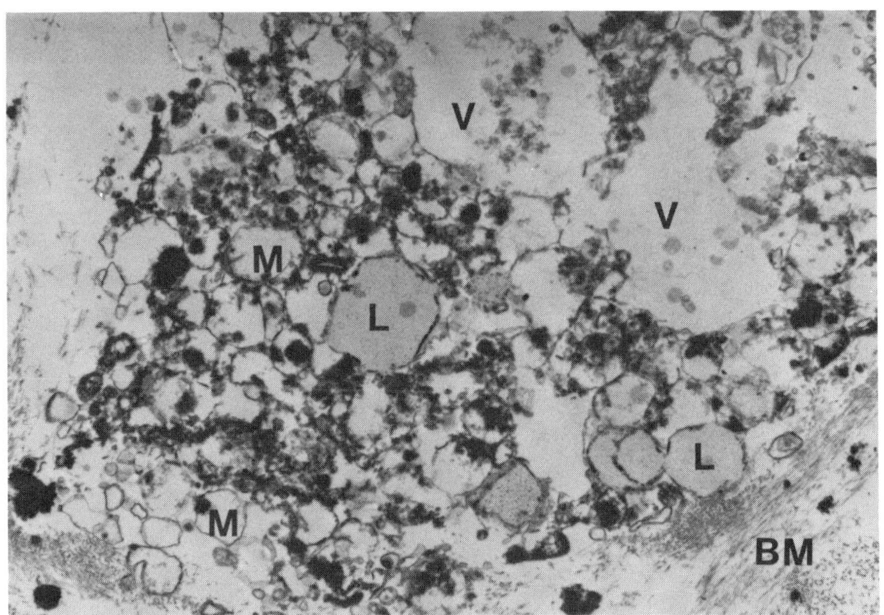

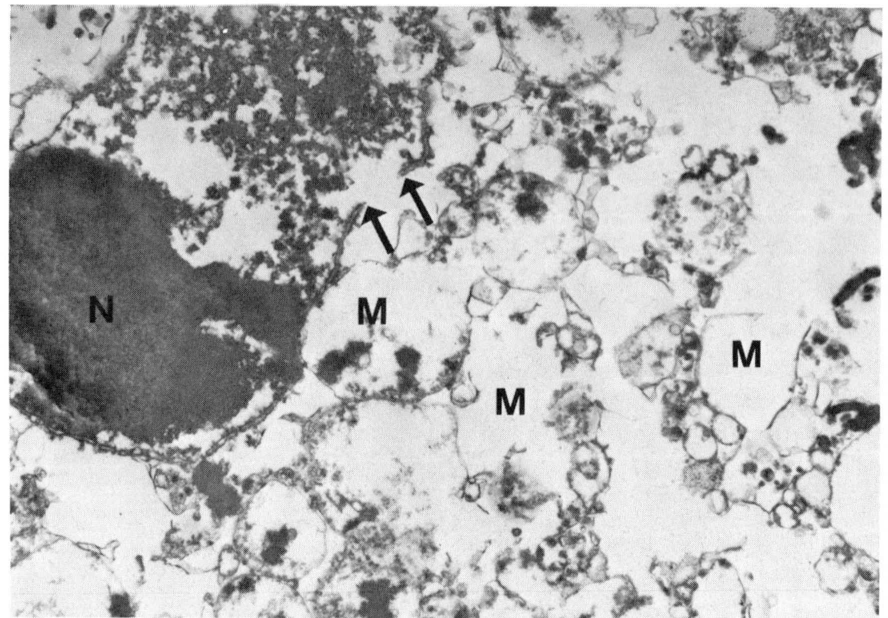

Figure 3-36. In this transmission electron micrograph of a tubule cell, there is conspicuous swelling of the mitochondria (M). The nucleus (N) reveals chromatin condensation and complete disruption of the nuclear membrane (arrows) (patient No. 7) (UA + LC, ×6,600).

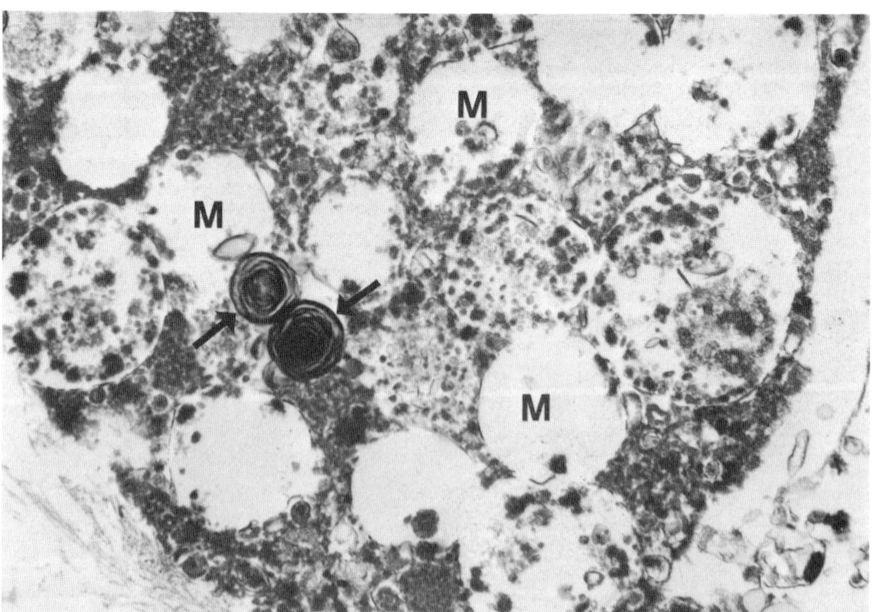

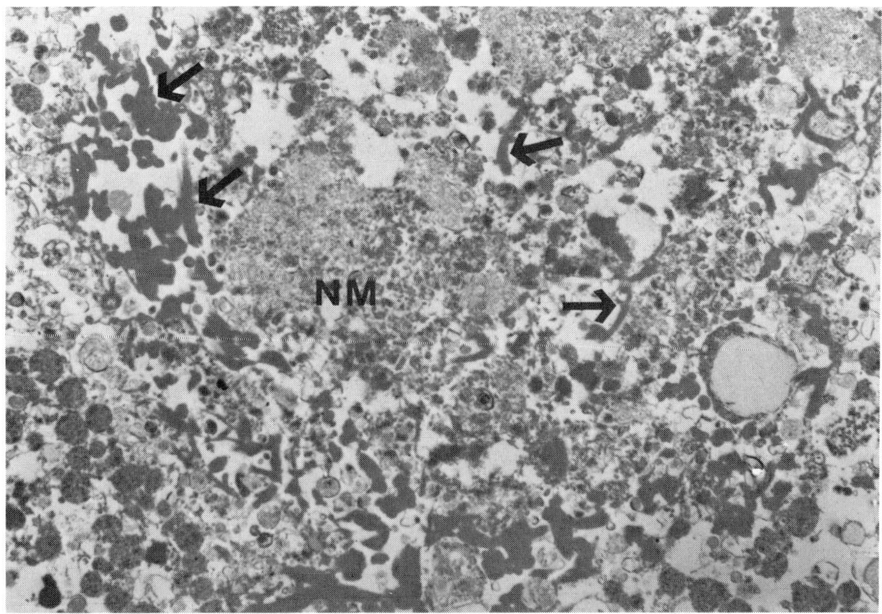

Figure 3-38.   In this tubule cell, masses of necrotic materials (NM) and large amounts of fibrin (arrows) are found (patient No. 7) (UA + LC, ×3,300).

mEq/liter). He became oliguric and was thought to have developed ARF. Hemodialysis was initiated. He also received cephalothin and gentamicin. During hemodialysis, he became hypotensive and an norepinephrine infusion was started to maintain blood pressure. On the second day of oliguria, a urine sample was collected for TEM analysis.

The TEM study of the urinary sediment revealed severe necrotic changes with intracellular edema in the renal tubule cells. The mitochondria were markedly swollen, with a complete loss of cristae in all of them and disruption of the membranes in some of them (Figs. 3-35–3-37). A few myeloid bodies were found in an occasional tubule cell (Fig. 3-37) and masses of necrotic materials and fibrin were also observed (Fig. 3-38).

Transmission electron microscopy of urinary sediments have demonstrated the ability of this technique to determine the severity of renal tubule changes as correlated with ARF outcome. A further analysis of TEM findings in sediments

Figure 3-37.   In this tubule cell, markedly swollen mitochondria (M) and two myeloid bodies (arrows) are found (patient No. 7) (UA + LC, ×8,300). From *Seminars in Nephrology,* Vol. 6, 1986, with permission

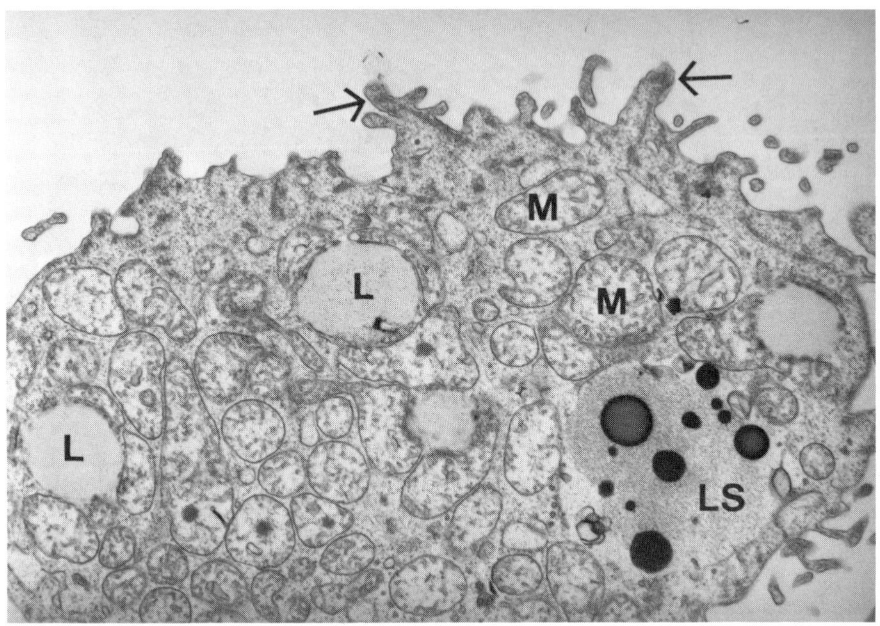

Figure 3-39.   In this tubule cell, which may be the distal segment of a proximal tubule, the mitochondria (M) are generally preserved. Some intact microvilli are still present (arrows); lipid droplets (L) and a lysosome (LS) can also be seen (UA + LC, ×4,800). From *Seminars in Nephrology,* Vol. 6, 1986, and *Kidney International,* vol. 28, pp. 58–63, 1985, with permission.

obtained from 31 patients with ATN, as shown in Table 3-1, permitted classification of three types of cells, based on the degree of ischemic changes exhibited by the tubule cells as outlined by Trump *et al.*[13] In classifying these cells, the appearance of the mitochondria and the integrity of the cell membranes were emphasized. Sediments were divided into three types: Type I sediment ($N = 11$); type II sediment ($N = 8$); and type III sediment ($N = 12$). *Type I sediment* consists of a homogeneous population of severely damaged tubule epithelial cells. In this type of sediment, uniformly necrotic cells and cellular fragments are seen. Mitochondria are swollen and devoid of cristae, with large flocculent densities usually called amorphous dark bodies, which are considered to represent irreversible cellular damage.[14] Nuclei generally are not present but, when present, breaks in their nuclear membranes and condensation of chromatin materials are seen (Fig. 3-36). Lysosomes are rarely seen.

Type II sediment consists of a homogeneous population of mild to moderately damaged tubule epithelial cells. Membranes encompassing the cells and subcellular organelles generally are intact. Mitochondria exhibit variable degrees

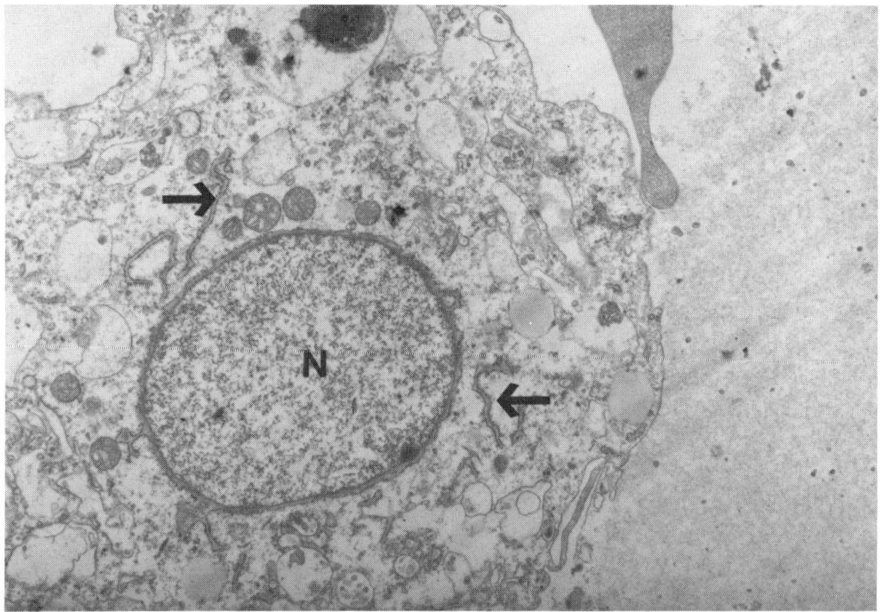

Figure 3-40.   In this tubule cell, the subcellular components, which include a nucleus (N), mitochondria, and rough-surfaced endoplasmic reticulum (arrows) are well preserved (patient No. 13, Table 3-1) (UA + LC, ×3,300).

of swelling but are otherwise normal in appearance. Nuclei and lysosomes are observed (Figs. 3-39 and 3-40).

Type III sediment consists of a heterogeneous population of cells, with findings seen in both type I and type II sediments. There is considerable intracellular variation in the degree of mitochondrial injury in type III sediment.

Recovery phase sediment obtained from patients are either negative or show only transitional epithelial cells (Fig. 3-34), as seen in patient No. 6.

URINARY SEDIMENT TEM ANALYSIS AND CLINICAL COURSE

Clinical profiles, along with dialysis intervention, renal recovery, and mortality rates, are shown in Table 3-1. As seen from the table, most, or all, of the patients with type II sediments and at least 50% of the patients with type III sediments recovered their renal function. No patients with type I sediment recovered renal function. The relationships between the sediment types seen and

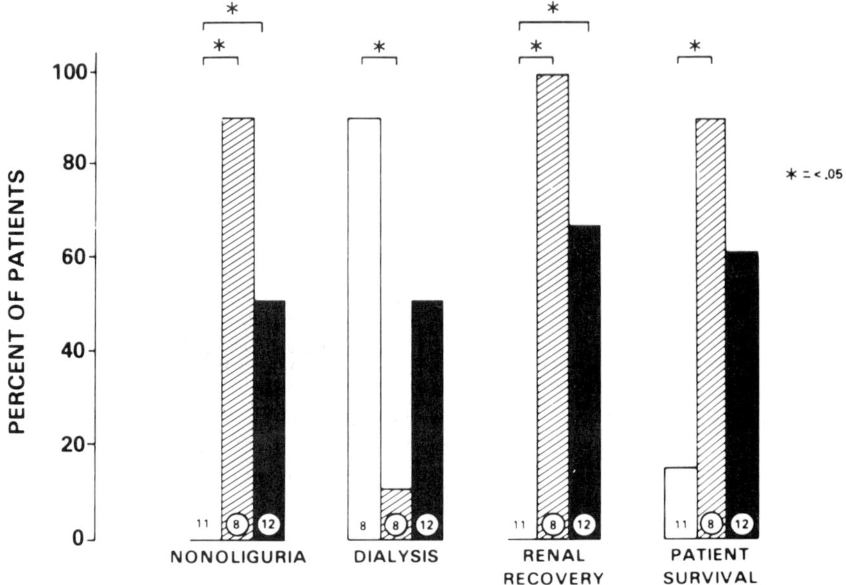

Figure 3-41.   This bar graph shows the relationship between types of urinary sediments and indices of the functional severity and clinical outcome of the underlying disease. Key: open bar, patients with type I sediments; hatched bar, patients with type II sediments; and closed bar, patients with type III sediments. The number of patients from each group included in each analysis is shown within the bars ($p < 0.05$). Reprinted from *Kidney International,* Vol. 28, pp. 58–63, 1985, with permission.

the various indices of the functional severity and clinical outcome of the underlying renal disease are depicted in Fig. 3-41.[10] As shown in this figure, none of the patients with type I sediments, 88% of the patients with type II sediments, and 50% of the patients with type III sediments were nonoliguric. In addition, 88% of the patients with type I sediments who survived beyond 48 hr of the onset of ARF required dialysis, but only 13% of patients with type II sediments and 50% of patients with type III sediments required dialysis. No patients with type I sediments recovered renal function, whereas all the patients with type II sediments and 67% of the patients with type III sediments recovered renal function. Finally, only 18% of the patients with type I sediments survived, whereas 88% of the patients with type II sediments and 58% of the patients with type III sediments survived.

In addition to the examples of TEM studies of urinary sediments presented here, there are other conditions under which TEM study of urinary sediment aid in the prognosis. One such condition is malignant hypertension, which can cause ARF. A rapid deterioration of renal function in a patient with malignant hyper-

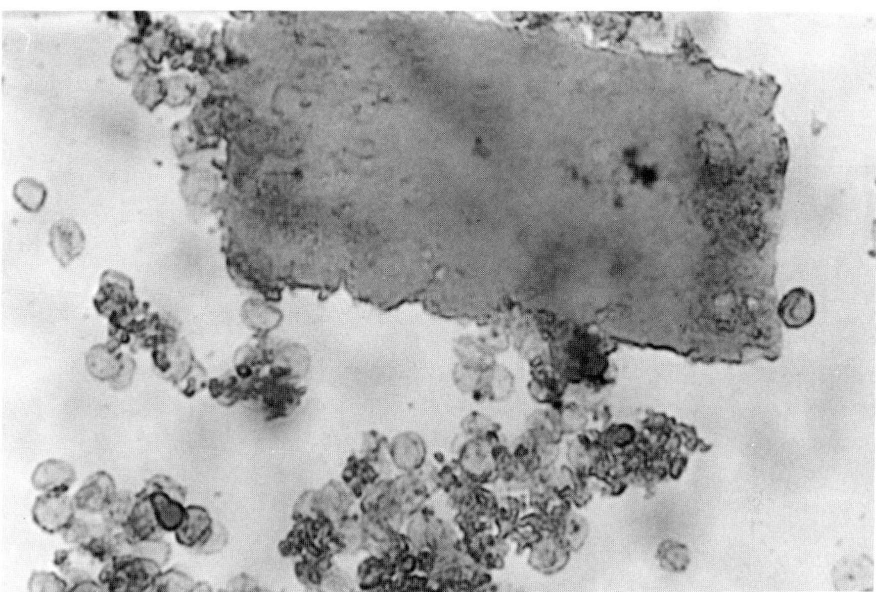

Figure 3-42. This light micrograph (patient No. 8) shows a broad cast, as is commonly seen in renal failure, with many attached leukocytes (unstained wet preparation, ×400).

tension and chronic renal insufficiency has been observed by the author.[15] Similarly, ATN has been reported by other investigators in patients with accelerated hypertension who developed ARF.[16] The TEM study of urinary sediment from a patient with malignant hypertension and renal failure is presented here to demonstrate that ATN does occur in malignant hypertension.

Patient No. 8, J. C., a 49-year-old black male, was admitted to the Veterans Administration Medical Center, Augusta, Georgia, on June 30, 1985, with a long history of headache, weakness, and progressive dyspnea on exertion before admission to the hospital. Family members stated that he was hypertensive for 10 yr or more and that he was not taking any antihypertensive drugs. His headaches had become frequent and recently had became more severe. Before being admitted, he had visited the emergency room of the University Hospital, Augusta, Georgia, where his blood pressure was found to be systolic 270 mm Hg and diastolic 150 mm Hg. He was treated with 10 mg of nifedipine orally and an intravenous infusion of nitroprusside and transferred to the Veterans Administration Medical Center, Augusta. An admission physical examination showed that he was in minimal distress; his blood pressure then was systolic 190 mm Hg and diastolic 100 mm Hg. The most remarkable physical finding was a bilateral papilledema with hemorrhages and exudates (grade IV retinopathy). Auscultation of the heart revealed S_3 and S_4 gallop. Rales were heard posteriorly over both lungs. Urinalysis showed numerous large hyaline

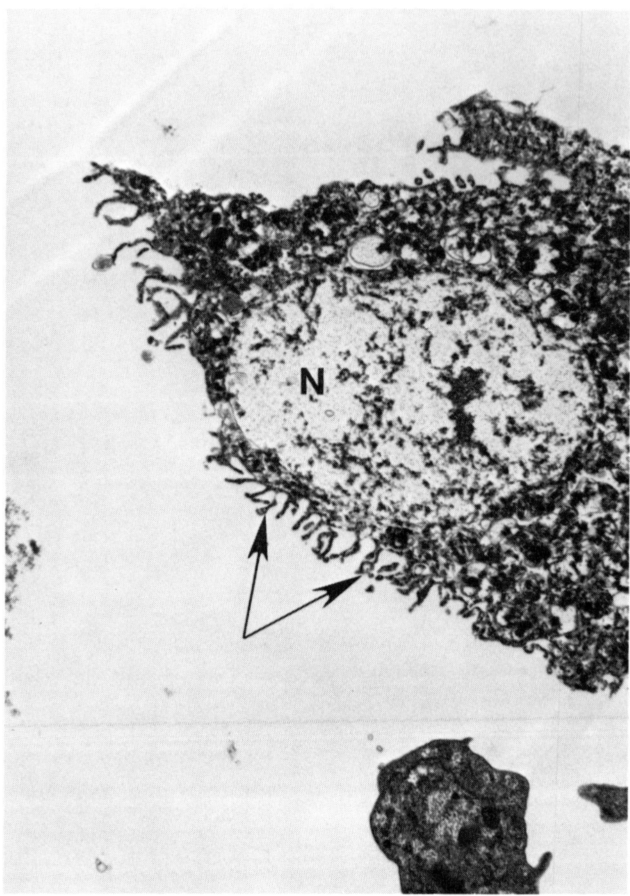

Figure 3-43.   In this transmission electron micrograph of urinary sediment from patient No. 8, a proximal tubule epithelial cell, with clear microvilli (double arrows), is seen. The nucleus (N), which shows complete dissolution of the chromatin material, has been displaced away from the basilar part of the cell because of widespread necrosis (UA + LC, ×5,000).

(broad or renal failure) casts (Fig. 3-42), granular casts, epithelial cells, red blood cells, and WBC. Serum chemistries revealed a sodium of 132 mEq/liter, potassium 2.7 mEq/liter, chloride 95 mEq/liter, bicarbonate 18.6 mEq/liter, urea nitrogen 112 mg/dl, creatinine 19.4 mg/dl, and phosphate 5.8 mg/dl. His hemoglobin and hematocrit were 8.9 g/dl and 26.4%, respectively. He was put on daily hemodialysis. His nitroprusside drip was discontinued on the third hospital day, and oral anithypertensive drug therapy was initiated. On July 1, 1985, a sample of urine was collected for TEM analysis. On July 2, 1985, his predialysis serum urea nitrogen and serum creatinine were 69 mg/dl and 12.8 mg/dl, respectively. In the early morning of July 4, 1985, he was found unresponsive by the nursing staff. He had an idioventricular rhythm, with a systolic blood pressure of 60 mm Hg. Attempts at resuscitation failed, and he was pronounced dead. Autopsy was not permitted. The TEM study of urinary sediment showed necrotic proximal and distal tubules (Figs. 3-43 and 3-44).

Comments: The necrotic tubule epithelial cells suggested ATN in this patient, though the mechanism(s) of ATN in malignant hypertension are unclear. One possibility is a marked decrease in renal blood flow as the result of a malignant lesion of the afferent arteriole, with excessive renin–angiotension activity.

DIAGNOSIS OF ACUTE RENAL FAILURE

Though this book has not the scope to discuss the diagnosis of ARF, diagnostic tests are presented briefly to support the findings of urinary sediment

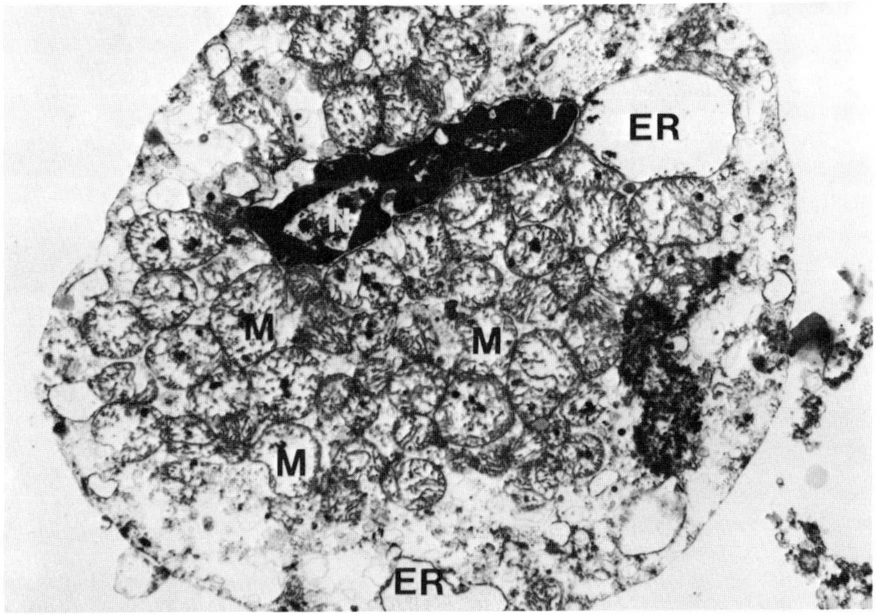

Figure 3-44.   In this transmission electron micrograph (patient No. 8), the anatomy of this necrotic tubule cell is obscured by the presence of many mitochondria (M) and dilated endoplasmic reticulum (ER); it seems to have originated from the proximal tubule. The mitochondria show discrete dark bodies, a sign of ischemia (UA + LC, ×7,500).

Table 3-2
Blood and Urinary Indices in Different Types of Acute Renal Failure[a]

Type of ARF	Urine protein	Urinary sediment	Urinary Na (60–100 mEq/liter)	FENa (1%)	SUN/Cr (ratio $\leq$20)	UOsm ($>$500 mOsm/kg)	U/P creatinine ratio(100$^+$)	Serum Osm (280–89 mOsm/kg)
Prerenal failure	0 to 1$^+$	Hyaline casts	<20 [may be 10]	<1%	$\geq$30	500+	$\geq$40	Normal or high
Acute intrinsic renal failure	1$^+$ to 2$^+$	Granular casts, epithelial casts, RBC, WBC, RBC cast (occ)	$\geq$40	$\geq$2%	<20	300–400	<20	Normal or high
Obstructive renal failure	0	0	$\geq$40	$\geq$2%	$\leq$20	Variable	$\leq$20	Normal or low
Acute glomeru-lonephritis	3$^+$ to 4$^+$	All types of casts, RBC, WBC	<20	<1%	$\geq$30	500+	$\geq$40	Normal or low

[a] Normal values are in parentheses.

studies. They include

1. Urinary sodium (UNa) and osmolality (Uosm)
2. Fractional excretion of sodium (FENa)
3. Serum urea nitrogen (SUN)
4. SUN/serum creatinine (Scr) ratio
5. Urinary (U) creatinine/plasma (P) creatinine ratio
6. Ultrasonography of the kidneys
7. A 24-hr urinary protein
8. Renal angiogram (arterial or venous)
9. Renal biopsy

Since it takes time to do a TEM study of urinary sediment, it is prudent to examine stained urinary sediment using conventional LM to determine whether the ARF is prerenal or is the result of acute tubular, tubulointerstitial, or glomerular lesions. When the diagnosis is in doubt, as it usually is, UNa, FENa, Uosm, SUN/Scr ratios, and U/P creatinine ratio can help distinguish between prerenal ARF and ATN (Table 3-2). These tests, however, do not substantiate such diagnoses as glomerulonephritis, glomerular necrosis, renal vein thrombosis, or obstructive uropathy.

When urine protein and urine LM are negative and UNa and Uosm are unrewarding, a renal sonogram to delineate the pelvicalyceal system and to rule out obstructive uropathy is essential. When the dipstick method demonstrates the presence of 3^+ to 4^+ protein, and there are numerous casts of different types, including red blood cell casts, further evaluation for glomerulonephritis is warranted. These evaluations include a 24-hr quantitative proteinuria, urine protein electrophoresis, and possibly, a percutaneous renal biopsy.

Urinary LM showing mainly RBC in a patient with sudden onset of ARF raises the possibility of renal artery embolism. The above features, along with a 4^+ protein by the dipstick method, leads to the suspicion of renal vein thrombosis. A renal sonogram may show kidney enlargement in renal vein thrombosis, whereas a isotope renogram will show no blood flow in renal artery embolism. In such cases, selective or bilateral renal venogram and arteriogram, respectively, will confirm the diagnosis.

MANAGEMENT OF ACUTE RENAL FAILURE

After obstructive uropathy and glomerular disease have been eliminated, the differential diagnosis resolves upon a prerenal type of ARF, ATN, and an intermediate or transition stage between prerenal failure and ATN. In such situations, it is appropriate to do a therapeutic test without delay. A schematic diagram of the management of ARF, including the therapeutic test, is shown in

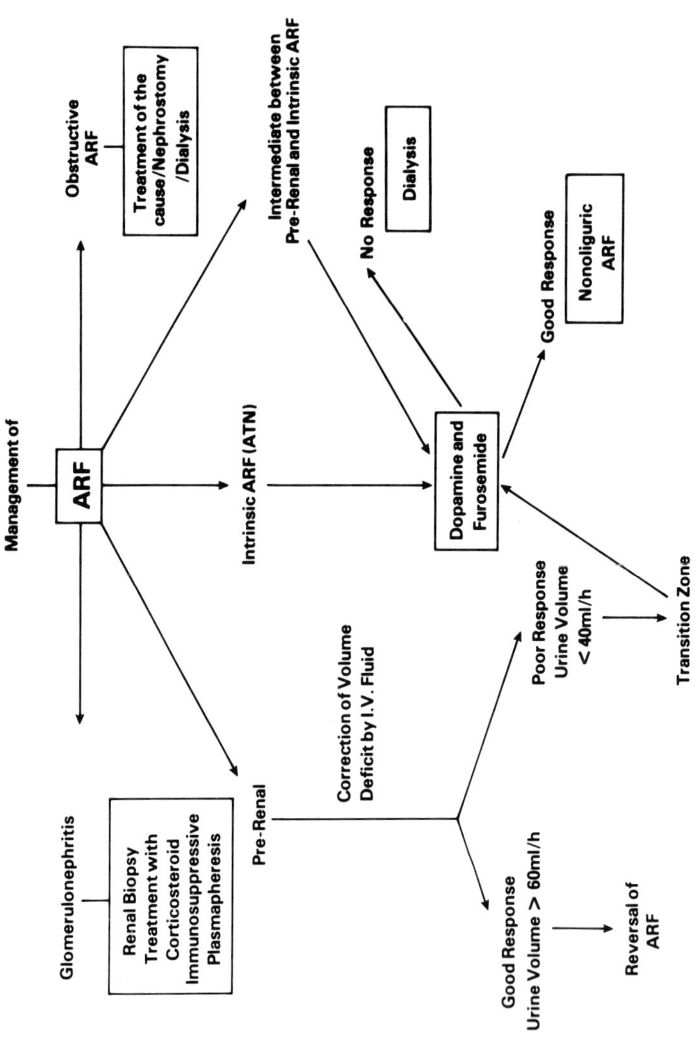

Figure 3-45. A schematic diagram of the management of acute renal failure. See the text for an explanation. From *JAPI*, Vol. 32, 1984, with permission.

Fig. 3-45.[17] The therapeutic test involves the rapid administration of normal saline (250 ml/hr) for 4 hr. A good response is characterized by a urine flow of greater than 60 ml/hr. The urine sodium will briskly increase, but the FENa will still be less than 2%; a poor response is associated with a urine flow of less than 40 ml/hr. There will be a less striking increase in urinary sodium, but the FENa may be greater than 2%. In patients with a poor response to fluid challenge, the possibilities of ATN and the intermediate or transition stage between prerenal failure and ATN are likely. At this time, it is logical to consider infusion of furosemide and dopamine in those patients with SUN and Scr of less than 100 mg/dl and 10 mg/dl, respectively, a normocatabolic state, and a stable general condition. If the goal is to induce diuresis to convert oliguric into nonoliguric ARF through the natriuretic and vasodilator effects of furosemide, it is more appropriate to infuse furosemide continuously than to administer it by intermittent boluses. Infusion of saline with furosemide is recommended, and the infusion rate is titrated to deliver 20 mg of furosemide in 60- to 120-ml saline/hr. Dopamine in low dose (1–3 Ug/min) acts as a vasodilator and can be delivered separately in a small volume of fluid. Infusions of both furosemide and dopamine are continued for 48 to 72 hr. If a good response, as defined earlier, occurs, the infusions should be continued for several days but with a more dilute solution of furosemide. When diuresis is sustained and the renal function is stabilized, the infusions are discontinued. A poor response, however, implies ATN and all the manipulations to induce natriuresis and diuresis are likely to be ineffective. Therefore, the infusions are discontinued and the patient is treated by conservative methods or dialysis. Infusions of furosemide and dopamine have converted oliguric ARF to nonoliguric ARF and modified the course of ARF in some patients (Fig. 3-30).[17]

In summary, the TEM study has made a significant contribution in complete understanding of the cellular changes in the urinary sediment. Since the cellular changes observed by TEM reflect those in renal tubules *in situ,* this study determines the severity of ATN and thereby aids in the assessment of prognosis. We have shown that the severity of changes in the tubule cells in the urinary sediment correlate remarkably with the need for dialysis, renal function recovery, and mortality. Mild change in the tubule cells denotes good renal recovery and no or slight mortality, while homogeneous population of severely necrotic cells in the urinary sediment signifies an overall poor outcome.[18]

REFERENCES

1. Anderson RJ, Schrier RW: Clinical spectrum of oliguric and nonoliguric acute renal failure. In *Acute Renal Failure,* Stein JH, Brenner BM (eds). New York, Churchill-Livingston, 1980, p 1.
2. Hou SH, Bushinsky DA, Wish DB, *et al:* Hospital acquired renal insufficiency. *Am J Med* 1983; 74:243–248.

3. Banomini V, Baldrati L, Scolari MP, *et al:* Acute renal failure: Ten years experience. In *Acute Renal Failure,* Eliahow HE (ed). London, John Libbey, 1982, p 149.

4. Butkus DE: Persistently high mortality in acute renal failure. *Arch Intern Med* 1983; 143:209–212.

5. Conger JD, Schrier RW: Renal hemodynamics in acute renal failure. *Ann Rev Physiol* 1980; 42:603–614.

6. Patak RV, Fadem SZ, Lifschitz MD, *et al:* Study of factors which modify the development of norepinephrine-induced acute renal failure in the dog. *Kidney Int* 1979; 15:–227–237.

7. Mauk RH, Patak RV, Fadem SZ, *et al:* Effect of prostaglandin E administration in nephrotoxic and vasoconstrictor model of acute renal failure. *Kidney Int* 1977; 12:122–140.

8. Cronin RE, deTorrente A, Miller PD, *et al:* Pathogenetic mechanisms in early norepinephrine-induced acute renal failure: Functional and histologic correlates of protection. *Kidney Int* 1978; 14:115–125.

9. Siegel NJ, Glazier WB, Chandry IH, *et al:* Enhanced recovery from acute renal failure by post ischemic infusion of adenine nucleotides and magnesium chloride in rats. *Kidney Int* 1980; 17:338–349.

10. Mandal AK, Sklar AH, Hudson JB: Transmission electron microscopy of urinary sediment in human acute renal failure. *Kidney Int* 1985; 28:58–63.

11. Mandal AK, Nordquist JA, Thigpen MW: Electron microscopy studies of papillary interstitial granules in normal human kidneys. *Ann Clin Lab Sci* 1979; 9:37–46.

12. Stein PD, Sabbah HN, Mandal AK: Augmentation of sickling process due to turbulent blood flow. *J Appl Physiol* 1976; 40:60–65.

13. Trump BF, Mergner WJ, Kahng MW, *et al:* Studies on the subcellular pathophysiology of ischemia. *Circulation* 1976; 53:117–126.

14. Jennings RB, Ganote CE: Structural changes in myocardium acute ischemia. *Circ Res* 1974; 34(suppl 111):156–168.

15. Mandal AK, Bell RD, Nordquist JA, *et al:* Anatomic pathology and pathogenesis of the lesions of small arteries and arterioles of the kidney in essential hypertension. In *Path Annu,* Sommers SC, Rosen PP (eds). Appleton-Century-Croft, New York, 1977, pp 331–371.

16. Sevitt LH, Evans DJ, Wong OM: Acute oliguric renal failure due to accelerated hypertension. *Q J Med* 1971; 40:127–144.

17. Mandal AK, Treat RC: Diagnosis and management of acute renal failure. *Jour Assoc Physicians India* 1984; 32:203–208.

18. Mandal AK: Transmission electron microscopy of urinary sediment in renal disease. *Sem Nephrol* 1986; 6:346–370.

4

Aminoglycoside Nephrotoxicity

Aminoglycosides are antibiotics and semisynthetic antibiotic derivatives obtained from cultures of Streptomyces or Micromonospora. The drugs in this group include streptomycin, kanamycin, gentamicin, tobramycin, amikacin, netilmicin, neomycin, and paromomycin. They are active against many aerobic gram-negative bacteria, mainly sensitive strains of Enterobacter, *Proteus, Pseudomonas,* and *Serratia;* and gentamicin, tobramycin, and amikacin are particularly active against *P. aeruginosa.*[1]

The aminoglycosides, especially gentamicin and tobramycin, are increasingly used to treat urinary tract infections and serious systemic infections in patients admitted to medical, surgical, and intensive care units. As more aminoglycosides are used, the incidence of nephrotoxicity or acute renal failure (ARF) has risen. The incidence of nephrotoxicity varies greatly from one report to another, ranging from 4% to 55%.[2–4] Some authors have reported nephrotoxicity in 36.3%[3] or as high as 55.2%[4] of patients treated with gentamicin. There are also reports of nephrotoxicity in as low as 4% of patients treated with gentamicin,[5] or somewhere in between these two extremes. Fong *et al.*[6] have reported definite nephrotoxicity in 10% of patients treated with gentamicin and 8% of patients treated with tobramycin. This wide discrepancy has not been explained. Some of the differences, however, may be attributable to serious primary illnesses, in which gram-negative infection often occurs as a terminal event. Our own study (see Clinical Studies) illustrates this.

Most reports, however, agree that tobramycin and amikacin are less nephrotoxic than gentamicin.[3–5] Plaut *et al.*[3] conducted a 3-yr prospective study to determine the incidence of nephrotoxicity with gentamicin, tobramycin, and amikacin. Beginning April, 1975, 170 adults admitted to two general hospitals in Buffalo, New York were selected for study. Patients were treated in acute care units and most of them had indwelling urinary catheters in place. Because of the method of selection the patients were mostly older with infections complicated by serious medical and surgical problems. Nephrotoxicity was defined by the rise of serum creatinine of 0.5 mg/dl or more during aminoglycoside therapy or up to 7 days thereafter. Nephrotoxicity was attributable to the aminoglycoside used, unless another cause, such as septic shock, was apparent. Tobramycin nephrotoxicity (22.8%) occurred significantly less often than did gentamicin nephrotoxicity (36.3%) ($p < 0.05$). There was no difference in the incidence of tobramycin and amikacin nephrotoxicity. The relative safety of tobramycin may result from its lower tissue accumulation. In this study, nearly one in five patients had bacterial superinfections, usually caused by resistant gram-negative rods, and superinfection contributed impressively to the overall mortality of 30%.[3]

Though aminoglycoside-induced ARF is very prevalent, clinically, reports of histopathological studies documenting renal lesions are seldom seen. A characteristic, but not totally specific morphological manifestation of aminoglycoside nephrotoxicity is the formation of numerous myeloid body-containing cytosegrosomes within the proximal tubule epithelium (Fig. 4-1). Sphingomyelinase enzyme activity is depressed by aminoglycoside antibiotics, and of all the aminoglycosides, gentamicin induces the most severe depression. Netilmicin has less of an effect, as does tobramycin, and amikacin has virtually no effect on the activity of this enzyme. This inhibition of sphingomyelinase activity appears to cause phospholipid accumulation and myeloid body formation. Therefore, the accumulation of myeloid bodies should not be considered the primary mechanism of cellular injury. Other morphological changes in tubule epithelial cells include mitochondrial swelling (the result of state 3 mitochondrial respiration inhibition), brush border disruption, and in severe cases, frank cell necrosis with the pathological features of toxic acute tubular necrosis.

Thus far, no technique, short of renal biopsy, revealed morphological changes in the renal tubule cells in ARF, whether aminoglycoside induced or not. Recently, however, we reported that transmission electron microscopy (TEM) of urinary sediments from patients with ARF provides useful information about the severity of changes in the renal tubules and that the severity of changes in the renal tubule cells correlate well with renal recovery and outcome in such patients.[7] The purpose of this chapter is to demonstrate that TEM of urinary sediments can be a useful tool in distinguishing aminoglycoside-induced ARF from other types of ARF. This chapter also presents evidence that successive TEM studies of urinary sediments is more meaningful than single sediment studies in marking the onset of aminoglycoside-induced ARF.

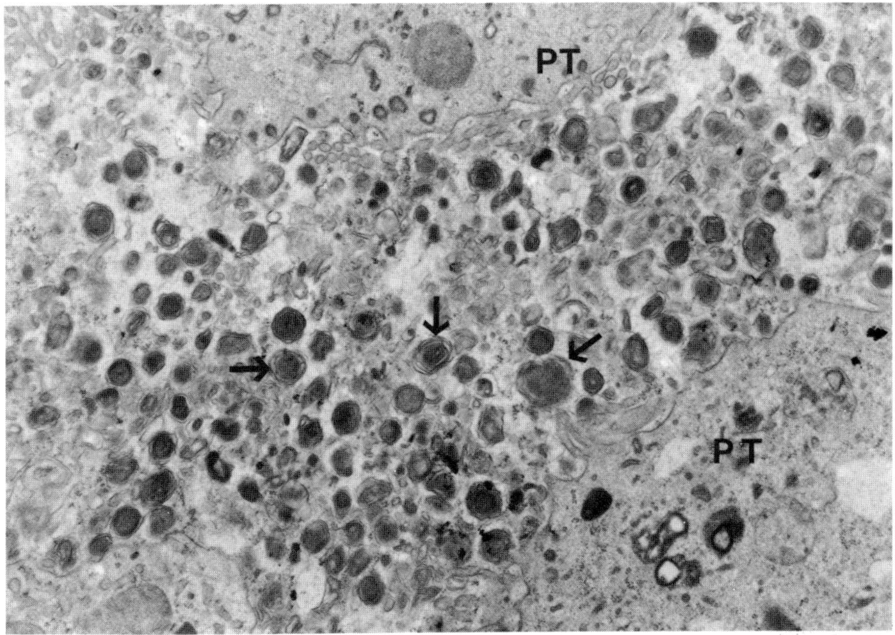

Figure 4-1.   This transmission electron micrograph shows numerous myeloid bodies (arrows) within the lumen of a proximal tubule. The apical part of the proximal tubule (PT) is shown (UA + LC, ×20,000).

URINARY MYELOID BODIES AND AMINOGLYCOSIDE NEPHROTOXICITY

This study on urinary sediment[8] was intended to quantitate the myelin figures and relate them to aminoglycoside-induced renal failure. In the study, 54 patients received aminoglycosides; 21 patients were controls. The myelin figures in the urinary sediment were quantitated into six groups, from 0 to V according to the number of figures. An analysis of this study shows three different correlations: (1) between the presence of myelin figures in the urine and aminoglycoside administration, (2) between the number of myelin figures and the accumulated dose of the aminoglycoside, and (3) between the number of myelin figures and obvious renal failure. The absence of urinary myelin figures in control subjects attests to their diagnostic value. The authors have stated that urinary sediment TEM to detect myelin figures appears to be a reliable technique to confirm cases in which the aminoglycoside was thought to be the cause of ARF. Also, this noninvasive method can be used in continuing studies.

CLINICAL STUDIES

TEM Analysis

In this study (by the author),[9] urine samples were collected from 21 patients (15 male, 6 female) who had been treated with aminoglycosides for periods of 3 to 20 days. Their ages varied from 23 to 74 years. Among these 21 patients, 16 received gentamicin and 5 tobramycin. Also, 17 patients received concomitantly one or more nonaminoglycoside antibiotics, and only 4 patients received gentamicin alone. The clinical and antibiotic profiles are presented in Table 4-1.

Serum creatinine levels were measured before (base line), during, and several days after termination of aminoglycoside therapy. Aminoglycoside nephrotoxicity (or ARF) in this study was defined, as in a previous study,[3] by the abrupt decline in renal function (rise in serum creatinine ≥ 0.5 mg/dl from baseline levels) in the absence of a known ischemic insult, and by two additional criteria: (1) the persistence of ARF after the correction of any recognized hemodynamic abnormalities and (2) the slow improvement in renal function after aminoglycoside therapy termination.

Urine samples for TEM studies were collected at intervals during and after aminoglycoside therapy. Urine samples were obtained from Foley catheters in all patients admitted to intensive care units, and spontaneously voided urine samples were collected from all other study subjects. Repeated urine samples were obtained from 11 patients (Nos. 3, 4, 5, 7, 8, 9, 10, 11, 16, 17 and 18). Urine samples (10 ml) were centrifuged immediately at 3,000 rpm in a table top centrifuge for at least 10 min. Sufficient amounts of sediment were not recovered uniformly in urine samples obtained from nonoliguric patients, and simultaneous centrifugation of several 10-ml samples was then required for adequate pellet formation. After centrifugation, the supernatant was pipetted out, leaving the sediment undisturbed. The sediment was suspended in a fixative of 4% glutaraldehyde in phosphate buffer and 10% formalin (7 : 3) (pH 7.4), and recentrifuged for uniform fixation. After overnight refrigeration, the sediment was postfixed in 2% osmium, dehydrated in alcohol solutions, and embedded in Spurr (block).

From the blocks, thick sections were cut, mounted on glass slides, and stained with epoxy tissue stain. The slides were examined by light microscopy (LM). The fields that contained large collections of coarse granularlike materials (myeloid bodies) and/or of cells (Fig. 4-2) were selected for TEM study. Thin sections (0.02–.03 μ) were prepared, mounted on copper grids, stained with uranyl acetate and lead citrate (UA + LC), and examined with a JEOL, JEM 100 cx, 1980 electron microscopy unit. Findings were analyzed from 8 × 10 inch photographic prints. The numbers of myeloid bodies and tubule epithelial

Table 4-1
Clinical and Antibiotic Profiles

Patient No.	Age/race/sex	Diagnosis	Aminoglycoside[a]	Duration (days)	Concomitant nonaminoglycoside antibiotic(s)	Urine collection relative to the duration of G or T therapy
1	72/W/M	Chronic lymphocytic leukemia, aspiration pneumonia	G	4	Penicillin; cefoxitin	3rd day of G
2	63/W/M	Motor vehicle accident, multiple fractures; sepsis, hepatic failure	G	8	Ampicillin; cefamandol	12 days after G discontinued
3	62/B/M	Right lower lobe pneumonia, acute respiratory failure	G	13	Penicillin; clindamycin	2 days after G discontinued
4	58/B/M	Squamous cell carcinoma of left lung, left pneumonectomy	G	10	Cefazolin; penicillin	2 days after G discontinued
5	69/W/M	Malnutrition, sepsis	G	19	Oxacillin; ampicillin	10th day of G
6	28/B/M	AIDS: *Pneumocystis cariini* pneumonia	G	11	None	11th day of G
7	28/W/F	Motor vehicle accident, splenectomy	G	19	Ampicillin	Last day of G
8	61/B/F	Abdominal abscess, sepsis, hepatic failure	T	21	Ampicillin; clindamycin	5th and 14th day of T

(*continued*)

Table 4-1
(*Continued*)

Patient No.	Age/race/sex	Diagnosis	Aminoglycoside[a]	Duration (days)	Concomitant nonaminoglycoside antibiotic(s)	Urine collection relative to the duration of G or T therapy
9	48/B/M	Alcoholic cirrhosis, *Pseudomonas* pneumonia	G	21	Nafcillin	19th and 20th day of G
10	65/W/M	Cardiac arrest	G	12	Cefoxitin	3rd and 6th day of G
11	23/B/F	Bacterial endocarditis, urinary tract infection	T	16	Vancomycin	2 days and 4 days after T completed
12	27/B/M	Metastatic disease, sepsis	G	3	Cefoxitin	10 days after G discontinued
13	56/B/M	Intracranial bleeding	G	8	None	6 days after G discontinued
14	63/W/M	Common duct stone, cholecystectomy	G	10	Cefoxitin	4th day of G
15	62/B/M	Fever, aspiration pneumonia	G	10	Piperacillin; ampicillin	5 days after G discontinued
16	40/W/M	Motor vehicle accident	T	10	Piperacillin	6th day of T and 5 days after T discontinued
17	72/B/F	Multiple myeloma	T	17	Ticarcillin	1 day before 3 days after T
18	35/B/F	Alcoholic pancreatitis	T	18	Cefoxitin	5th and 10th day of T
19	27/W/F	Multiple sclerosis, chronic urinary tract infection	G	8	None	5th day of G
20	74/B/M	Syringomyelia, right lower lobe pneumonia	G	5	None	2 days after G discontinued
21	70/B/M	Dementia, Alzheimer's disease, pneumonia	G	12	Cefoxitin; penicillin	7th day of G

[a] G, gentamicin; T, tobramycin.

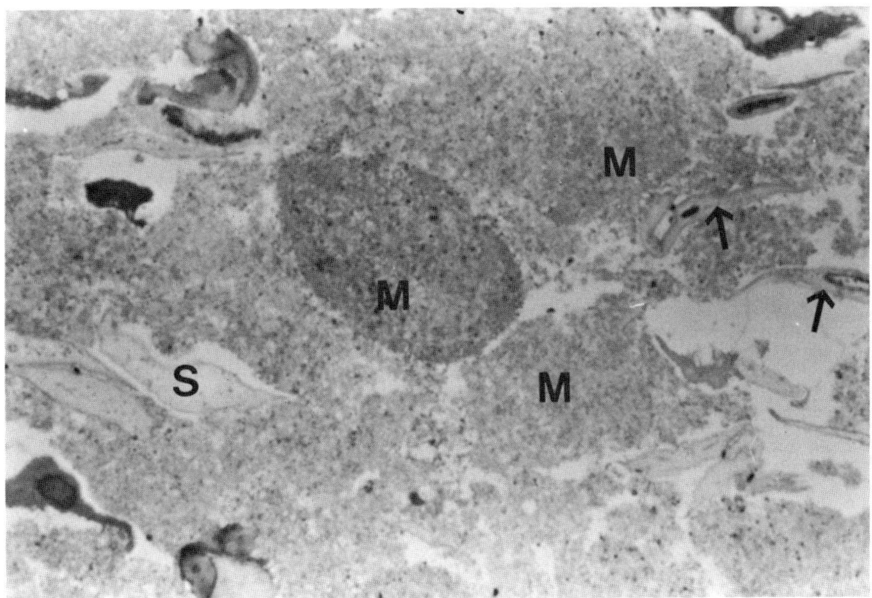

Figure 4-2.   A thick-section light micrograph demonstrates masses of finely granular material that appears to be myeloid bodies (M). Note squamous (S) or transitional (arrows) epithelial cells (epoxy tissue stain, ×200).

cells in the urinary sediment were semiquantitified from + through +++ (where +, few; ++, moderate; +++, numerous).

Serum creatinine levels, TEM analyses of urinary sediments, and follow-up studies are presented in Table 4-2. From Table 4-2, it can be seen that 12 of 21 patients (57%) developed aminoglycoside nephrotoxicity or ARF and 9 patients did not develop ARF. Analyses that showed the differences between the two groups with and without ARF are presented in Table 4-3. From Table 4-3, it will be seen that 11 of 12 patients with ARF were receiving nonaminoglycoside antibiotics concomitantly, whereas 6 of 9 patients without ARF received nonaminoglycoside antibiotics concomitantly. The difference, however, was not significant. Similarly, there was no significant difference in the duration of aminoglycoside therapy between the two groups. Of the patients with ARF, 10 of 12 had myeloid bodies and necrotic renal tubule cells. In one patient with ARF (No. 12), the sediment was negative. This negative finding may be attributed to the fact that this patient received gentamicin for 3 days and that the urine was examined 10 days after termination of gentamicin therapy. In one patient with ARF, the pellet was inadequate, but an adequate pellet for TEM study was found in eight of nine patients without ARF. Myeloid bodies were found in the urinary

Table 4-2
Renal Function and Urinary Sediment Studies and Outcome[a]

| Patient No. | Serum creatinine levels (mg/dl) | | | ARF | TEM Urinary sediment | | Renal function recovery | Outcome (follow-up urinary sediment) |
	Baseline	During AM	Post AM		Myeloid bodies	Necrotic RTC		
1	1.0	2.1	1.8(2)	Yes	+ + +	+	Improvement	Died (respiratory arrest)
2	1.3	2.2	6.6(16)	Yes	+	+ +	No recovery	Died (sepsis, hepatic failure)
3	1.3	2.7	1.7	Yes	+ + +	+ +	Recovered	Discharged [2 weeks urinary sediment (myeloid bodies only)]
4	1.2	2.4	1.1	Yes	+ + +	+ +	Recovered	Discharged (5 weeks urinary sediment negative)
5	0.6	1.6	0.8	Yes	+ +	+	Recovered	Nursing home (4 weeks urinary sediment negatives)
6	0.6	2.2	2.5(7)	Yes	Inadequate pellet		No recovery	Died
7	0.7	1.5	Not available	Yes	+ + +	+	Recovered	Discharged (1 week only myeloid bodies)

8	2.1	4.1	6.5(aminoglycosides)	Yes	+ + +	+ +	No Recovery	Died [sepsis (TEM of urinary sediment: myeloid bodies and RTC)]
9	0.4	1.7	1.5(9)	Yes	+ +	+ +	Improvement	Died (respiratory arrest)
10	1.8	3.2	2.7(9)	Yes	+ + +	+ +	No recovery	Died (respiratory arrest)
11	1.0	2.8	1.0	Yes	+	+	Recovered	Discharged
12	0.3	1.1	0.8(13)	Yes	0	0	Recovered	Died (respiratory arrest)
13	0.8	0.9	1.1	No	Inadequate pellet		No ARF	Discharged
14	1.2	0.7	1.3	No	+ + +	+	No ARF	Discharged
15	1.3	0.7	0.7	No	+ +	0*	No ARF	Discharged
16	0.7	0.9	0.8	No	+ +	0*	No ARF	Discharged
17	0.9	1.0	1.0	No	+	+	No ARF	Discharged
18	1.1	0.5	1.0	No	+ +	0*	No ARF	Discharged
19	0.8	0.4	0.6	No	0	0	No ARF	Discharged
20	1.0	0.4	0.7	No	0	0*	No ARF	Discharged
21	1.2	1.3	1.3(13)	No	0	0*	No ARF	Died (respiratory arrest)

[a] Key: *, only transitional epithelial cells; ARF, acute renal failure; AM, aminoglycosides; ( ), Death (number of days) (after aminoglycoside therapy discontinued); RTC, renal tubule cell; +, few; + +, moderate; + + +, too numerous to count; 0, none.

Table 4-3
Patients Who Developed versus Patients Who Did Not Develop Acute
Renal Failure Following Aminoglycoside Therapy

	Acute renal failure	p values	Nonacute renal failure
Total patients (N)	12	NS[a]	9
Average age of patients (years)	50.3	NS	55.4
Concomitant nonaminoglycoside antibiotic(s) used	11	NS	6
Average duration of aminoglycoside administration (days)	11.8	NS	9.2
Adequate pellet for TEM study	11	NS	8
Myeloid bodies present	10	NS	6
Renal tubule cells present	10	<0.01	2

[a]NS, nonsignificant.

sediments of five patients, whereas few necrotic renal tubule cells were present in two of these five. Though no difference was found in the incidence of myeloid bodies between the two groups, the appearance of necrotic renal tubule cells in the two groups differed greatly ($p < 0.01$).

Follow-up Studies of ARF Patients. Follow-up studies showed that six patients (Nos. 3, 4, 5, 7, 11, and 12) (50%) recovered completely. The renal function of an additional four patients (Nos. 1, 6, 9, and 10) who died of primary or intercurrent illnesses had either improved or stabilized their renal function at the time of death. The renal function of the remaining two patients (Nos. 2 and 8) progressively deteriorated. These two patients had associated severe liver disease, which could account for their progressive renal failure. Follow-up sediment studies showed myeloid bodies only in two patients (Nos. 3 and 7) and myeloid bodies and necrotic renal tubule cells in one patient (No. 8). Follow-up urinary sediments were negative in two patients (Nos. 4 and 5).

The TEM studies of urinary sediments from several individual patients illustrate the validity of this technique in assessing aminoglycoside nephrotoxicity.

Patient No. 1, E. O., a 58-year-old black male, was admitted to the Veterans Administration Medical Center, Augusta, Georgia, on February 6, 1984, with the complaint of coughing blood for 2 weeks before hospital admission. He admits to two-pillow orthopnea, paroxysmal nocturnal dyspnea, and a 98-pack a year smoking history. Except for a thoracotomy scar on the right, the physical examination was negative. A chest X-ray showed a left hilar fullness and a bronchoscopy with bronchial biopsy documented a squamous cell carcinoma in the left upper lobe. On March 9, 1984, left pneumonectomy was performed.

The details of antibiotic regimen, serial urine output, serum urea nitrogen (SUN), and serum creatinine (Scr) levels are shown as follows.

Date (1984)	Antibiotic(s) (dosage and duration)	Urine output (ml/24 hr)	SUN (mg/dl)	Scr (mg/dl)
February 6	None	Not available	11	0.9
March 9	Cefazolin 1 g IV q 6 hr	1055[+]	14	1.2
March 14	As above	1190[+]	32	2.1
	(intravenous fluid administration increased; fever of unknown origin)			
March 15	Gentamicin 150 mg stat, then 120 mg q 12 hr	3243	30	1.6
March 19	Cefazolin and gentamicin	1587	61	2.8
	(nephrology consultation sought/cefazolin and gentamicin discontinued)			
	(urine sample collected for TEM study)			
March 26				
March 29	None	3020	28	2.0
April 2	None	5950	16	2.2
April 23	None	1735	11	1.4
May 9	(discharged from the hospital)			
May 18	(follow-up visit/physical examination normal; urine sample collected for TEM study)			

The data presented substantiate that this patient developed ARF secondary to cefazolin or gentamicin or more likely to the combination of these antibiotics. The ARF was nonoliguric, however, cephalothin might have potentiated aminoglycoside in producing ARF in this patient.[10] This was further confirmed by the complete reversal of ARF upon antibiotic withdrawal.

Figures 4-3 through 4-8 are from the TEM studies of Patient No. 1. In the TEM analysis of the first urinary sediment, excessive numbers of myeloid bodies had become densely aggregated in the form of a cast (Fig. 4-3). In addition to myeloid bodies casts, there were numerous free myeloid bodies (Fig. 4-4). Whorl formation was more conspicuous in the free myeloid bodies than in those in the cast. Some tubule epithelial cells containing intralysosomal myeloid bodies were found (Fig. 4-5). In some tubule epithelial cells, the subcellular components were largely replaced by whorl membranes (Fig. 4-6).

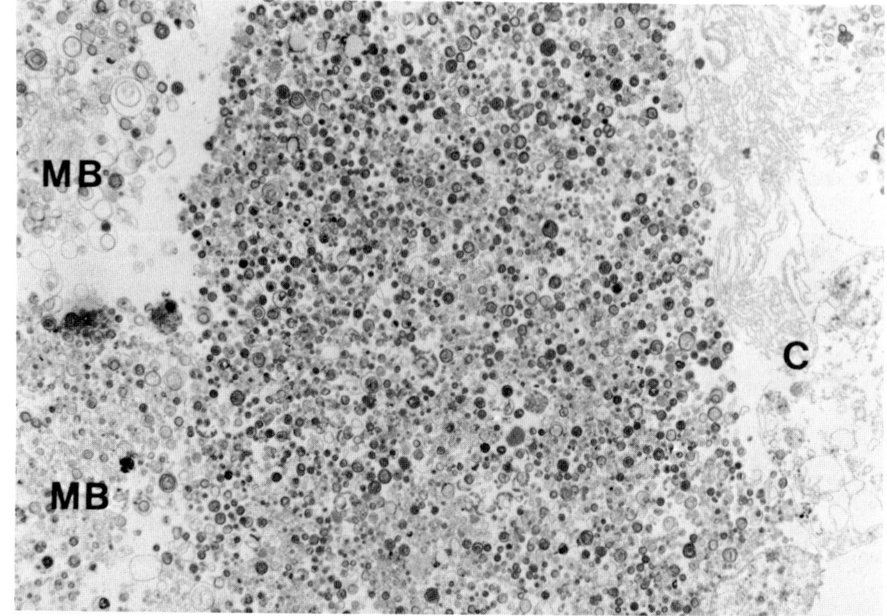

Figure 4-3. This transmission electron micrograph shows a myeloid body cast. At the margin of the cast, a necrotic tubule cell (C) and free myeloid bodies (MB) are seen (UA + LC, ×2,000). From *Seminars in Nephrology,* Vol. 6, 1986, with permission.

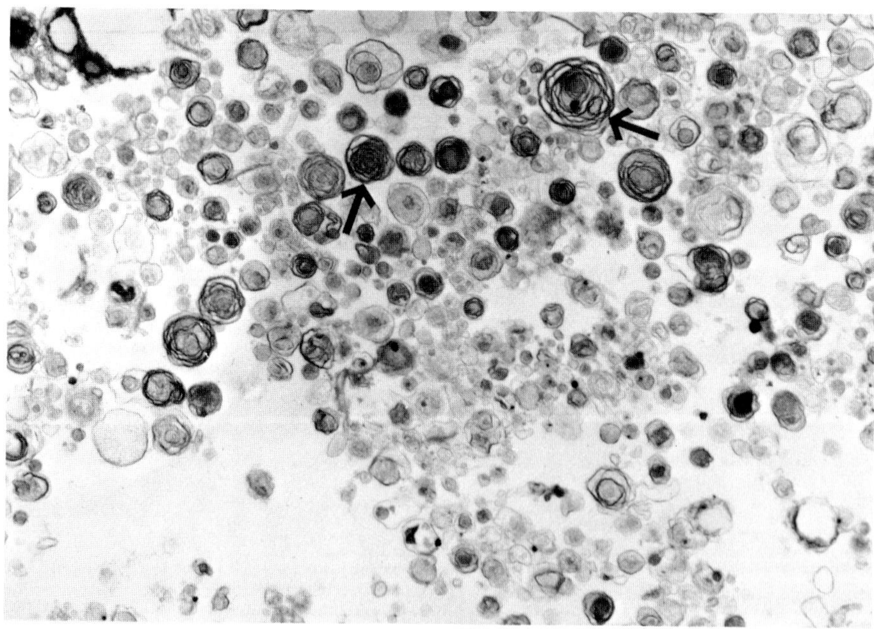

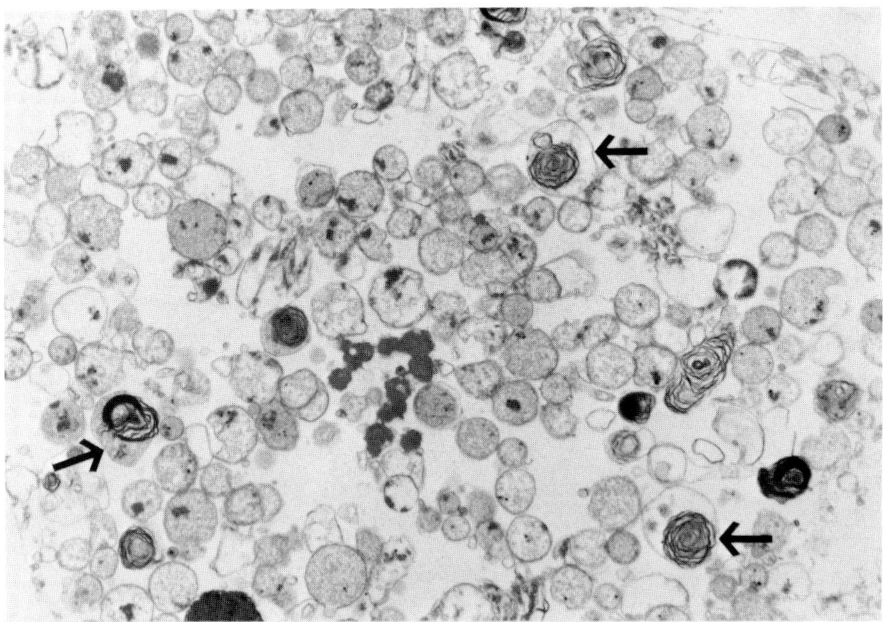

Figure 4-5.   This transmission electron micrograph shows the dissolution of mitochondria and many intralysosomal whorls or myeloid bodies (arrows) (UA + LC, ×5,000).

Most of the proximal and distal tubule epithelial cells demonstrated swelling of the mitochondria with loss of cristae and amorphous dark bodies, but a few cells had less affected or unaffected mitochondria and nuclei (Figs. 4-7 and 4-8). The follow-up urinary sediment study was negative.

Comments: These urinary sediment findings parallel the morphological changes in the kidneys, as described for aminoglycoside nephrotoxicity. It is not clear, however, where all the myeloid bodies were formed—at the luminal membrane or microvilli of the cells or within the lysosomes in the cell since sediment findings provided evidence for all these sites. It is also difficult to explain the ischemic changes in the tubule cells since there was no evidence of an ischemic insult in this patient. The cellular changes, however, appeared to be reversible.

Figure 4-4.   In this transmission electron micrograph, many free myeloid bodies of different sizes and with typical whorl formation (arrows) are seen (UA + LC, ×6,600). From *Seminars in Nephrology,* Vol. 6, 1986, with permission.

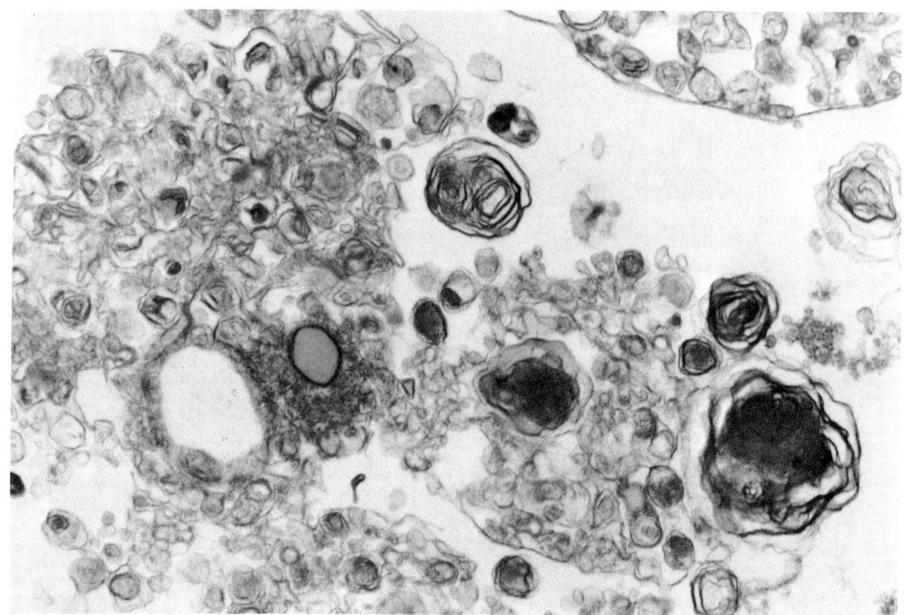

Figure 4-6.   In this transmission electron micrograph, the tubule cell membranes are disrupted, with conglomeration and large whorl formation (UA + LC, ×13,000).

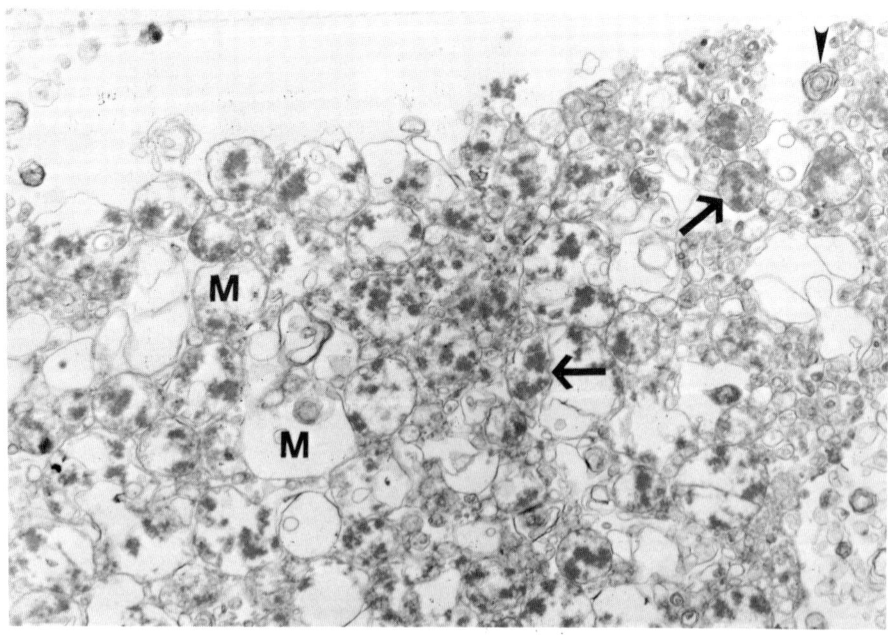

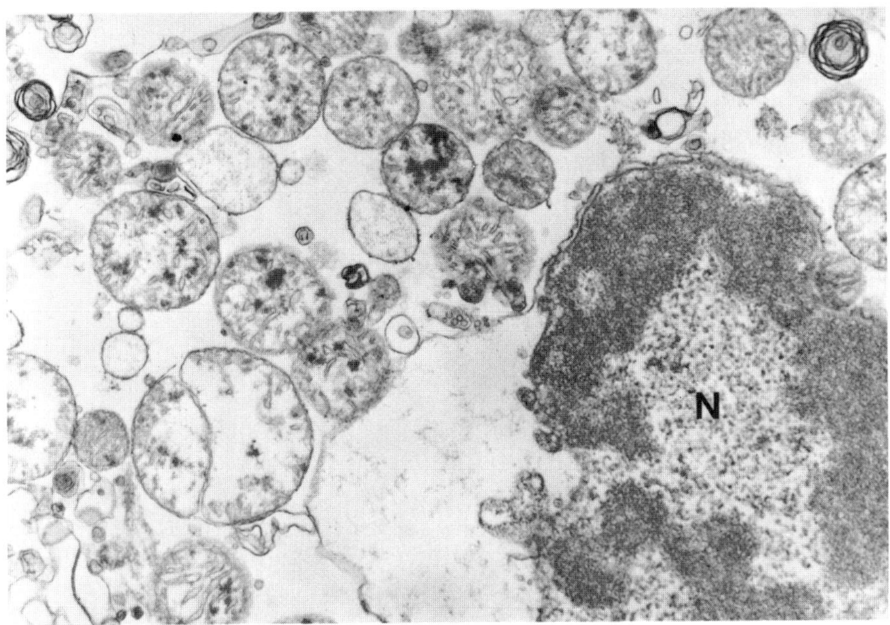

Figure 4-8.   This tubule cell shows relatively less affected subcellular structures. The nucleus (N) does not appear to be severely damaged, but some mitochondria are swollen, with loss of cristae, whereas others are less affected (UA + LC, ×8,300).

This TEM assessment of the urinary sediment was supported by the complete reversal of ARF in this patient. Furthermore, complete healing of the renal lesion was corroborated by negative findings in a follow-up urinary sediment study.

Patient No. 2, C. O., a 62-year-old black male, was admitted to the Veterans Administration Medical Center, Augusta Georgia, on May 6, 1984, with acute respiratory failure secondary to pneumonia. He also exhibited features of mild volume depletion. A

Figure 4-7.   A tubule cell is shown by transmission electron microscopy. The nephron segment from which this cell originated cannot be determined, but because of the presence of numerous mitochondria and a few apical pits, the cell might be of proximal tubule origin. The mitochondria (M) are either swollen, with loss of cristae, or show amorphous dark bodies (arrows). The luminal membrane is lost, but an intracellular myeloid body can be seen (arrowhead).

chest X ray showed right lower lobe infiltration. The antibiotic regimen and the serial
serum urea nitrogen (SUN) and serum creatinine (Scr) levels were as follows.

Date (1984)	Antibiotic (dosage and duration)	SUN (mg/dl)	Scr (mg/dl)
May 6	Penicillin 1 million units q 4 hr	51	1.9
May 11	Gentamicin 80 mg q 8 hr	21	1.3
May 17	Gentamicin	14	1.2
May 23	Gentamicin	22	2.7
	(gentamicin discontinued)		
May 25	Clindamycin	23	3.3
	(urine sample collected for TEM analysis)		
May 31	None	45	4.1
June 6	None	33	2.4
June 13	None	15	1.9
	(urine sample collected for TEM analysis)		
June 19	None	16	1.4

The first urinary sediment TEM revealed mainly myeloid bodies casts (Figs. 4-9 and
4-10), remnants of acellular necrotic tubules (Fig. 4-11), in which the cellular structure
might have been replaced by myeloid bodies (Fig. 4-12). The second urinary sediment
TEM showed small numbers of free myeloid bodies only.

Comments: The urine sediment findings in patient No. 2 are similar to those
of patient No. 1, except that fewer necrotic tubule epithelial cells were found.
The sediment findings, therefore, seemed to indicate less extensive renal lesions,
which was confirmed by a complete reversal of ARF in this patient. The presence
of myeloid bodies only in the follow-up urinary study, when the renal function
had returned to normal, argues in favor of the myeloid bodies as a marker of
the aminoglycoside effect, rather than the aminoglycoside-induced ARF.

Patient No. 3, D. J., a 61-year-old black female, was admitted to the Medical
College of Georgia Hospital on July 9, 1984, with a history of abdominal abscess. Her
medical history also included diabetes mellitus and hypertension.

Figure 4-10.   In this myeloid body cast (patient No. 2), it appears as if whorls are embedded
within a whole tubule cell. A portion of the tubule (T), with many lysosomes and protein
precipitates (arrows), is shown (UA + LC, ×3,300).

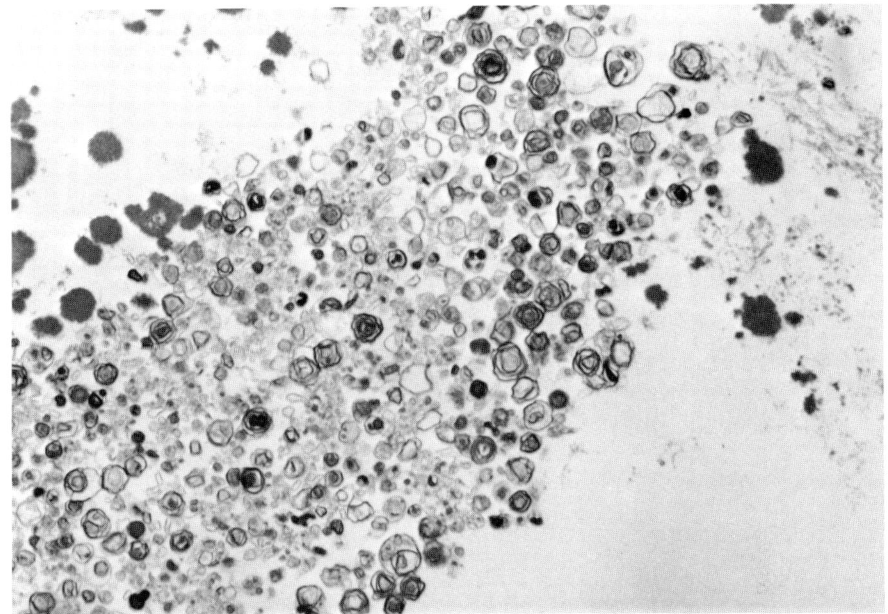

Figure 4-9.   This transmission electron micrograph shows a myeloid body cast in the urinary sediment of patient No. 2. Note the matrix, which appears to be made up of fragments of tubule cells in which whorls are embedded (UA + LC, ×5,000).

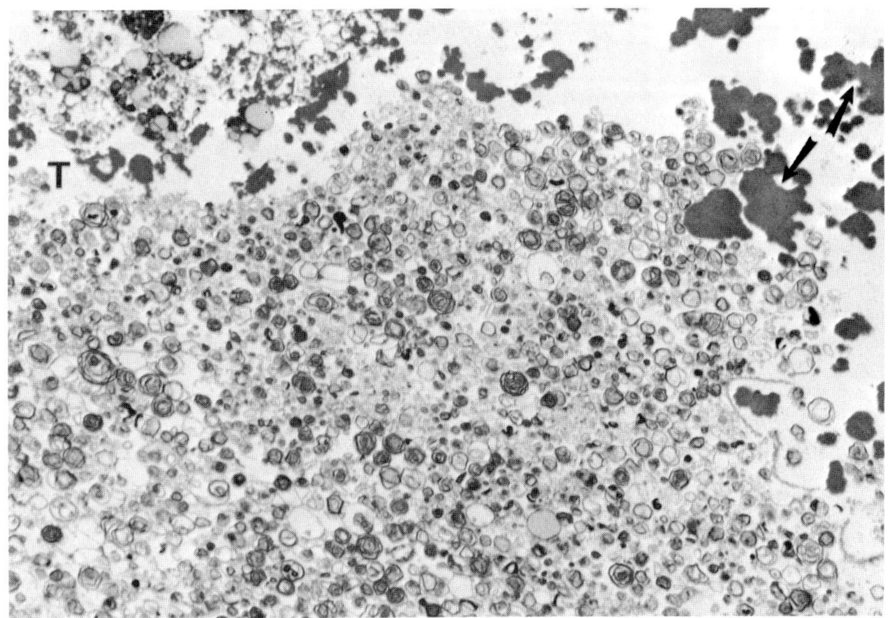

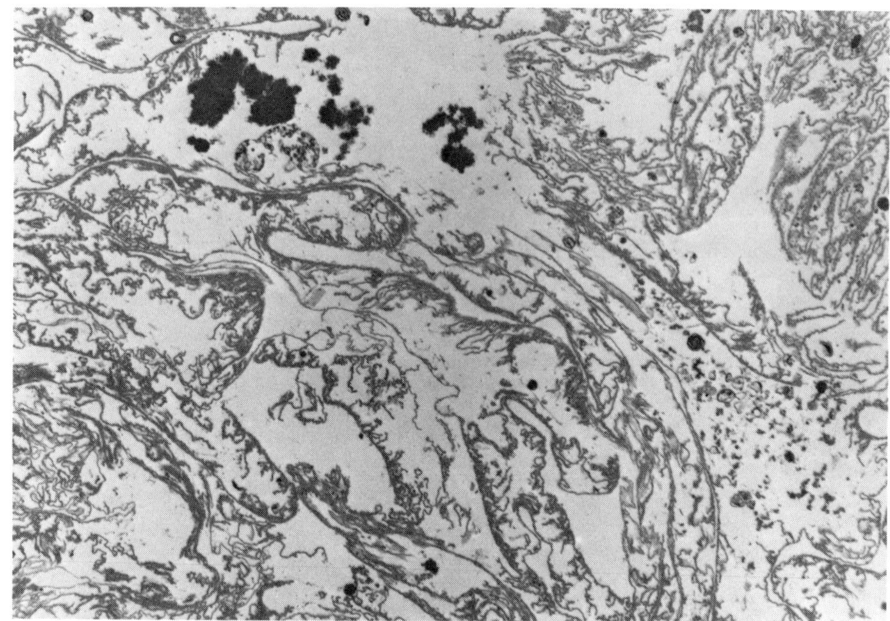

Figure 4-11.   This micrograph shows what may be the remnants of the basement membranes of acellular tubules (UA + LC, ×2,600).

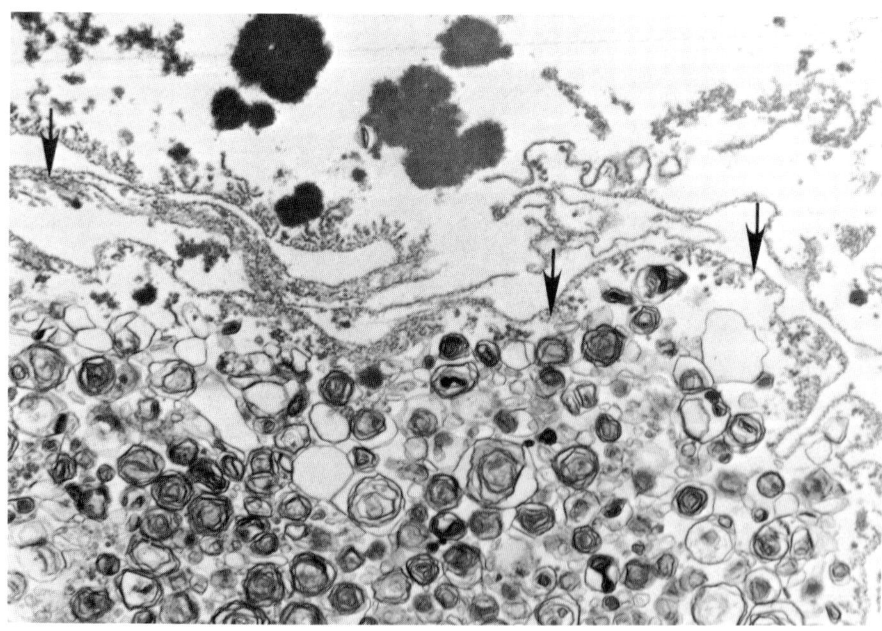

The antibiotic regimen, serial urine output, serum urea nitrogen (SUN), and serum creatinine (Scr) were as follows.

Date (1984)	Antibiotics (dosage and duration)	Urine output (ml/24 hr)	SUN (mg/dl)	Scr (mg/dl)
July 9	Tobramycin 80 mg q 8 hr	Not available	22	2.1
July 12	As above + ampicillin 2 g q 6 hr	1356	27	2.0
	(urine sample collected for TEM analysis)			
July 16	Tobramycin	2695	58	2.7
July 22	Tobramycin	688	74	4.1
	(urine sample collected for TEM analysis)			
July 23	Tobramycin		97	6.5

On July 23, the serum bilirubin level was 33.3 mg/dl; on July 29, the patient died. The final diagnosis at autopsy was abdominal abscess, necrotizing fascitis, sepsis, and ARF.

The first urinary sediment TEM from July 12, 1984, showed many free myeloid bodies. Few tubule epithelial cells were observed, but intracellular whorls were found (Fig. 4-13). There were, however, many transitional epithelial cells. The second urinary sediment TEM, from July 22 (when renal function had decreased), revealed many necrotic tubule epithelial cells (Figs. 4-14 and 4-15) but few myeloid bodies.

Comments: The urinary sediment studies in this patient demonstrated that the appearance of necrotic tubule epithelial cells, but not of myeloid bodies in the urine, coincided with the decrease of renal function.

Patient No. 4, J. W., a 48-year-old black male, was admitted to the Medical College of Georgia Hospital on July 7, 1984, with a history of gastrointestinal bleeding from ruptured esophageal varices. He was known to have alcoholic cirrhosis. Upon admission, he was also found to have a *Pseudomonas* pneumonia.

Figure 4-12. This transmission electron micrograph shows a tubule devoid of cells but packed with myeloid bodies. The basement membrane (arrows) of the tubule can be seen (UA + LC, ×6,600).

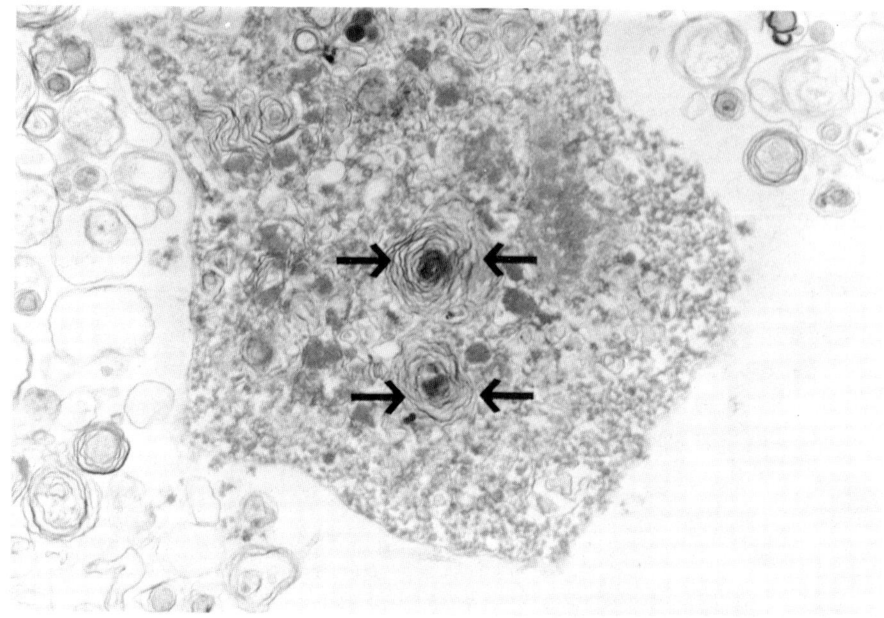

Figure 4-13. This transmission electron micrograph (patient No. 3) shows a tubule epithelial cell with several intracellular myeloid bodies (between arrows) and many free myeloid bodies around the cell (UA + LC, ×10,000). From *Seminars in Nephrology,* Vol. 6, 1986, with permission.

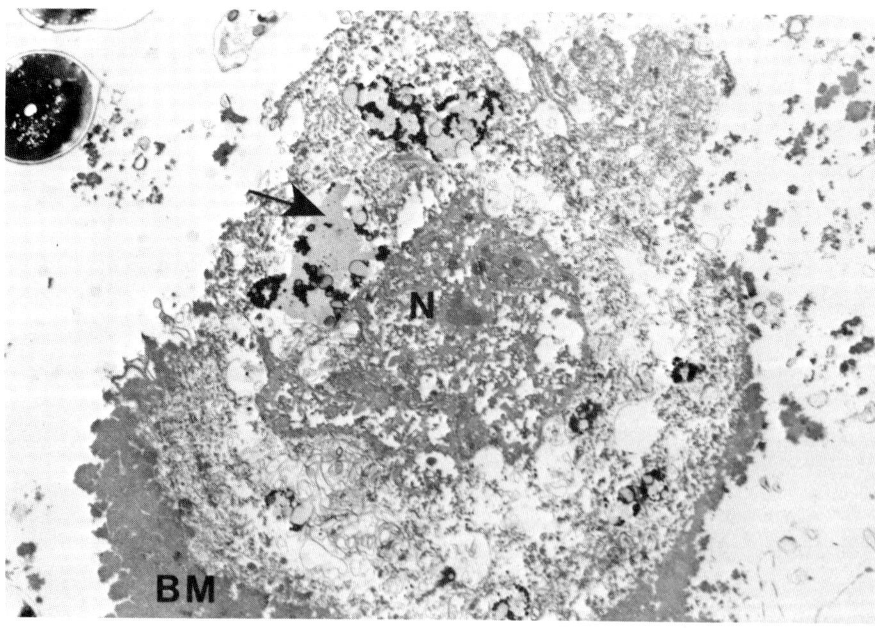

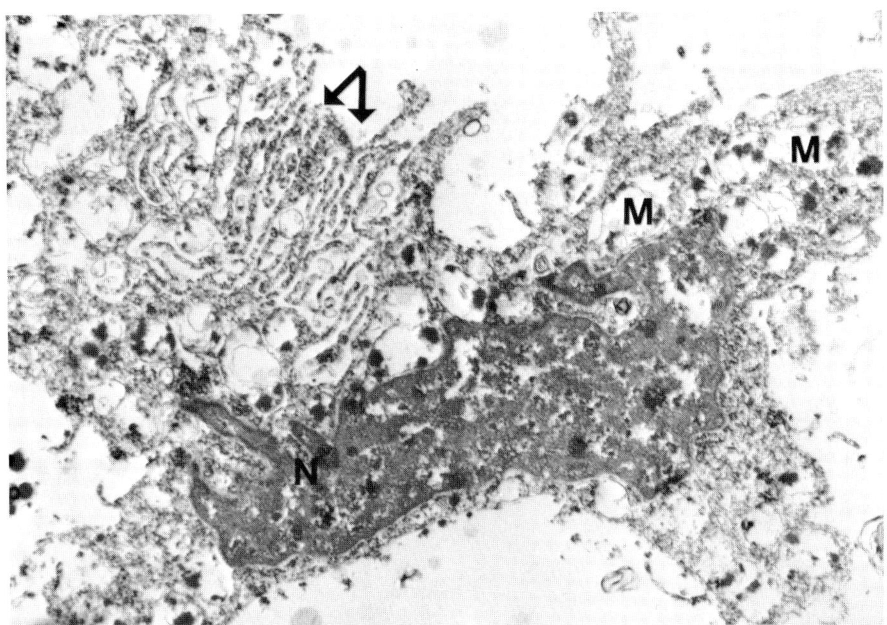

Figure 4-15.   This proximal tubule cell (patient No. 3) is characterized by many disrupted microvilli (arrows), swollen mitochondria (M) with amorphous dark bodies, and a large nucleus (N). The nucleus is displaced toward the cell apex (UA + LC, ×6,600).

The antibiotic regimen and the serial serum urea nitrogen (SUN) and serum creatinine (Scr) levels were as follows.

Date (1984)	Antibiotic regimen (dosage and duration)	SUN (mg/dl)	Scr (mg/dl)
July 7	None	2	0.4
July 10	Gentamicin 90 mg q 8 hr	Not available	Not available
July 18	As above	6	0.4
	(urine sample collected for TEM study)		
July 23	As above	16	0.5
July 30	As above	54	1.7
	(urine sample collected for TEM study)		
August 3	Tobramycin 200 mg q 12 hr		
August 4		89	1.6

Figure 4-14.   In this necrotic tubule epithelial cell, dissolution of the nucleus (N) and a homogeneous condensation of the basement membrane (BM) are seen. Many lysosomes (arrow) can be found (UA + LC, ×2,600).

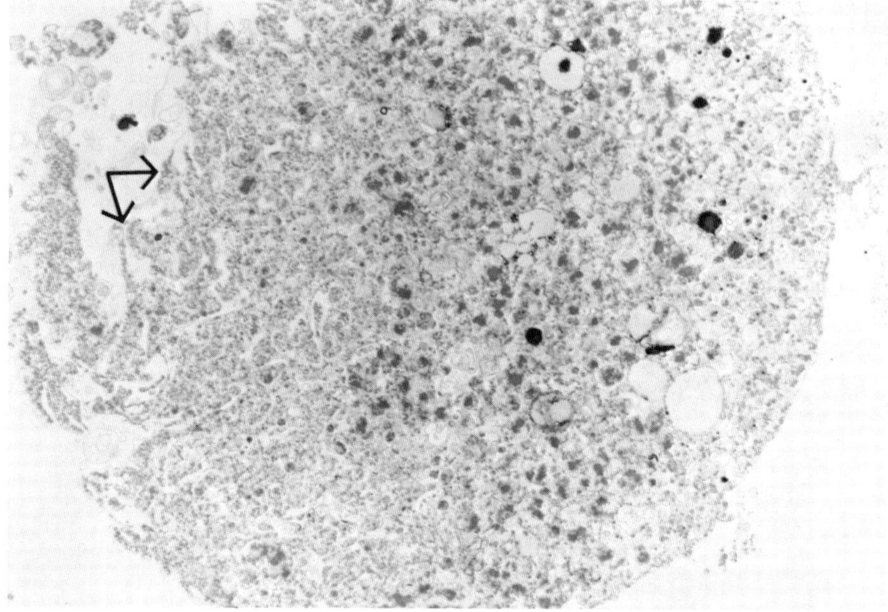

Figure 4-16. A severely necrotic proximal tubule cell, with still recognizable microvilli (arrows), is seen in this transmission electron micrograph (patient No. 4). This cell contains many intracellular myeloid bodies and lysosomes (UA + LC, ×3,300).

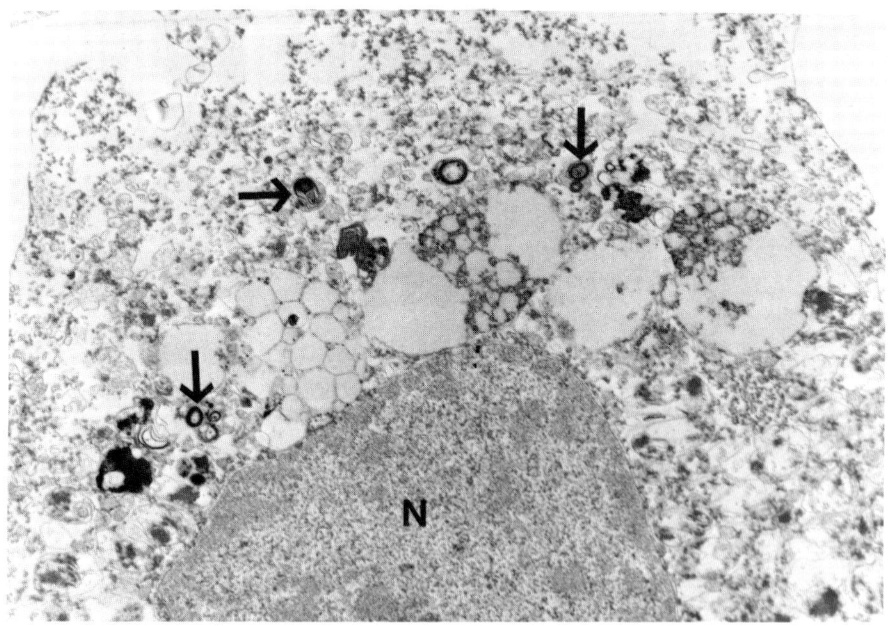

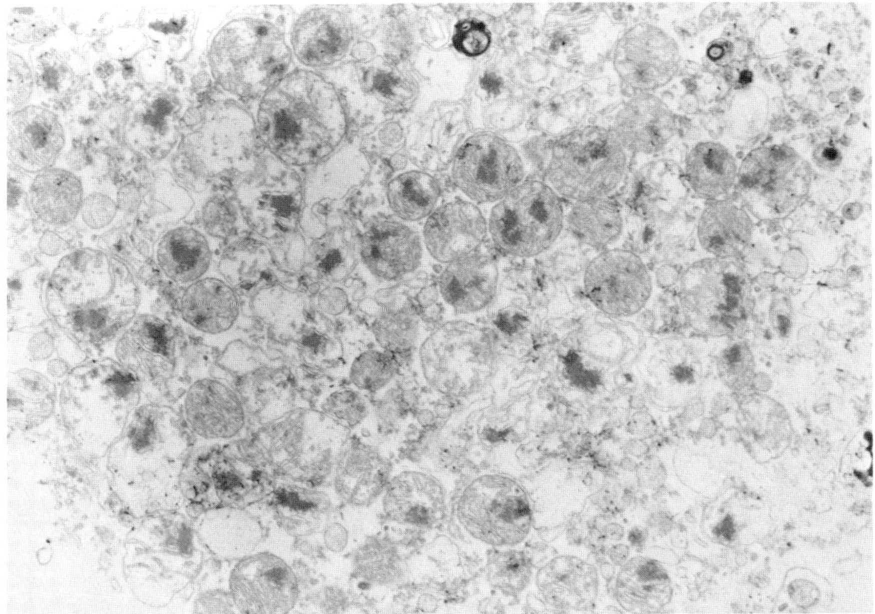

Figure 4-18. This cell shows ischemic damage characterized by the appearance of amorphous dark bodies within the mitochondria (patient No. 4) (UA + LC, ×6,600).

The patient died on August 9. The first urinary sediment TEM from July 18, 1984, revealed only free myeloid bodies; the second sample from July 30, 1984, many tubule epithelial cells. The origin of some of the cells appeared to be the proximal tubule (Figs. 4-16 and 4-17); the origin of other cells could not be determined. In general, the cells demonstrated variable changes: In some cells, microvilli were disrupted and the mitochondria almost replaced by amorphous dark bodies (Fig. 4-16); in other cells, damage to the mitochondria was less severe (Fig. 4-18).

Comments: The initial urinary sediment showed only myeloid bodies, suggesting an aminoglycoside effect; the second urine sample showed many necrotic tubule cells, which coincided with the decrease in renal function.

Patient No. 5, R. G., a 35-year-old black female, was admitted to the Medical College of Georgia Hospital on June 23, 1984, with a history of alcohol abuse and a diagnosis of acute pancreatitis. One week before her admission, her SUN was 5 mg/dl.

Figure 4-17. A reasonably well-preserved cell characterized by an intact nucleus (N) and many intralysosomal myeloid bodies (arrows) is shown (patient No. 4) (UA + LC, ×5,000).

Her antibiotic regimen and the serial serum urea nitrogen (SUN) and serum creatinine (Scr) levels were as follows.

Date (1984)	Antibiotic regimen (dosage and duration)	SUN (mg/dl)	Scr (mg/dl)
June 26	Tobramycin 80 mg q 8 hr		
	(temp, 38.4° C; peripheral WBC count, 20,800)		
June 27	As above	4	0.6
June 29	As above	6	0.5
July 6	As above	9	0.6
July 9	(urine sample collected for TEM analysis)		
July 20	(tobramycin discontinued)		
July 26	(tobramycin 80 mg) q 8 hr		
July 28	(tobramycin discontinued)		
July 30		20	0.9
	(urine sample collected for TEM analysis)		

The first urinary sediment TEM showed transitional epithelial cells, neutrophilic leukocytes, small numbers of myeloid bodies, and no tubule epithelial cells (Fig. 4-19). The second urinary sediment study, three weeks after the first sediment study, revealed an increasing number of myeloid bodies but no tubule epithelial cells (Fig. 4-20).

Comments: Both urinary sediment studies revealed only myeloid bodies. Neither specimen showed necrotic tubule epithelial cells, which suggested preservation of renal function. This was confirmed by the absence of clinical ARF.

An additional patient (not included in Table 4-1), is presented to show that TEM analysis of urinary sediment can demonstrate aminoglycoside nephrotoxicity in a patient who is receiving aminoglycoside but who apparently develops ARF from another cause.

Patient No. 6, M. B., a 34-year-old white male, developed quadriplegia following a gunshot wound in the neck on August 24, 1985, and was admitted to a hospital in Athens, Georgia. He was transferred to the Veterans Administration Medical Center, Augusta, Georgia, on September 23, 1985. The patient had an esophageal perforation, mediastinitis, and numerous infections. He received gentamicin from January 23 through February 5, 1986, which was followed by amikacin from February 5 through February

Figure 4-20. Increasing numbers of myeloid bodies are found in the second urinary sediment from patient No. 5, but no tubule epithelial cells are seen (UA + LC, ×5,000). From *Seminars in Nephrology,* Vol. 6, 1986, with permission.

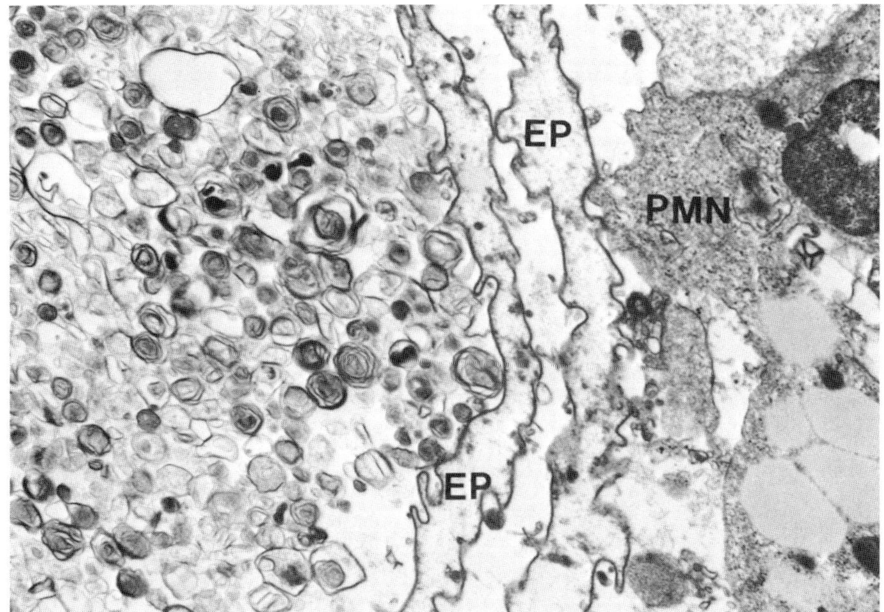

Figure 4-19. This transmission electron micrograph (patient No. 5) shows myeloid bodies along with transitional epithelial cells (EP) and a portion of a polymorphonuclear neutrophil (PMN) (UA + LC, ×6,600). From *Seminars in Nephrology,* Vol. 6, 1986, with permission.

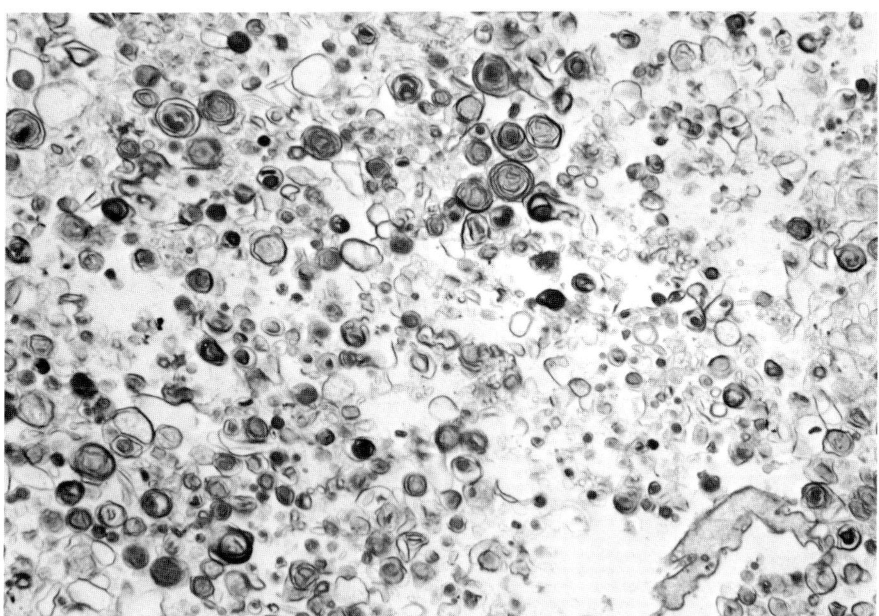

16, 1986. On February 14, 1986, a sigmoidoscopy was done as a part of the work-up for diarrhea of two weeks' duration. Twenty-four hours later, he developed severe abdominal pain and hypotension (80/50 mm Hg). He remained hypotensive with essentially no urine output for 24 hr. On February 16, 1986, a flat film of the abdomen revealed free air in the abdomen and organ perforation was suspected; he was immediately taken for surgery, and a perforated duodenal ulcer was found and repaired. Following surgery, he was placed on dopamine drip (4 μg/kg per min) and his urine output increased promptly and markedly. On February 18, 1986, a renal consultation was sought for an elevated serum urea nitrogen and serum creatinine levels of 31 mg/dl and 3.8 mg/dl, respectively. A diagnosis of aminoglycoside nephrotoxicity was made; but ischemic acute tubular necrosis (ATN), on the basis of prolonged hypotension, could not be ruled out. Daily examination of the urinary sediment by LM showed epithelial cells, epithelial casts, and granular casts; this, however, did not discriminate between aminoglycoside nephrotoxicity and ATN. In addition to aminoglycosides, the patient received clindamycin and subsequently cimetidine, which was initiated on January 23, 1986. His peripheral blood eosinophil count progressively increased to reach a maximum of 14% on February 21. On the following day, his serum creatinine peaked at 4.9 mg/dl. A urine sediment (Wrights stain) was reported to be positive for eosinophils. Thus, peripheral eosinophilia, accompanied by eosinophiluria, suggested a third diagnosis of Tagamet-induced acute interstitial nephritis. Tagamet was discontinued upon the recommendation of the nephrology team. A sample of urine was collected for TEM analysis on February 26, 1986. From February 25, the patient's renal function improved, and in about five weeks, he had had an almost complete recovery of renal function.

This patient's serial serum urea nitrogen (SUN), serum creatinine (Scr) levels, and urine output are shown below.

Date (1986)	SUN (mg/dl)	Scr (mg/dl)	Urine output (ml/day)
February 2	12	0.4	Not available
February 14	9	1.0	Not available
February 16	26	3.1	1,900
February 17	31	3.9	3,100
February 20	34	4.3	3,150
February 22	41	4.9	5,600
February 25	42	4.4	3,900
February 26		(urine sample collected for TEM analysis)	
February 28	40	3.1	Not available
March 3	38	2.4	Not available
March 10	22	1.9	Not available
March 20	15	1.7	1,600
April 2	11	0.8	Not available

From the above data, it should be noted that, on February 14, the patient had a more than 0.5 mg/dl increase in serum creatinine level from February 2. Therefore, according to our definition, the patient had developed aminoglycoside nephrotoxicity on February 14, though the Scr level was still within normal limits. Two days later, the patient manifested an overt nonoliguric ARF, which is consistent with aminoglycoside nephro-toxicity. The urinary sediment TEM showed necrotic segments of tubules or necrotic tubule cells studded with myeloid bodies (Figs. 4-21 and 4-22) and cellular casts containing numerous myeloid bodies (Fig. 4-23). Although some tubule cells were severely necrotic, others were not (Fig. 4-24). Many neutrophils but few lymphocytes were found (Fig. 4-24); an occasional plasma cell was also found (Fig. 4-25). No eosinophils were observed.

Comments: This patient received two aminoglycosides—gentamicin, fol-lowed by amikacin—for a total period of 25 days. On February 14, after 23 days of one or the other aminoglycoside, his serum creatinine was elevated by more than 0.5 mg/dl. On February 16, his overt renal insufficiency coincided with duodenal perforation, hypotension, and surgery; thus, these factors may be more responsible, etiologically, for the ARF than the aminoglycosides. Though urinary sediment was not studied by TEM until 10 days after the aminoglycoside was discontinued, the sediment findings by TEM analysis indicated aminogly-coside nephrotoxicity. Furthermore, a rapid and complete recovery of renal function favors aminoglycoside nephrotoxicity over ischemic ATN.

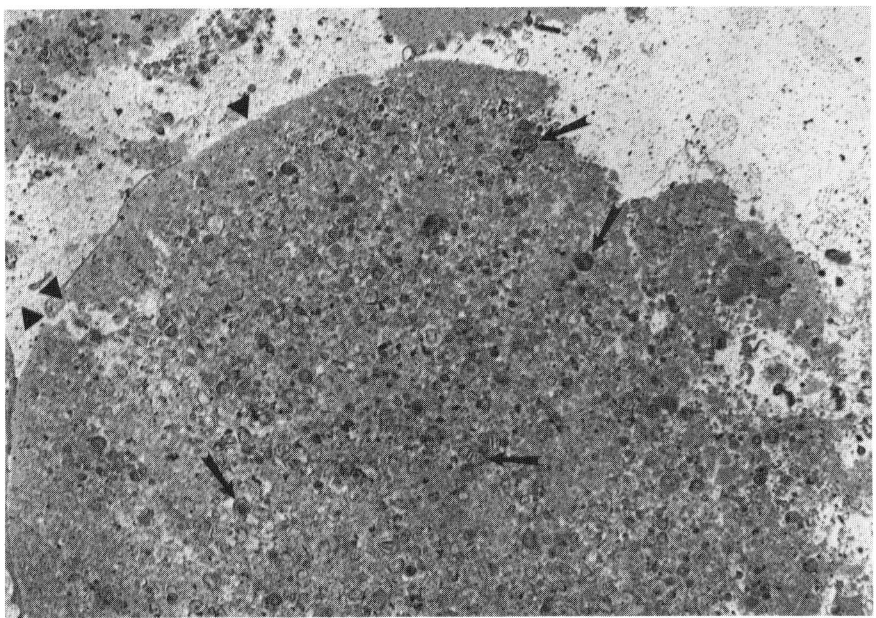

Figure 4-21.   Abundant myeloid bodies (arrows) are embedded within a totally necrotic renal tubule segment. The peripheral part of the necrotic segment (arrowhead), with disruption in the basement membrane (double arrowheads), is shown (UA + LC, ×3,000).

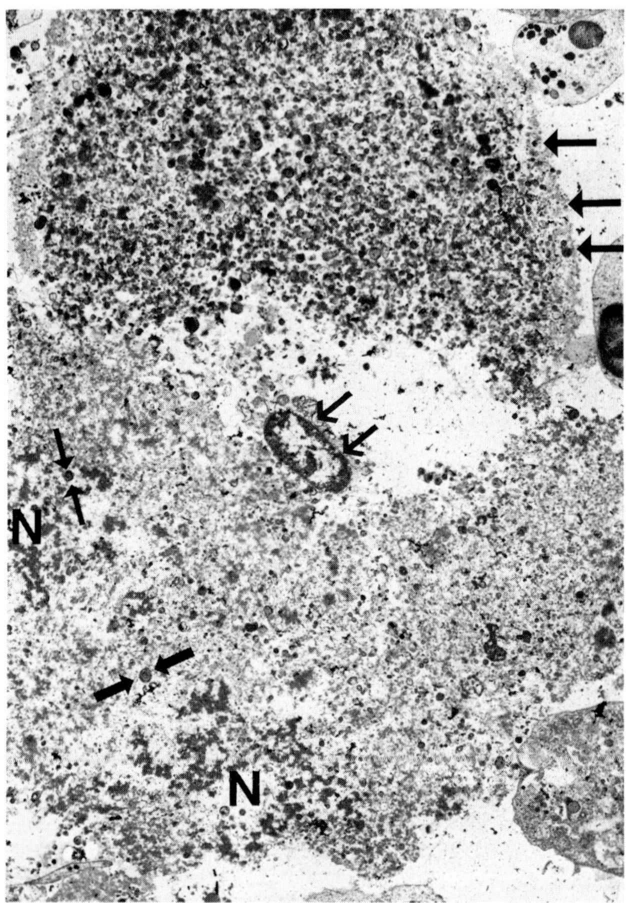

Figure 4-22.   One of the necrotic cells shown here by transmission electron microscopy is studded with myeloid bodies (arrows); in the other necrotic cell, a nucleus with a few mitochondria (double arrows), has been pushed out of the cell. Remnants of other nuclei (N) are shown. The cell is too necrotic for the segment of origin to be recognized. Intracellular myeloid bodies (between arrows), however, are still evident (patient No. 6) (UA + LC, ×2,000).

The results of two successive urinary sediment studies in four patients with ARF (Nos. 8, 9, 10, and 11) and three patients without ARF (Nos. 16, 17, and 18) are shown in Table 4-4. In the four ARF patients, the first specimens showed predominantly myeloid bodies with few or no necrotic renal tubule cells, whereas the second specimens showed decreasing numbers of myeloid bodies with in-

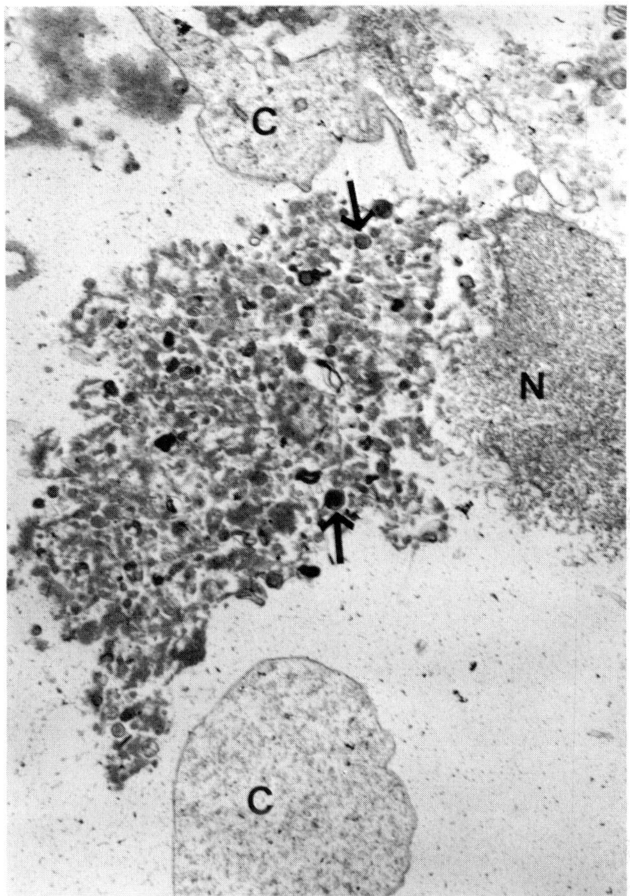

Figure 4-23.   In this myeloid body cast (patient No. 6), myeloid bodies (single arrows) are shown. The nucleus (N) and fragments of cells (C) from necrotic cell(s) can also be seen (UA + LC, ×7,500).

creasing numbers of necrotic renal tubule cells that coincided with the rise in serum creatinine. In contrast, urinary sediments from three patients without ARF showed mainly myeloid bodies throughout the course. Furthermore, in aminoglycoside non-ARF patients, the number of myeloid bodies was significantly ($P < 0.005$) lower, tubule epithelial cells were fewer, and severely necrotic renal tubule cells were rare. Tubule cells containing intracellular myeloid bodies were never found in urinary sediments of patients with aminoglycoside non-ARF.

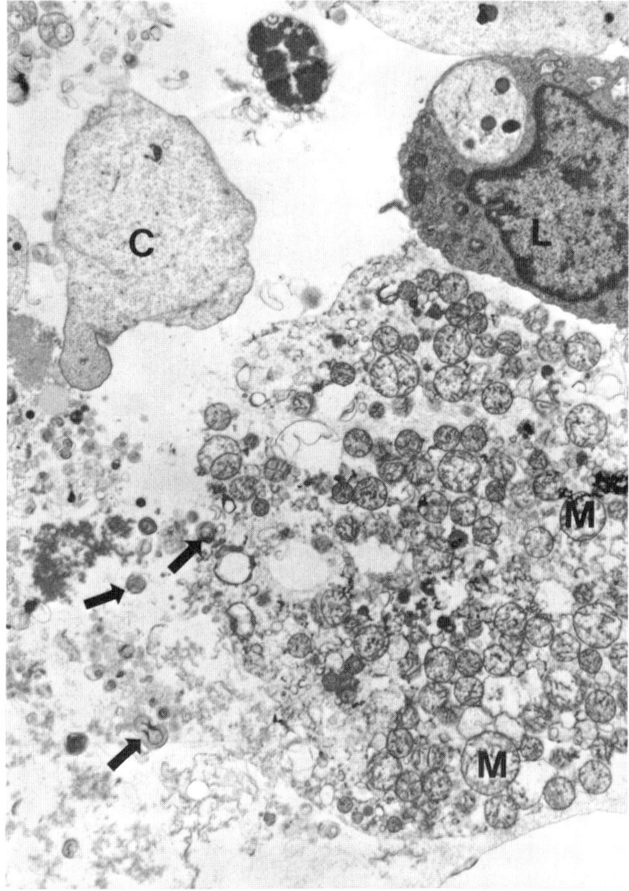

Figure 4-24. In this transmission electron micrograph (patient No. 6), a portion of a necrotic cell is seen. Some mitochondria (M) are swollen with disruption of cristae; other mitochondria appear to be intact. The intraluminal cellular membrane cannot be seen, but there are many myeloid bodies adjacent to the cell (arrows), with a portion of a lymphocyte (L) and a necrotic cell fragment (C) (UA + LC, ×5,000).

All aminoglycosides accumulate in the kidney, especially in the renal cortex as compared to the renal medulla. Renal accumulation of the antibiotic depends on the dose administered, the frequency of administration, and the total time of treatment. The degree of renal accumulation of the antibiotic and the extent of renal lesions or the severity of the renal functional impairment, however, are not related. The accumulation depends on the affinity of the aminoglycoside for the membrane receptors of the proximal tubule cell microvilli and on the en-

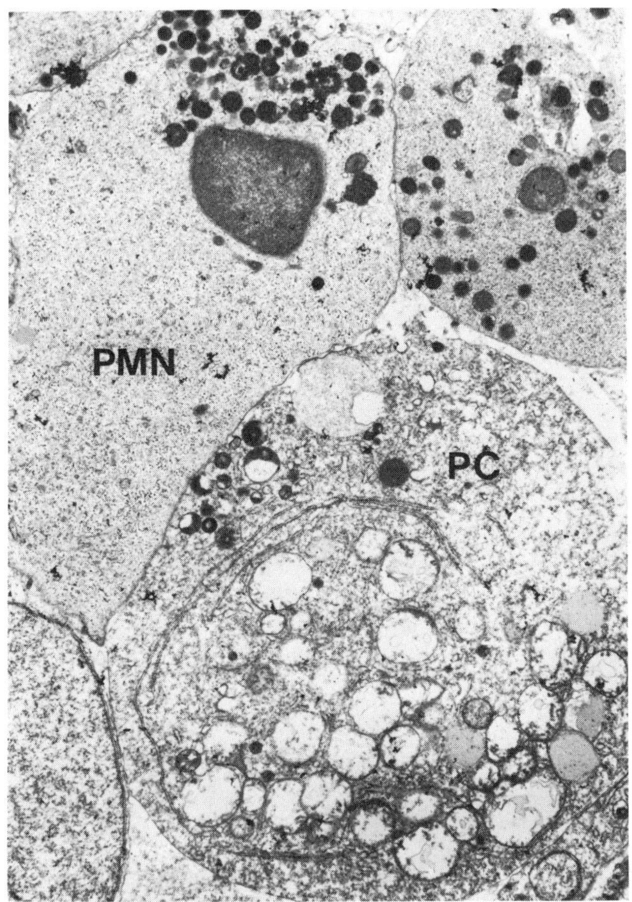

Figure 4-25. In this transmission electron micrograph, portions of neutrophil leukocytes (PMN), and a plasma cell (PC) can be found (patient No. 6) (UA + LC, ×5,000).

docytic activity of the cell.[2] The half-life of aminoglycosides in renal tissue exceeds 100 hr, and the excretion of the drug from renal tissue depends upon the glomerular filtration rate. It has been observed that nephrotoxic patients accumulate the drug in large amounts before any change in kidney function occurs.[11]

After treatment with any aminoglycoside, changes in the proximal tubules can be observed by TEM. Lysosomal changes appear early, and some investigators have hypothesized that as aminoglycosides accumulate within lysosomes, the first apparent morphological change is myeloid body formation.[12] The ap-

Table 4-4
Two Consecutive Urinary Sediment Studies

	Acute renal failure				No acute renal failure		
Patient No.	8	9	10	11	16	17	18
Date	7/12/84	7/18/84	7/26/84	4/10/84	7/23/84	7/26/84	7/9/84
Serum creatinine (mg/dl)	2.1	0.4	1.8	1.0	0.7	0.9	1.1
Urinary sediment							
Myeloid bodies	+ + +	+ +	+ + +	+ +	+	+	+
Necrotic renal tubule cells	+	0	0	0	0	+	0
Date	7/22/84	7/30/84	7/30/84	4/15/84	7/30/84	7/30/84	7/14/84
Serum creatinine (mg/dl)	4.1	1.7	3.2	2.8	0.9	1.0	1.0
Urinary sediment							
Myeloid bodies	+ +	+	+ +	+	+ +	+	+ +
Necrotic renal tubule cells	+ +	+ +	+ +	+	0	+	0

pearance of myeloid bodies within the lysosomes in Figs. 4-5 and 4-17 supports this hypothesis. These investigators, and others, have also proposed that during an aminoglycoside course, lysosomes in the proximal tubules continuously take up the aminoglycoside, which leads to a progressive increase in lysosome size.[12,13] The function of these giant lysosomes is not known. It is possible that lysosomes store myeloid bodies and release their contents into the extracellular environment by exocytosis.[14] This may explain the presence of free myeloid bodies in the luminal aspects of tubule cells and in the urine.

URINARY SEDIMENT TEM ANALYSIS IN AMINOGLYCOSIDE NEPHROTOXICITY

Observations of urinary sediments studied by TEM in patients treated with aminoglycosides are important in understanding the pathogenesis and diagnosis of aminoglycoside-induced ARF.

Pathogenesis

First, aminoglycosides inhibit the enzyme sphingomyelinase in tubule cells, which leads to an accumulation of phospholipids or myeloid bodies.[2] Phospholipids are constituents of all cellular membranes, which are abundant in the proximal tubule cells.[13] Since the proximal tubule has more membranes and mitochondria, this segment is more vulnerable to the aminoglycoside effect than the distal tubule. Like other membranes, mitochondrial membranes are apt to be adversely affected by aminoglycoside. The appearance of dark bodies within the mitochondria, shown in Figs. 4-7 and 4-18, indicates that ischemic changes are taking place. When most of the mitochondria are severely affected, the cell undergoes lysis. Though, theoretically, nephrotoxicity should demonstrate tubule changes of toxic ATN, the eventual pathological change observed in aminoglycoside-induced ARF may be ischemic ATN. One difficulty in elucidating the toxicity mechanism is the focal character of the tubular necrosis. Moreover, it is not easy to determine whether the ultrastructural changes seen in subnecrotic cells, for example, at the lysosomal membrane level, are the causes or the consequences of such necrosis.[15]

Second, myeloid bodies are formed only when the tubule cell is normal or near normal and the plasma membrane is reasonably intact at the time aminoglycoside therapy is initiated. Myeloid bodies, therefore, are most likely to be found in the urinary sediment of a patient whose renal function was normal, or stable with chronic renal insufficiency, at the time of aminoglycoside therapy. Conversely, there may be no or few myeloid bodies in the urinary sediment of a patient who has developed ATN from another cause before aminoglycoside therapy. This is exemplified by the results of our previous study,[7] in which myeloid bodies were conspicuously absent in the sediments of patients with ATN, though many of these patients had received aminoglycosides during the course of ARF.

Third, large numbers $(+ + +)$ of myeloid bodies in the urine indicate excessive myeloid body formation in renal tubule cells. Heavy accumulation of myeloid bodies in the renal tubule cells, as shown in Figs. 4-12 and 4-21 through 4-23, is thus likely to be followed by cellular disintegration or ATN.

Diagnosis

First, myeloid bodies can be found by TEM examination in the urinary sediment in a high percentage (80%) of patients treated with aminoglycosides, though a few free myeloid bodies have little or no clinical significance. The persistence of or a slight increase in the number of myeloid bodies without the appearance of tubule cells in the serial sediment studies does not indicate overt renal insufficiency.

Second, it has been proposed that prominent myeloid bodies in renal tubules appear to be a sensitive marker of gentamicin toxicity.[16] Since we did not find a significant difference in the appearance of myeloid bodies between aminoglycoside ARF and aminoglycoside non-ARF groups, we believe that myeloid bodies are more specific for aminoglycoside accumulations in the kidneys than for nephrotoxicity. This has been reported by other investigators.[15,17] In one study of 90 patients without myeloid bodies, none had received gentamicin within six weeks of tissue examination.[17] Nonetheless, we found a significantly ($p < 0.05$)

greater number of myeloid bodies in the aminoglycoside ARF group than the aminoglycoside non-ARF group. The presence of excessive numbers of free myeloid bodies, intracellular myeloid bodies (Figs. 4-13 and 4-16), or myeloid body casts accompanied by necrotic tubule cells is likely to be associated with progression to clinical nephrotoxicity or ARF.

Third, the presence of + + necrotic tubule cells accompanied by + + to + + + myeloid bodies in first samples, or the appearance of + + necrotic tubules in second samples preceded by + + to + + + myeloid bodies in first samples, tends to coincide with the increase in serum creatinine or the onset of aminoglycoside ARF.

Fourth, in the diagnosis of aminoglycoside nephrotoxicity, it is prudent to state that, from our observations, repetitive urinary sediment studies are more useful than single sediment studies in predicting renal changes and the appearance of aminoglycoside-induced ARF. Thus, in this study, the author concludes that the presence of necrotic renal tubule cells in the urinary sediment indicates ARF, and that when these cells are preceded or accompanied by + + to + + + myeloid bodies, an aminoglycoside-induced ARF is indicated. This noninvasive technique is worth examining and reexamining to establish its application in clinical practice.

Management

The management of aminoglycoside nephrotoxicity is essentially prevention, that is, the cautious use of aminoglycosides. Because urinary sediments were rarely obtained from amikacin- and tobramycin-treated patients and because no urinary sediments were obtained from netilmicin-treated patients, our observations do not allow us to suggest that one aminoglycoside is safer than another. From our review of the literature, it is difficult to draw firm conclusions that tobramycin or amikacin or netilmicin is safer than gentamicin. Therefore, it is more important to minimize or control the factor(s) that induce aminoglycoside nephrotoxicity than to choose one aminoglycoside over another. These factors include regulating the dosage according to age and renal function and limiting the aminoglycoside course to 10 days. In old patients, dosage must be reduced by two-thirds to one-half the adult dose. Fluid and electrolyte balance must be maintained and the use of other potentially nephrotoxic substances, such as a radiocontrast material, should be avoided. Serum potassium levels should also be monitored. In hypokalemic patients, potassium supplements should be given to raise the serum potassium to normal levels. Gentamicin can cause potassium wasting and hypokalemia; conversely, hypokalemia may aggravate gentamicin nephrotoxicity.[18] The cause-and-effect relationship between these two factors is unclear, though it is known that hypokalemia causes vacuolation of the proximal tubules. Since the aminoglycosides accumulate in the proximal tubules, one wonders if vacuolar changes in the proximal tubules might predispose to the necrotic lesions induced by aminoglycosides.

The dose levels of aminoglycosides that can lead to aminoglycoside nephrotoxicity are not known, nor is the effect of concomitant use of another antibiotic, especially cephalothin or penicillin.

Irrespective of the meticulous use of aminoglycosides, nephrotoxicity can occur, but when it does, it is usually mild and reversible. Once nephrotoxicity is recognized clinically, it is recommended that the drug be discontinued. Judgment must be used, however, so that the drug is not discontinued in the absence of aminoglycoside nephrotoxicity, when ARF is the result of, for example, ischemic ATN in a patient with sepsis. In such a case, discontinuation of the aminoglycoside would be a disaster. In some patients, it can be a very difficult task to determine whether the ARF is the result of sepsis or aminoglycoside administration. In such critical situations, urinary sediment TEM can facilitate the differential diagnosis.

In cases of aminoglycoside nephrotoxicity, the renal failure usually reverses spontaneously upon withdrawal of the antibiotic, but the return of base-line renal function may take several weeks. Dialytic intervention seldom, if ever, is warranted in the management of aminoglycoside nephrotoxicity. In our study, no patient required dialysis.

REFERENCES

1. McEvoy GK, McQuarrie GM (eds): Aminoglycosides, in *Drug Information; American Hospital Formulary Service*, American Society of Hospital Pharmacists, 1986, pp 50–66.
2. Fillastre JP, Hemet J, Tulkens P, *et al:* Comparative nephrotoxicity of four aminoglycosides: Biochemical and ultrastructural modifications of lysosomes, in *Advances in Nephrology*, Hamburger J, Grognier J, Grunfield JP, et al (eds), Vol 12, Chicago, Year Book Medical Publishers, Inc., 1983, pp 253–275.
3. Plaut ME, Schentag JJ, Jusko WJ: Aminoglycoside nephrotoxicity: Comparative assessment in critically ill patients. *J Med* 1979; 10:257–266.
4. Kumin GD: Clinical nephrotoxicity of tobramycin and gentamicin. A prospective study. *JAMA* 1980; 244:1808–1810.
5. Jackson GG: Present status of aminoglycoside antibiotics and their safe effective use. *Chemotherapy* 1977; 1:200–215.
6. Fong IW, Fenton RS, Bird R: Comparative toxicity of gentamicin versus tobramycin: A randomized prospective study. *J Antimicrob Chemother* 1981; 7:81–88.
7. Mandal AK, Sklar AH, Hudson JB: Transmission electron microscopy of urinary sediment in human acute renal failure. *Kidney Int* 1985; 28:58–63.
8. Coulon G, Saint-Hillier Y, Carbillet JP, *et al:* Myeloid bodies in urine and nephrotoxicity of aminoglycosides. *Nephrologie* 1984; 5:107–116.
9. Mandal AK, Mize GN, Birnbaum DB: Transmission electron microscopy of urinary sediment in aminoglycoside nephrotoxicity. *Renal Failure*, in press.
10. Wade JC, Smith CR, Petty BG, *et al:* Cephalothin plus an aminoglycoside is more nephrotoxic than methicillin plus an aminoglycoside. *Lancet* 1978; 2:604–606.

11. Schentag JJ, Lasezkay G, Plaut ME, *et al:* Comparative tissue accumulation of gentamicin and tobramycin in patients. *J Antimicrob Chemother* 1978; 4:23–30.
12. Whelton A, Solez K: Aminoglycoside nephrotoxicity: A tale of two transports. *J Lab Clin Med* 1982; 99:148–155.
13. DeBroe ME, Paulus GJ, Verpooten GA, *et al:* Early effects of gentamicin, tobramycin, and amikacin on the human kidney. *Kidney Int* 1984; 25:643–652.
14. Deduve C, Wattiaux R: Function of lysosomes. *Annu Rev Physiol* 1966; 28:435–495.
15. Tulkens PM: Experimental studies on nephrotoxicity of aminoglycosides at low doses. *Am J Med* 1986; 80(suppl 6B)105–114.
16. Kosek JC, Mazze RI, Cousins MJ: Nephrotoxicity of gentamicin. *Lab Invest* 1974; 30:48–57.
17. Houghton DC, Campbell-Bowell MV, Bennett WM: Myeloid bodies in the renal tubules of humans: Relationship to gentamicin therapy. *Clin Nephrol* 1978; 10:140–145.
18. Brinker KR, Bulger RE, and Dobyan DC, *et al:* Effect of potassium depletion on gentamicin nephrotoxicity. *J Lab Clin Med* 1981; 98:292–301.

5

Bacteriuria and Pyuria

Basab K. Mookerjee, M.D., and Saleem Khan, M.D.*

Significant progress has been made in the area of bacteriuria and pyuria in the last two decades. The development of quantitative bacteriological techniques helped define various types of bacteriuria. This made it possible to follow large numbers of bacteriuric patients and led to a clearer understanding of the natural history of bacteriuria. It is now clear that a significant proportion of healthy adult females have asymptomatic bacteriuria, which can follow a highly variable course in becoming persistent, in resolving spontaneously for good, or in relapsing frequently. We now know that the development of end-stage renal failure in such individuals (bacteriuric patients who have structurally and functionally normal urinary tracts) is extremely unusual. Therefore, interest has been justifiably switched to urinary tract infections in infancy and in childhood and to those infections that occur in association with renal scars and anatomical or functional abnormalities of the genitourinary tract. In this brief chapter, we will review some of these issues, but the limited scope will not permit exhaustive discussion of research literature or of controversial issues. The interested reader is directed to the appropriate articles as listed in the references.

SIGNIFICANT BACTERIURIA

Significant bacteriuria is defined as the presence of bacteria in the urine that is not the result of contamination of the urine during the collection process,

* Basab K. Mookerjee, M.D., and Saleem Khan, M.D., Section of Nephrology, Department of Medicine, Veterans Administration Medical Center and State University of New York at Buffalo, Buffalo, New York 14215.

for example, fecal or vaginal contamination from the prepuce or contamination from collection vessels or urinary catheters. Precise knowledge of the site and manner in which urine is collected and the quantitative evaluation of the microorganisms present in the urine sample are essential for establishing significant bacteriuria. There is general agreement that when the "clean voided" method of urine collection is used, the presence of 100,000 organisms/ml, or more can be used operationally to define the presence of significant bacteriuria. Kass *et al.* demonstrated that about 95% of the patients having proven clinical urinary tract infection had counts of this magnitude, whereas in most cases when the urine was contaminated, the counts were rarely in excess of 1,000/ml.[1,2] Very few samples had intermediate counts. About 75% of patients with true bacteriuria have much higher counts, in excess of 10^6/ml or more, and counts of this magnitude are usually not due to contamination.[1,2]

It should be understood that these bacterial counts are not absolutely diagnostic in themselves, but rather they constitute a statistical probability of infection or of contamination. Thus, a count of 10^5/ml in a single random voided specimen indicates significant bacteriuria at a 80% confidence level; this means that in one of five such individuals, the bacteriuria is the result of contamination. If two successive urine specimens have counts of 10^5/ml or above, the confidence level for the diagnosis of significant bacteriuria increases to 95%. Similarly, a count of 10^3/ml (or less) indicates contamination with a confidence level of 80%, although 20% of such individuals will subsequently provide a urine speciman that will yield 10^5 colonies/ml or more. While urine is in the bladder, it is sterile, but it is an excellent culture medium if bacteria are introduced. The bacterial count of early morning specimens are generally higher than random samples drawn at other times through the day, since microorganisms, if present, are afforded a longer growth period in the bladder. Bacteriuria is detectable when such urine is voided in the morning after intravesical multiplication of the bacteria, to give a generally higher colony count than where urine is contaminated during collection.[3,4]

The concept of significant bacteriuria, as formulated by Kass, applies to asymptomatic individuals generally infected with gram-negative bacilli (Fig. 5-1). The confidence limits in symptomatic individuals or populations who are infected with different bacteria, however, may be quite different.

It follows that bacterial counts below 10^5/ml can occur in patients having true bacteriuria. Such low counts are considered valid when they are persistent, reproducible, and lead to the growth of the same organism every time. Quantitative methods have been devised to establish the presence of significant bacteriuria in difficult or borderline cases. Lampert and Berlyne have found that the bacterial excretion rate measured by timed collections of clean voided urine and quantitative cultures is often diagnostically helpful when the concentration of bacteria in urine is less than 10^5/ml.[5] In their study of 40 patients, the excretion

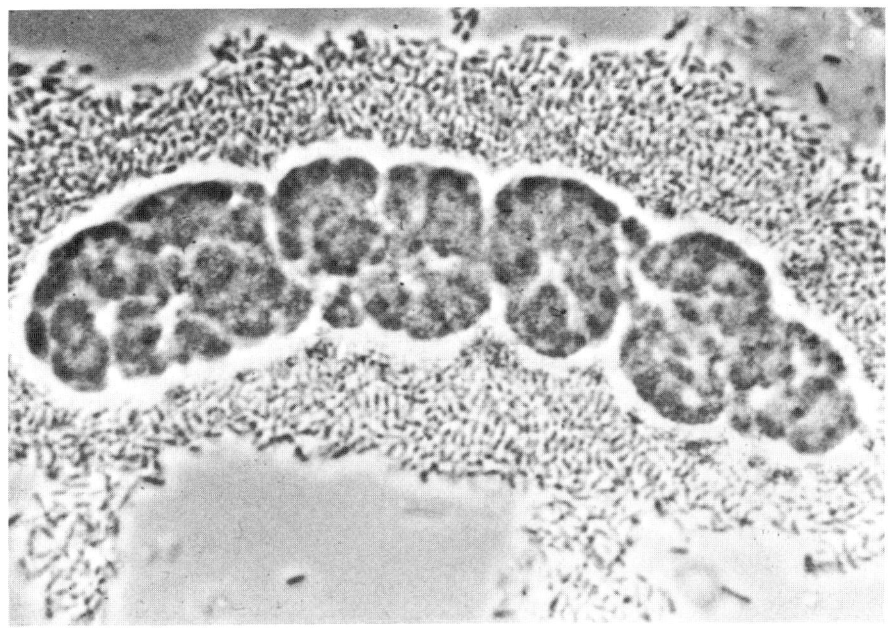

Figure 5-1.   This light micrograph shows a urinary cast of mixed (epithelial and white blood) cells surrounded by gram-negative rods. This phenomenon is often observed in patients with severe renal parenchymal infections (UA + LC stains, ×1,940).

of 10,000 bacteria/min invariably indicated significant bacteriuria.[5] Dontas *et al.* found significant bacteriuria in borderline cases by oral water loading or after intravenous furosemide followed by quantitative cultures.[6] However, these tests are cumbersome, have limited usefulness, and are not generally accepted in clinical practice.

DIAGNOSIS AND BACTERIOLOGY

An accurate bacterial count in urine is crucial to the diagnosis of bacteriuria. Its reliability depends entirely on the method used for speciman collection. Thus, strict adherence to well-established protocols for urine collection is necessary so that the collection method does not reduce the confidence level at which the clinician can distinguish true bacteriuria from contamination. In the male, a midstream sample should be collected from free flowing urine in a sterile container after retraction of the foreskin. In the females, the labia are held apart and the periurethral area cleaned with soap followed by drying with clean swabs. The use of antiseptics in washing is fraught with the risk of contamination of

Table 5-1
Microorganisms Isolated in Patients with Asymptomatic Bacteriuria[a]

	Newcastle-upon-Tyne research group[36]	Kunin et al.[12]
Escherichia coli	91.7	83.6
Klebsiella (sp.)	5.2	9.8
Proteus (sp.)	1.2	0.8
Staphylococcus	0.8	3.3
Others	1.1	2.5

[a] Percent of total number of patients.

the sample with the chemical preparation, which may lead to falsely low bacterial counts. A midstream sample is then collected in a sterile container. These collection techniques, however, are not reliable in infants and young children. Adhesive urine collection bags are often used for these patients, but such samples usually come in contact with the skin of the prepuce or the perineum and the samples are also not midstream. It has been shown that for such patients, a percutaneous suprapubic aspiration of urine is both safe and reliable.[7] Suprapubic aspiration has also been shown to be a useful technique in bacteriuria in adults and can be safely performed during pregnancy or purperium.[8,9]

Specimens should be inoculated into cultures within 2 hr of collection, but if this is not possible, they may be stored at 4°C for up to 48 hr. Culture bacterial counts can be rigorously estimated quantitatively by pour plate or surface colony counting methods. Since quantitation is time consuming, expensive, and not cost-effective for large populations, semiquantitative methods carefully calibrated against specimans containing known numbers organisms are widely used. Many semiquantitative methods using bacteriological techniques have been devised; these include swabs, filter paper strips, dip-spoon, dip-slide, roll tube, and standard loop techniques. Other semiquantitative methods use chemicals. Among these are the nitrite test that depends on bacterial conversion of urinary nitrate to nitrite and the tetrazolium test that depends on reduction of the colorless triphenyl tetrazolium to insoluble red formazan by bacterial action. Some tests depend on bacterial utilization of the low concentration of glucose (up to 6 mg%) in normal urine. Other methods combine bacteriological and chemical techniques, such as the "pad culture" method (Microstix, Ames Laboratories). Bacteriological or combined methods are preferred to chemical methods, in light of the high incidence of false negatives with the latter. False negatives are unusual with bacteriological methods, unless the patient is on antimicrobial chemotherapy, a fact easily established when the history is taken. False positives do occur when bacteriological methods are used, but primarily because of errors in urine collection; and they can easily be resolved by repeating the test. Culture methods have been detailed by Kunin.[10]

Between 80 to 90% of the isolates from patients with asymptomatic bacteriuria are *Escherichia coli* species (Table 5-1[11,12]). A single organism is cultured out in the majority of cases. Other organisms rarely isolated include *Proteus*, *Staphylococcus*, and *Klebsiella* species. In patients having symptomatic urinary tract infection (UTI), the bacteriology is similar, but the number of *E. coli* infections is much lower (about 50%). Kunin *et al.*[13] and Gruneberg *et al.*[14] have clearly shown that, in cases yielding *E. coli*, an overwhelmingly large proportion of cases involved organisms belonging to a relatively small group of O-serotypes. Gruneberg *et al.* have presented evidence of correspondence of serotypes between urinary and fecal strains in patients with UTI.[14] In asymptomatic bacteriuria, however, such correspondence has not been universally shown.[15] It is still considered likely that the serotype profile in asymptomatic bacteriuria reflects the distribution of the organisms in normal fecal flora at an earlier point in time, presumably when the urinary tract was colonized. Alter-

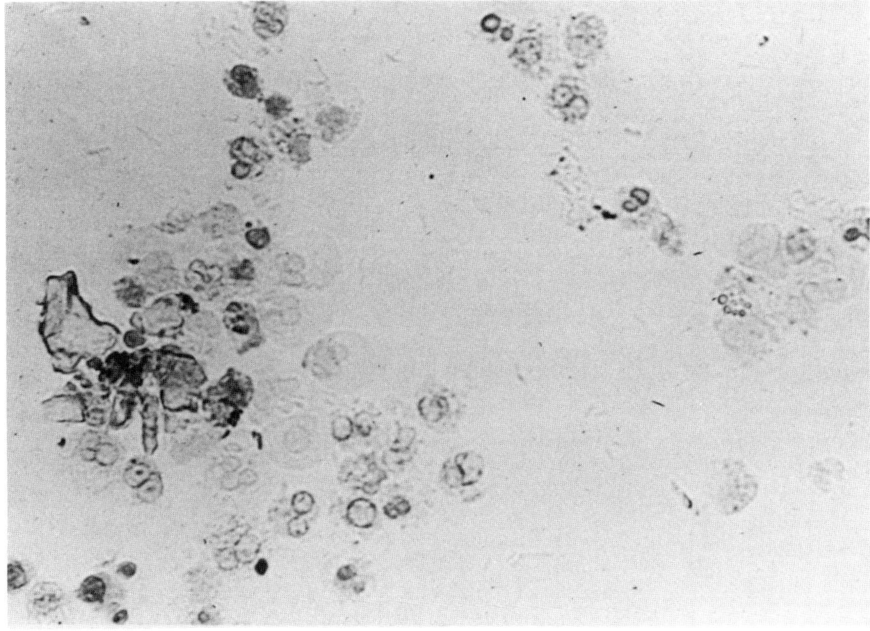

Figure 5-2.   These pus cells, or polymorphonuclear leukocytes (PMN), shown by light microscopy of urinary sediment, often appear larger than normal, with swollen, pale cytoplasm (Wright stain).

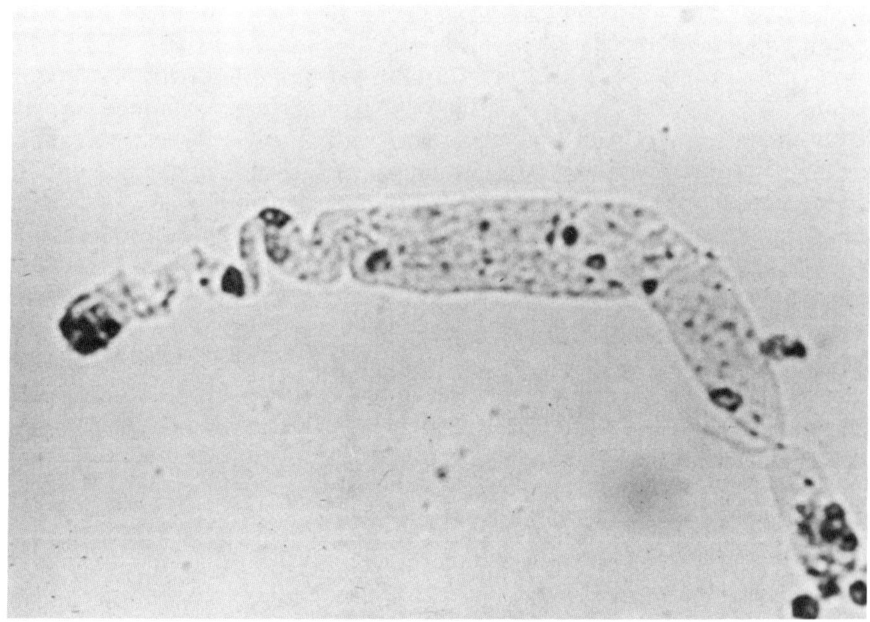

Figure 5-3.   In this white blood cell cast, the WBC are seen at the ends of the cast; a few are also embedded in the body of the cast, which has a predominantly hyaline matrix (Wright stain).

natively, certain serotypes of *E. coli* may have increased pathogenicity for the urinary tract of susceptible individuals. The presence of significant number of pus cells in the urine has been traditionally considered to be the hallmark of active UTI (Fig. 5-2). The presence of more than five pus cells in a high-power field in centrifuged urinary sediment is considered significant; though a quantitative excretion rate of pus cells of 200,000 to 400,000/hr is considered to be definitive. It should be pointed out that less than half of the patients with significant bacteriuria will have more than five pus cells in a high-power field, and white blood cell casts (Fig. 5-3) are rarely found in such urines, in the absence of severe active infection.[1] The white cell cast can be used as a marker in clinical situations clearly suggestive of acute pyelonephritis to distinguish between a lower urinary tract infection and an upper urinary tract renal parenchymal infection. Though white blood cells (WBC) embedded in a cast clearly indicate upper urinary tract renal parenchymal infection in this clinical context, white blood cell casts can also be seen in conditions other than infection, such as glomerulonephritis or tubulointerstitial nephritis. Glitter cells (leukocytes that show brownian movement of their cytoplasmic organelles) are not specific for the presence of infection; the effect is the result of low osmolality. A number of provocative tests, using various preparations of corticosteroids or endotoxin, induce pyuria in patients suspected of having urinary tract infection. These tests, however, are not widely used in current urological or nephrological practice.[10]

Pyuria may occur in the absence of bacteriuria (Table 5-2). Indeed, sterile pyuria used to be considered to be strongly suggestive of renal tuberculosis. Tubulointerstitial nephritis, analgesic nephropathy, and membranous glomerulonephritis are other conditions commonly associated with a sterile pyuria. The presence of polymorphonuclear eosinophillic leukocytes is often diagnostic of allergic tubulointerstitial nephritis, especially accompanying acute renal failure (ARF), fever, rash, peripheral eosinophilia, and the use of certain drugs, particularly the semisynthetic penicillins.

EPIDEMIOLOGY OF BACTERIURIA

Bacteriuria in infants is more common in boys than in girls. The method of urine collection used is critical in evaluating data, since suprapubic bladder puncture is considered to be more reliable than urine collection by the plastic "strap-on" device. Using the suprapubic puncture technique, Edelman *et al.* have reported a prevalence of bacteriuria of 0.7% in full term and of 2.9% in premature infants.[16] Approximately half of the neonates who were further studied with voiding cystourethrograms were shown to have vesicoureteral reflux. A somewhat higher incidence (3.6%) has been reported in studies performed by using the strap-on bag device.[17] A majority of authorities, however, believe that collection of urine for culture in such bags is unreliable, except as a screening device. When positive cultures are obtained using similar devices, repeated

Table 5-2
Isolated Bacteruria and Pyuria

A.   Pyuria without bacteria
1. Tubulointerstitial nephritis (drug allergy), nephrotoxic, analgesic nephropathy
2. Growth inhibited by *in vivo* use of antibacterial agents, antibiotics, or specimen contaminated *in vitro* with antibacterial or antiseptic agents
3. Genitourinary tuberculosis
4. Bladder or vaginal irritative conditions
5. Membranous glomerulonephritis

B.   Bacteriuria without pyuria
1. Urinary tract infection
2. *In vitro* contamination of urine (urine left at room temperature in nonsterile environment, etc.)

culturing or even suprapubic aspiration may be necessary to confirm significant bacteriuria in this age group.

Symptomatic UTI is common in preschool children, being 10 to 20 times more frequent in girls than in boys. Episodes of fever and symptomatic UTI may call attention to the problem; in other cases, such subtle symptoms as dysuria, pain on voiding, or foul smelling urine noticed by the mother may be the only presenting features. In this age group, the nitrite dip strip test, conducted by mothers at home, has been shown to be a most practical, effective screening device.[10] Kunin *et al.* studied 1,573 preschool girls (3–5 years old) by this method and concluded that the true incidence of bacteriuria in this age group is approximately 1.5%.[10]

In school-age children, bacteriuria is 30 times more common in girls (prevalence 1.2%) than in boys.[18] The prevalence rate may only represent cases found colonized at one point in time, and it has been estimated that approximately 5% of school-age girls will have at least one episode of significant bacteriuria or symptomatic UTI before they graduate. For the most part, aerobic, gram-negative bacilli of fecal origin are responsible for the vast majority of these cases, suggesting an "ascending" route of these infections from fecal sources.[18]

In preschool and school-age children, asymptomatic bacteriuria or clinical UTI should be taken with utmost seriousness, in view of their association with renal scars and vesicoureteral reflex and their tendency to cause problems later.[18,19] In a study reported by Kunin *et al.*, approximately 20% of school girls who were first discovered to have asymptomatic bacteriuria were shown to have vesicoureteral reflex.[10] Lindberg has reported, in a study done in Sweden, that approximately 30% of such girls will have symptomatic UTI.[20]

The prevalence of bacteriuria in adult women varies with age and sexual activity. In young nuns, it is 0.5%, rising to about 1% when the age of 35–44 is reached.[21] Unmarried women tend to have lower rates of bacteriuria compared with married women, in whom it increases with parity.[22] The prevalence of both bacteriuria and frank UTI increases with age in females and may reach 10% in elderly women. The term *honeymoon cystitis* has been used to describe symptomatic UTI associated with sexual activity in young women.

The clearest evidence linking asymptomatic bacteriuria with the subsequent development of frank UTI is found in pregnant women.[23] Significant bacteriuria occurs in 2 to 6% of pregnant women in the first trimester. Symptomatic UTI, however, usually occurs in the third trimester and is much more common, occurring in 30% of pregnant women known to be bacteriuric. Furthermore, the effective treatment of bacteriuric women during the early part of pregnancy with antimicrobial agents dramatically lowers the incidence of symptomatic UTI by 80 to 90%. It also appears that the risk of premature births is significantly higher in untreated bacteriuric women and in women with intractable, recurrent UTI.[23,24]

In males, bacteriuria and UTI are rarely seen before the age of 50 years, in the absence of congenital defects of instrumentation. Infection in boys is rare, and is more frequently associated with the *Proteus* species, compared to girls who usually have *E. coli*.[25] *Proteus* is readily encountered in the prepucial sac.[10] In older man, prostatic enlargement, or other anatomical abnormalities that lead to instrumentation, favor colonization. Infection tends to persist when a significant residual volume of urine remains in the bladder or diverticuli. Bacteriuria has been reported in 3.5% of men over age 70 and may be as high as 15% in hospitalized elderly men. Adult diabetics tend to have higher rates of bacteriuria and UTI than nondiabetic adults. In the presence of indwelling urinary catheters, virtually all patients develop significant bacteriuria after 72 hr.

NATURAL HISTORY OF BACTERIURIA

Bacteriuria is significantly associated with symptomatic UTI attacks. Sussman, in a study of 107 pregnant women with asymptomatic bacteriuria and 88 matched controls,[26] found that bacteriuric women had a significantly higher incidence of symptomatic UTI. Gillenwater *et al.* performed an extensive study of patients found to have bacteriuria up to 18 years previously.[27] During an 8-yr follow-up, episodes of significant bacteriuria occurred in 70% of 60 bacteriuric patients but in only 39% of 38 controls without previously documented bacteriuria.[10] Hospitalization for acute UTI was required in 10 patients but in only 1 woman in the control group.

The occurrence of renal scars, shrinkage, or progressive deterioration of renal function is extremely rare in bacteriuric patients with structurally normal urinary tracts. Aascher *et al.* performed long-term follow-up of adult bacteriuric women.[28] Though the bacteriuric women developed symptomatic UTI more frequently than their controls, there was no evidence that bacteriuria leads to *de novo* renal scarring or to elevated blood pressure or serum urea nitrogen. Thus, in the absence of preexisting renal damage or renal scars, asymptomatic bacteriuria is a relatively benign condition, complicated from time to time by symptomatic UTI.

The prognosis of bacteriuric patients with structural abnormalities of the genitourinary tract, however, is not always benign. Women with bacteriuria and renal scars have been found to date the onset of symptoms to their early childhood more frequently than bacteriuric women with structurally normal kidneys.[3] It appears that kidneys of growing children are more susceptible to scarring, which results in a distortion of the anatomy during ascending infections.[3,28] It is now clear that bacteriuria that is first detected in childhood is not entirely benign, that it is frequently associated with anatomical abnormalities of the genitourinary

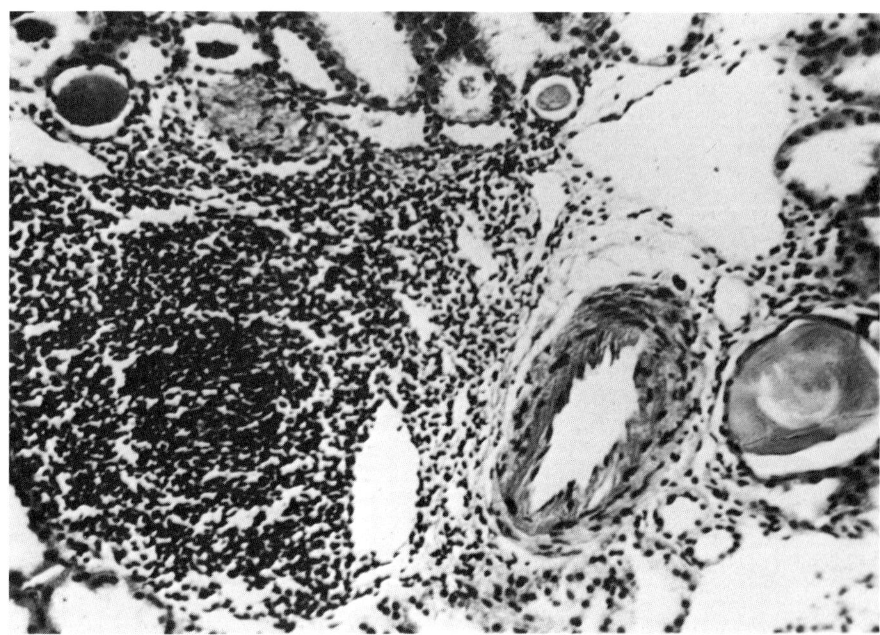

Figure 5-4. A section from a renal biopsy specimen from a patient with a parenchymal renal infection (pyelonephritis), in which a chronic inflammatory exudate (microabscess) is seen (left). There is a necrotic renal tubule at its edge. Around this, are other renal tubules, some with WBC-filled casts (H & E stain).

tract and that it can lead to renal scarring and a significant decrease in renal function.

Several studies have documented the association between bacteriuria and structural renal damage in this age group (Fig.5-4). In a 10-yr study of bacteriuric schoolgirls, Kunin *et al.*[18] showed that not only was symptomatic UTI more common but that 18.9% had vesicouretral reflux and 13% had evidence of renal scars or shrinkage. Similar conclusions have been reached by the Newcastle Asymptomatic Bacteriuria Research Group.[3,11] It is not clear if effective treatment of bacteriuria can prevent or arrest progressive renal damage in children having structural abnormalities. It appears prudent to apply preventive measures during the first five years of life and to correct any abnormalities that could lead to renal damage later in life.

Persistent bacteriuria does not appear to play an important role in the pathophysiology of hypertension, since large-scale epidemiological studies only established an association of borderline statistical significance.[2] Even in paraplegics with long-standing bacteriuria, hypertension is uncommon until end-stage renal failure develops.

Thus, the groups who are at risk for higher morbidity are bacteriuric patients with recurrent or intractable UTI, patients with structural abnormalities of the urinary tract, patients with renal contraction scars, newborns, preschool children, pregnant females, and diabetics. End-stage renal failure, or hypertension, develops rarely, but it is more likely to occur in the presence of functional or anatomical abnormalities that can often be corrected surgically. Since it is not possible to predict the morbid outcomes in individual patients accurately, it seems prudent to eradicate infection by the safest treatment modalities available, while reserving intensive follow-up and invasive corrective measures to high-risk groups.

DETECTION OF BACTERIURIA

Though it is reasonably well established that treatment of bacteriuria in individual patients will reduce morbidity from urinary infections, the cost-effectiveness of a mass population screening program in diminishing morbidity and mortality in each age- and sex-related population at risk is not well established. The logistical and technical problems inherent in mass screening are serious, with collection and processing of samples under exact prescribed conditions, data analysis, follow-up, and record keeping, etc., and it is not clear that the expense involved in such screening of the entire population would be justified by the expected return. For these reasons, certain priorities are generally set in order to maximize the benefits; these are accrued by focusing on high-risk groups in situations in which mass screening is practical and high standards of follow-up and care are assured.

Routine screening of the newborn for bacteriuria is not generally recommended except of those infants who fail to thrive or who are febrile and septic. Abbott *et al.*[29] have pointed to the relatively high frequency of major anatomical abnormalities in neonates having significant bacteriuria. Though a negative culture or a low bacterial count in a clean voided specimen or one collected with a strap-on device can be considered to be evidence against UTI, a positive quantitative culture should be repeated. Samples obtained by suprapubic puncture techniques are most dependable.

Screening, however, is recommended as part of the routine evaluation of preschool children, since the literature clearly indicates that symptomatic UTI is frequent at this age, especially in girls, and since UTI at this age is often associated with correctable urinary tract abnormalities. Since preschoolers are available only to the pediatrician in large numbers, the physician's office constitutes the only practical setting for such screening. Dip slides and nitrite test strips provided to the mother have also been used effectively. Because of the problems inherent in collecting urine from young children, repeated cultures are strongly recommended for those children who test positive initially. For school-age children, it has been shown that mass screening of girls can be conducted cost-effectively with relative ease, but the yield in boys is too low to include them in mass screening. The emphasis should be placed on young children during the first three years of school so that urological abnormalities can be detected and corrected early. It is most economical to test new girls entering school and retest them a year later; thus, all the first- and second-graders are screened each year. It must be pointed out that it is essential to combine screening with the availability of well-motivated pediatricians, urologists, and field personnel with the "ability to provide high standard of urological diagnosis and care." If such back-up is not assured, no mass screening program should be performed. In the light of Gillenwater's data,[27] it is crucial to follow children who prove positive and to alert their parents as to the possibilities of future morbidity before sexual activity and/or marriage or pregnancy.

All pregnant women should be screened for bacteriuria on their initial visit and periodically thereafter. Catheterization before delivery should be avoided if possible. Appropriate antibiotics should be prescribed to suppress or eradicate bacteriuria or UTI. Pregnant women are among the groups at highest risk. Adult diabetics, patients known to have structural lesions of the genitourinary tract, elderly subjects with bladder neck or prostatic problems, hospitalized or other patients with indwelling catheters or in need of frequent instrumentation are other high-risk populations. The urinary tract is one of the most common primary sources of contamination in patients presenting with gram-negative septicemia and shock, a condition with a high mortality rate.

MANAGEMENT OF SYMPTOMATIC URINARY TRACT INFECTIONS

In symptomatic UTI, the goals are to prevent (or treat) systemic sepsis, eradicate sequestered infection, reduce long-term sequelae, and relieve symptoms. Superficial mucosal infections (bladder or urethra) can easily be cured by delivery of effective concentrations of antibiotics in urine only. For treatment of infection in deeper tissue (kidney or prostate), however, effective serum concentrations of antibiotics are necessary.

All bacterial UTIs have been traditionally treated with one to two weeks of antimicrobial therapy, administered two to four times daily, in divided doses. Such treatment in women and children has been associated with a 10 to 20% failure rate, poor compliance, and a high incidence of side effects. In adult males, relapse rates close to 50% have been reported.[30,31] Most relapsing infections with the same organism occur in patients with prostatic or renal tissue invasion, whereas infection with new strains or organisms usually occurs in superficial mucosal infections of the bladder. These facts have led many to believe that conventional therapy is inadequate for patients with renal or prostatic tissue infections and is unnecessary for superficial bladder or other mucosal infections. This has led to the development of single-dose antimicrobial therapy.

For symptomatic bacteriuria in adult women, the following treatment plan is suggested (Table 5-3). For the first diagnosed episode of cystitis (colony count usually greater than 10^5/ml) or urethral syndrome (colony count often around 10^3 to 10^4/ml), single-dose treatment offers easier patient compliance and fewer side effects and is cost-effective.[32] In addition, a single-dose treatment is less apt to alter the perineal flora, whereas extended courses of antibiotics often foster the overgrowth of drug-resistant organisms. Two to three double-strength tablets of trimethoprim–sulfamethoxazole (Bactrim, Septra) can be used. Alternatives are 2 to 3 g amoxicillin or 1 to 2 g of Gantrisin orally. Cure rates of 87 to 94% have been reported with single-dose therapy. Nearly all patients in whom bacteriuria recurs experience symptoms within a few days of the cessation of therapy. This suggests the existence of infection in the upper urinary tract. A 10-day

Table 5-3
Treatment Plan for Cystitis or Urethral Syndrome

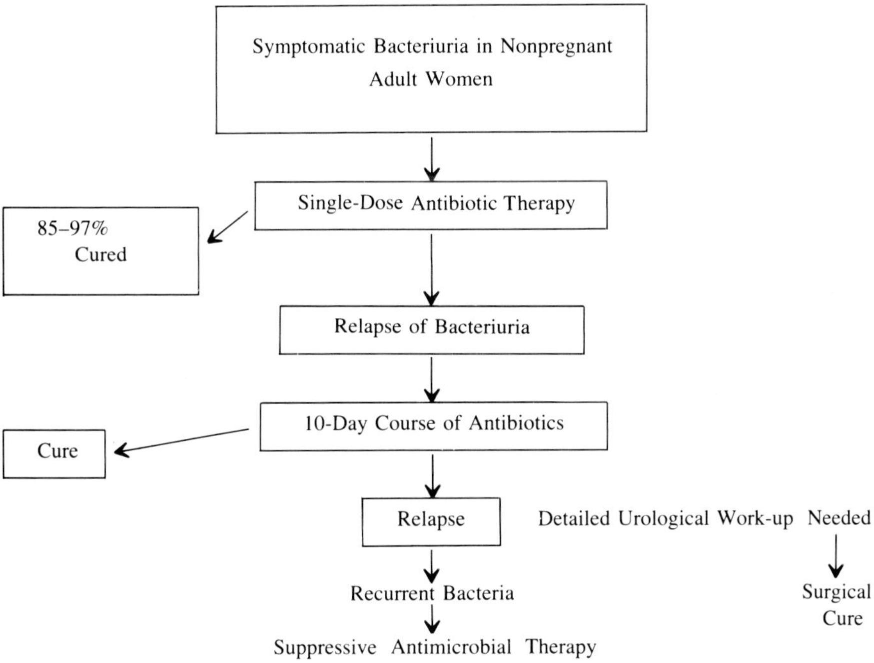

Symptomatic Bacteriuria in Nonpregnant Adult Women

↓

Single-Dose Antibiotic Therapy → 85–97% Cured

↓

Relapse of Bacteriuria

↓

10-Day Course of Antibiotics → Cure

↓

Relapse   Detailed Urological Work-up Needed

↓   ↓

Recurrent Bacteria   Surgical Cure

↓

Suppressive Antimicrobial Therapy

course of antibiotics is then suggested. This includes one of three choices: double-strength tablets of Bactrim or Septra, bid; 1 g of amoxicillin orally; or 1 g of Gantrisin orally bid. If symptoms recur after this second course of treatment, a detailed urological investigation is recommended.[33]

Patients with recurrent bacteriuria should be given chronic suppressive antimicrobial therapy.[34] Most such relapsing infections in women are the result of upper urinary tract foci; in older men, obstructive lower urinary tract problems are usually responsible. One-half of a single-strength tablet of trimethoprim–sulfamethoxazole at bedtime every night is recommended as suppressive therapy. For patients who cannot tolerate this treatment, low-dose nitrofurantoin (Macrodantin), 50 mg orally daily is effective. Patients treated with nitrofurantoin should be watched for the development of side effects, especially hepatitis and neuritis.

It is generally agreed that asymptomatic bacteriuria in pregnant women merits aggressive antimicrobial therapy. Random screening urine cultures should be obtained throughout pregnancy. If a culture is positive, a one- to two-week course with a nontoxic agent (ampicillin, cephalexin, or amoxicillin) should be instituted. Tetracycline should be generally avoided throughout pregnancy. Because of the risks of kernicterus, sulfonamides must be avoided in the last trimester of pregnancy. Preliminary evidence suggests single-dose therapy may also be effective in asymptomatic bacteriuria during that pregnancy, but until more evidence validates this approach, it is not recommended.[35] Similar management considerations apply to children.

Treatment of asymptomatic bacteriuria in nonpregnant women is somewhat controversial. The majority of clinicians prefer not to treat, since the evidence for long-term ill effects in this population is minimal and the condition itself is not associated with severe morbidity. It is, however, not unreasonable to make one attempt to eradicate such an asymptomatic bacteriuria with short-term, oral, nontoxic antibiotic therapy. Aggressive treatment with potentially toxic antibiotics is not indicated.

In urinary catheter-associated bacteriuria, the infections are ascending, originating from the site of junction of the urethral meatus and the catheter. Systemic antimicrobial agents have limited usefulness when indwelling catheters are in place longer than a few days to one week. In the absence of systemic sepsis, prophylactic antibiotic therapy in situations when indwelling catheters stay in for longer periods not only does not reduce incidence of infections but also favors selection of resistant organisms. Whenever indwelling catheters are in place for more than three days, a urine culture should be done upon withdrawal of the catheter. If the patient has normal lower urinary tract anatomy and function, the bacteriuria will usually clear spontaneously. If the initial culture is positive, it should be repeated two weeks later. If this second culture is positive, an appropriate antimicrobial agent should be selected, based on sensitivity results, and a 10-day course be given, followed by culture at day 14. Recurrence of bacteriuria indicates the need for a detailed urological investigation.

When systemic signs of sepsis develop in a situation in which indwelling catheterization is essential, aggressive therapy with antibiotic(s) chosen on the basis of culture sensitivity data is indicated.

CASE SUMMARY

Patient No. 1, L.S., a 67-year-old white female, was referred for evaluation of acute myelocytic leukemia. She was admitted on March 6, 1985, and was in her usual state of health until December 30, 1985, when she presented to a local physician with fever, shortness of breath, and weakness. She had a history of being treated chronically with Septra for urinary tract infection.

A urine culture on March 10, 1986, showed a count of over 100,000 *Enterobacter*. A urinalysis showed a few clumps of WBC and gram-negative rods upon gram staining. A urinary sediment from this patient was fixed for TEM analysis (Fig. 5-5 and 5-6).

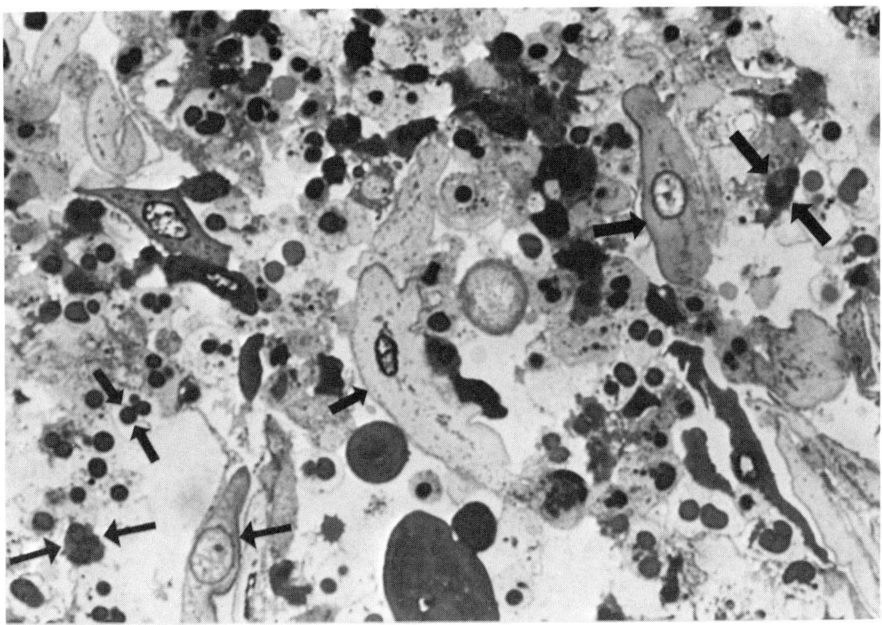

Figure 5-5.   This light micrograph of a semithin section of patient No. 1 shows polymorphonuclear leukocytes (PMN) (between two arrowheads) and squamous epithelial cells (single arrows) (epoxy tissue stain, ×400).

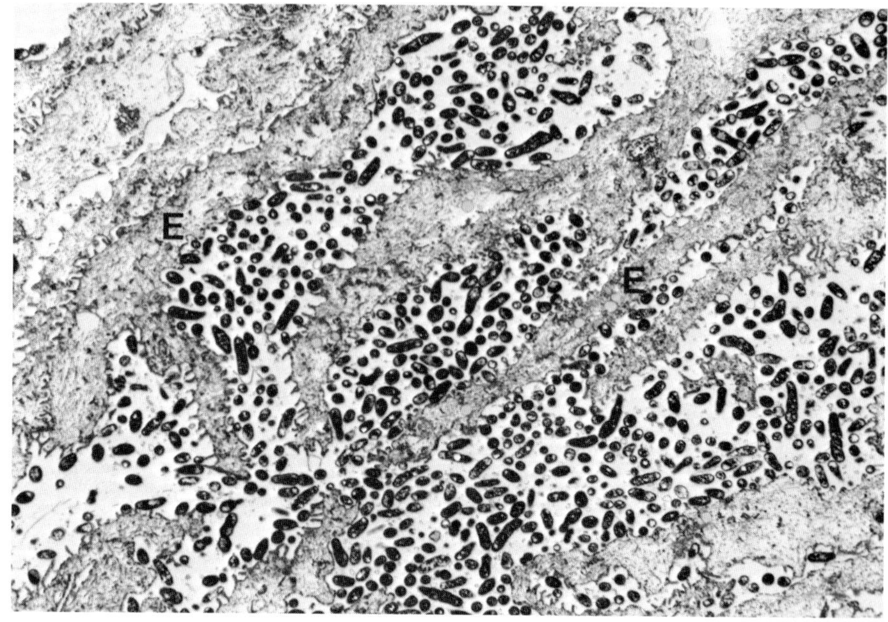

Figure 5-6.   Abundant numbers of bacteria can be seen adhering to the transitional epithelial cells (E) in this electron micrograph (epoxy tissue stain, ×2,500).

Acknowledgment: This work was supported by designated grants of the U.S. Veterans Administration. Figures 5-1–5-4 were reprinted with permission of Medcom, Incorporated (copyright 1969) from material of Dr. George E. Schreiner, M.D. We thank Dr. A. K. Mandal for Figs. 5-5 and 5-6.

REFERENCES

1. Kass EH: Asymptomatic infections of the urinary tract. *Trans Amer Assoc Physicians* 1956; 69:56–64.
2. Kass EH, Savage W, Santamarina BA: The significance of bacteriuria in preventive medicine, in Kass EH (ed): *Progress in Byelonephritis,* Philadelphia, FA Davis, 1965, pp 3–10.
3. Aascher AW, Chick S, Radford N, Waters WE, Sussman M, Evans J, McLachlan M, Williams J: Natural history of asymptomatic bacteriuria in non-pregnant women, in Brumfitt W, Aascher AW (ed): *Urinary Tract Infection.* London, Oxford University Press, pp 52–61.
4. Aascher AW, Sussman M, Waters WE, Chick S: Urine as a medium for bacterial growth. *Lancet* 1966; 2:1037–1041.
5. Lampert I, Berlyne GM: Bacterial excretion rates in the diagnosis of urinary tract infections. *Lancet* 1971; 1:51–52.

6. Dontas AS, Kasviki-Charvati P: Significance of diuresis provoked bacteriuria. *J Infec Dis* 1976; 134:174–180.

7. O'Doherty N: Urinary tract infection in the neonatal period and later infancy, In O'Grady F, Brumfitt W (ed): *Urinary tract infection*, London, Oxford University Press, 1968; pp 113–121.

8. Bailey RR, Little PJ: Suprapubic bladder aspiration in diagnosis of urinary tract infection. *Brit Med J* 1969; 1:293–294.

9. Cohen S, Kass EH: A simple method for quantitative urine culture. *N Engl J Med* 1967; 277:176–180.

10. Kunin CM: Principles of urinary bacteriology and Immunology, in Kunin CM (ed): Detection, Prevention and Management of Urinary Tract Infections, Philadelphia, Lea and Febiger, 1979, pp 91–152.

11. Sussman M, Aascher AW: Watters, WE, Evans J, Campbell H, Evans K, Williams J: Asymptomatic significant bacteriuria in non-pregnant women - 1. Description of the population, *Brit Med J* 1969; 1:799–803.

12. Kunin CM, Deutscher R, Paquin A: Urinary tract infection in school children: An epidemiologic, clinical and laboratory study. *Medicine* 1964; 43:91–130.

13. Kunin CM: Asymptomatic bacteriuria. *Annu Rev Med* 1966; 17:383–406.

14. Gruneberg RN, Leigh D, Brumfitt W: *E. Coli* serotypes in urinary tract infections, In O'Grady F, Brumfitt W (eds): London, Oxford University Press, pp 68–79.

15. Roberts AP: Micrococcaceae from the urinary tract in pregnancy. *J Clin Path* 1967; 20:631–632.

16. Edelman CM, Jr, Ogwo J, Fine BP: The prevalence of bacteriuria in full term and premature newborn infants. *J Pediatr* 1973; 82:125–132.

17. Randolph MF, Morris KE, Gould EB: The first urinary tract infection in the female infant. *J Pediatr* 1975; 86:342–348.

18. Kunin CM: A ten-year study of bacteriuria in school girls; Final report of bacteriologic, urologic and epidemiologic findings. *J Infec Dis* 1970; 122:362–393.

19. Kunin CM: Epidemiology of bacteriuria and it's relation to pyelonephritis. *J Infec Dis* 1969; 120:1–9.

20. Lindberg U, Claesson I, Hanson LA: Asymptomatic bacteriuria in schoolgirls: I. Clinical and laboratory findings. *Acta Pediatr Scand* 1975; 64:425–431.

21. Kunin CM: McCormack RC: An epidemiologic study of bacteriuria and blood pressure among nuns and working women. *N Engl J Med* 1968; 278:635–642.

22. Kunin CM, Southall I, Paquin A: Epidemiology of urinary tract infections. *N Engl J Med* 1960; 263:817–823.

23. Gruneberg, RN, Leigh DA, Brumfitt W: Relationship of bacteriuria or pregnancy to acute pyelonephritis, prematurity and faetal mortality. *Lancet* 1969; 1:1–3.

24. Bryant RE, Windorn RE, Vineyard, Jr. JP: Asymptomatic bacteriuria of pregnancy and it's relation to prematurity. *J Lab Clin Med* 1964, 63:224–231.

25. Silverberg DS: City wide screening for urinary abnormalities in schoolboys. *Can Med Assoc J* 1974; 111:410–412.

26. Sussman M, Aascher AW, Waters WE, Evans JAS, Campbell H, Evans KT, Williams JE: Asymptomatic significant bacteriuria in the nonpregnant woman. I. Description of the population. *Brit Med J* 1969; 1:799–803.

27. Gillenwater JY: Diagnosis of urinary tract infections: Appraisal of diagnostic procedures. *Kidney Int* 1975; (suppl 4):53–54.

28. Aascher AM, Sussman M, Waters WE, Evans JA, Campbell H, Evans KT, Williams, JE: Asymptomatic significant bacteriuria in the nonpregnant woman II. Response to treatment and follow up. *Brit Med J* 1969; 1:804–806.

29. Abbott GD: Neonatal bacteriuria: A prospective study in 1460 infants. *Brit Med J* 1972; 1:267–269.

30. Turck M, Anderson KN, Petersdorf RG: Relapse and reinfection in chronic bacteriuria. *N Engl J Med* 1966; 275:70–74.

31. Fang LST, Tolkoff-Rubin NE, Rubin RH: Efficacy of single dose and conventional anoxicillin therapy in urinary tract infection localized by the antibody-coated bacteria technique. *N Engl J Med* 1979; 298:413–416.

32. Stamm WE: Prevention of urinary tract infections. *Am J Med* 1984; 76:148–153.

33. Schultz HJ, MacCaffery LA, Keys TF, Nobrega FT: Acute cystitis; a prospective study of laboratory tests and duration of therapy. *Mayo Clin Proc* 1984; 59:391–397.

34. Stamey TA, Condy M, Mihara G: Prophylatic efficacy of nitrofurantoin and trimethoprim–sulphasoxazole in urinary infections. *N Engl J Med* 1977; 296:780–783.

35. Bailey RR: Single dose therapy of bacteriuria of pregnancy, in Bailey RR (ed): *Single dose therapy of urinary tract infections*. Sydney, Australia, Aids–Health Science Press, 1983, page 73.

36. Newcastle Asymptomatic Bacteriuria Research Group: Asymptomatic bacteriuria in school children in Newcastle-upon-Tyne. *Arch Dis Childhood* 1975; 50:90–102.

6

Renal Transplant Rejection

Many patterns of allograft function may be seen after renal transplantation. These range from no function to immediate function. Oliguria in the early posttransplant period may be the result of hypovolemia, mechanical obstruction to urine flow, urinary leakage, decreased blood flow (renal artery or renal vein thrombosis) to the allograft, acute tubular necrosis (ATN), or graft rejection. In transplant recipients, a diagnosis of ATN is made by the exclusion of other causes of oliguria; it may be extremely difficult, however, to distinguish ATN from acute rejection. Laboratory tests such as urinary sodium and radioisotope renal scan are helpful but are not specific for either condition. Hitherto, renal biopsy has remained the only viable method to of distinguishing between rejection and ATN.

Recently, we have shown that transmission electron microscopy (TEM) of urinary sediment can be used to obtain information about the morphological changes in the kidneys of patients with ATN. We have demonstrated that TEM urinary sediment study can indicate the severity of renal changes in patients with ATN[1] and is capable of differentiating ATN from aminoglycoside-induced acute renal failure (ARF).[2]

Data on TEM studies of urinary sediments from several renal transplant patients follow. The method of urine collection sample processing, and the study techniques are the same as described in earlier chapters. Our observations have shown that urinary sediment TEM can lead to a reliable diagnosis of rejection without renal biopsy. This technique is especially useful, given the frequent administration of cyclosporine, which is often nephrotoxic. Furthermore, it is often difficult to distinguish cyclosporine nephrotoxicity from allograft rejection.[3] Herewith are clinical profiles and urinary sediment studies of several patients.

141

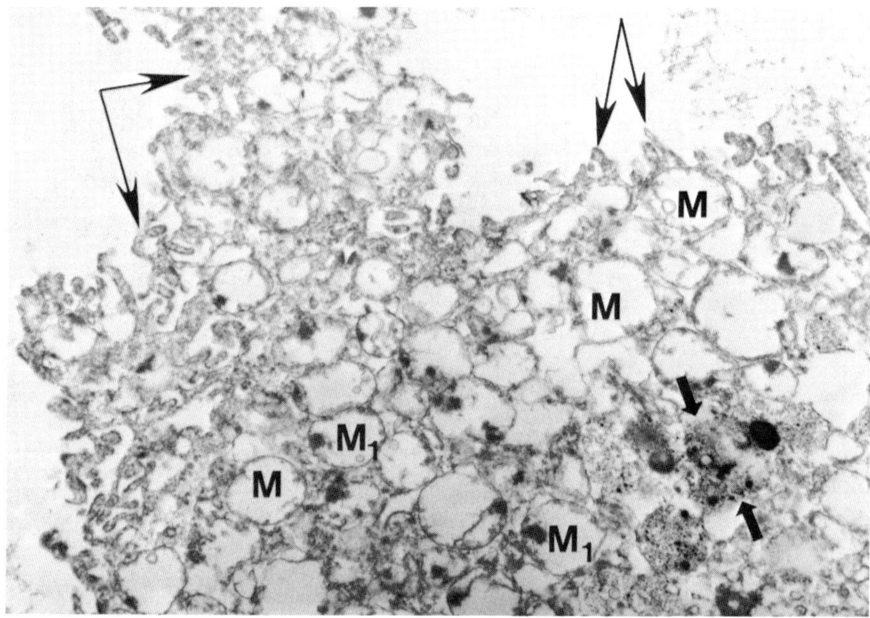

Figure 6-1.   A proximal tubule cell is characterized by remnants of microvilli (arrows) and many mitochondria (M), which are swollen and devoid of cristae, though some mitochondria (M$_1$) contain amorphous dark bodies. An occasional lysosome (between arrows) is shown (patient No. 1) (UA + LC, ×6,000). From *Seminars in Nephrology,* Vol. 6, 1986, with permission.

Patient No. 1, C. B., a 23-yr-old black male, received a kidney donated by a relative at the Medical College of Georgia Hospital, Augusta, Georgia, on March 28, 1984. The grafted kidney functioned well until May 8, 1984, when the patient was readmitted for evaluation of deteriorating renal function. His admission serum creatinine was 3.7 mg/dl, though urine volume was normal. A sample of urine was collected for TEM analysis. The patient was treated with cyclosporine, but his renal function continued to deteriorate rapidly. His serum creatinine was 12.9 mg/dl on May 29, 1984, when hemodialysis was started. Hemodialysis was continued until his death, August 18, 1985.

The TEM analysis of urinary sediment showed necrotic proximal and collecting tubule cells (Figs. 6-1 and 6-2), an epithelial cast (Fig. 6-3), abundant fibrin in the peritubular capillary (Fig. 6-4), and acute and chronic inflammatory cells (Figs. 6-5 and 6-6a).

Comments: The TEM findings demonstrated both necrotic tubule cells and fibrin and inflammatory cells that suggested acute cellular and humoral rejection.

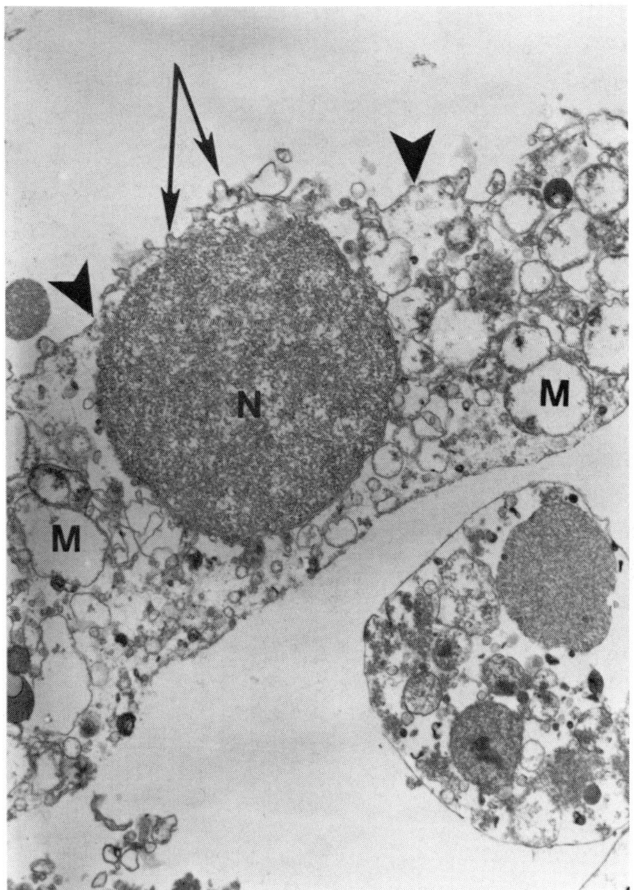

Figure 6-2.   In this micrograph, a collecting tubule cell is characterized by the cuboidal shape of the cell; the position of the nucleus (N), toward the apex of the cell; a few rudimentary microvilli (arrows); and sparse mitochondria (M). The nuclear chromatin material is condensed. There are fewer mitochondria (M), which are swollen and devoid of cristae; and the luminal membrane (arrowheads) is intact (UA + LC, ×5,000). From *Seminars in Nephrology,* Vol. 6, 1986, with permission.

These findings were confirmed by renal biopsy that showed acute cellular rejection (Fig. 6-6b).

Patient No. 2, E. L., a 42-yr-old black male, received a kidney donated by a relative at the Medical College of Georgia Hospital on February 22, 1984. A sample of urine

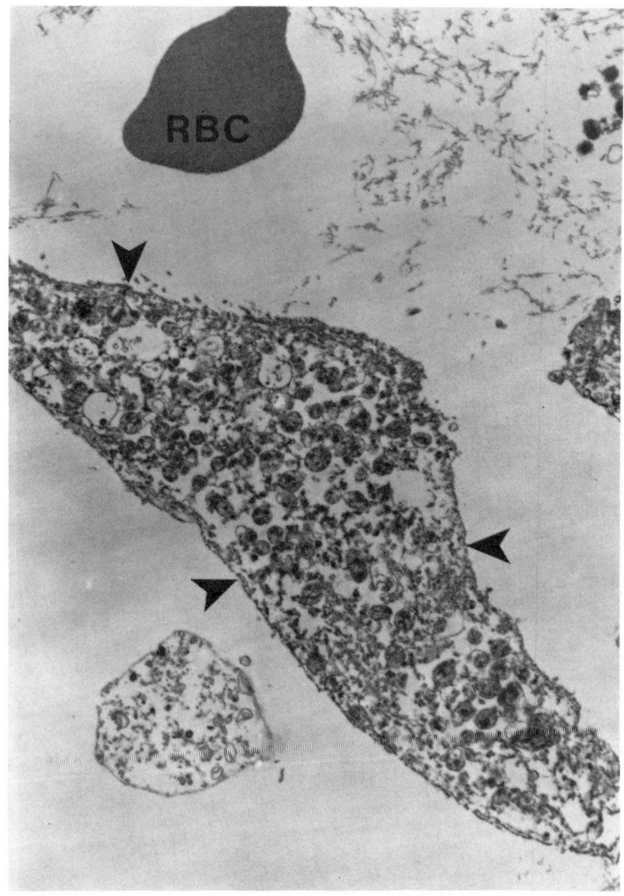

Figure 6-3. In this epithelial cast, the mitochondria appear intact. The cellular membranes (arrowheads) are preserved, and a red blood cell (RBC) is shown (UA + LC, ×3,300).

was collected immediately after the transplant for TEM analysis. During a routine visit to the transplant clinic on March 23, 1984, the patient's serum creatinine was found to be 2.5 mg/dl; hence, he was admitted for evaluation and treatment. Clinically rejection of the grafted kidney was suspected. He was treated with pulse therapy of methylprednisolone, but his renal function rapidly deteriorated. The following table shows this patient's serial serum urea nitrogen (SUN), serum creatinine (Scr), urine output, and the immunosuppressive drugs given.

Date (1984)	SUN (mg/dl)	SCr (mg/dl)	Urine output (ml/day)	Immunosuppressive therapy
March 23	60	2.4	Not available	Azathioprine, prednisone
March 29	33	2.5	Not available	Cyclosporine
April 1	47	3.6		Azathioprine discontinued
April 7	90	8.2		
April 15	57	10.2	300	
April 24	50	13.0	400	
May 9	49	15.4		

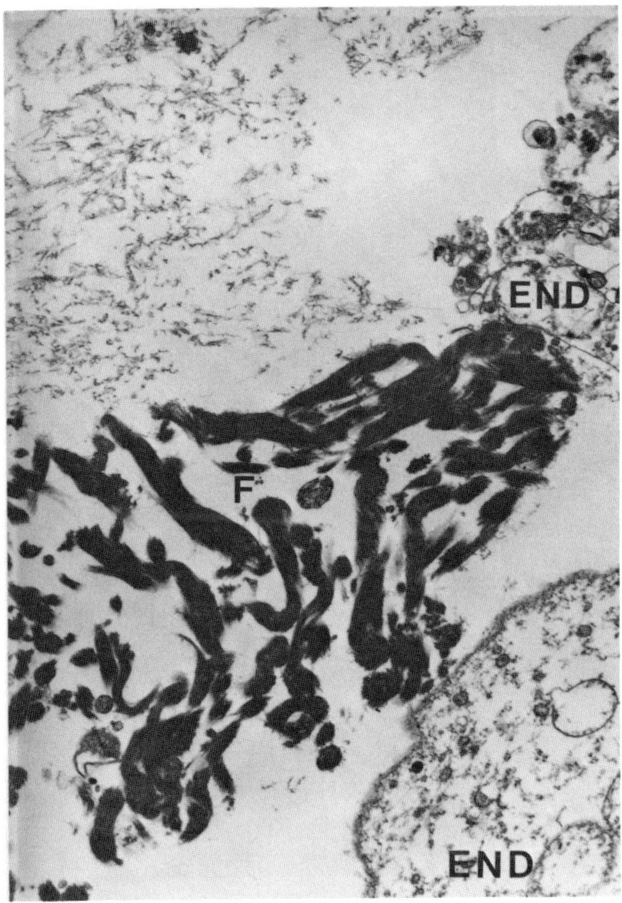

Figure 6-4.   A large amount of fibrin (F) is shown in the lumen of the peritubular capillary. The endothelial cells (END) appear to be necrotic (UA + LC, ×6,600). From *Seminars in Nephrology,* Vol. 6, 1986, with permission.

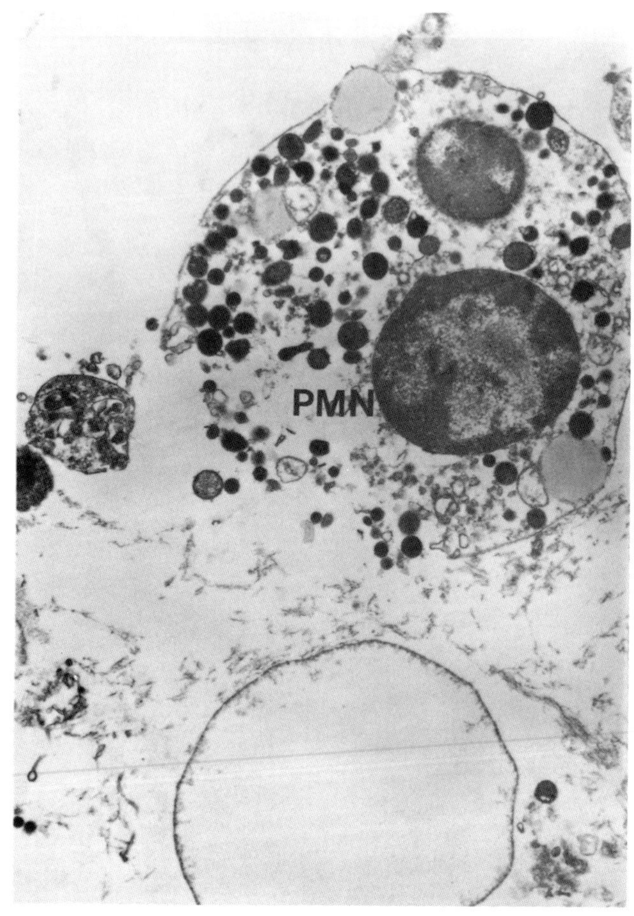

Figure 6-5.   A neutrophilic leukocyte (PMN), possibly within the peritubular capillary, is seen (UA + LC, ×5,000).

The patient was discharged from the Medical College of Georgia Hospital on May 9, 1984, to begin hemodialysis treatment in another facility three times a week. He also had hypertension, which was treated with propanolol and hydralazine.

The TEM analysis of urinary sediment showed many tubule epithelial cells, but their origin could not be determined, though they appeared to be proximal tubule cells (Figs. 6-7 and 6-8). Inflammatory cells, fibrin, and fibroblasts were seen in the interstitium (Figs. 6-9 and 6-10). Tubule cells were necrotic, with swollen mitochondria and amorphous dark bodies and loss or condensation of nuclear chromatin.

Comments: The urinary sediment findings were consistent with transplant rejection, which was supported by the serum creatinine level of 1.9 mg/dl on March 16, 1984. The grafted kidney had never functioned normally. A month after transplantation, the patient's renal function had irreversibly deteriorated. Thus, it can be concluded that the results of the urinary sediment TEM predicted rejection and renal function deterioration.

Patient No. 3, D. C., a 35-yr-old black male, received a cadaveric renal transplantation on February 28, 1984, at the Medical College of Georgia Hospital. A urine sample

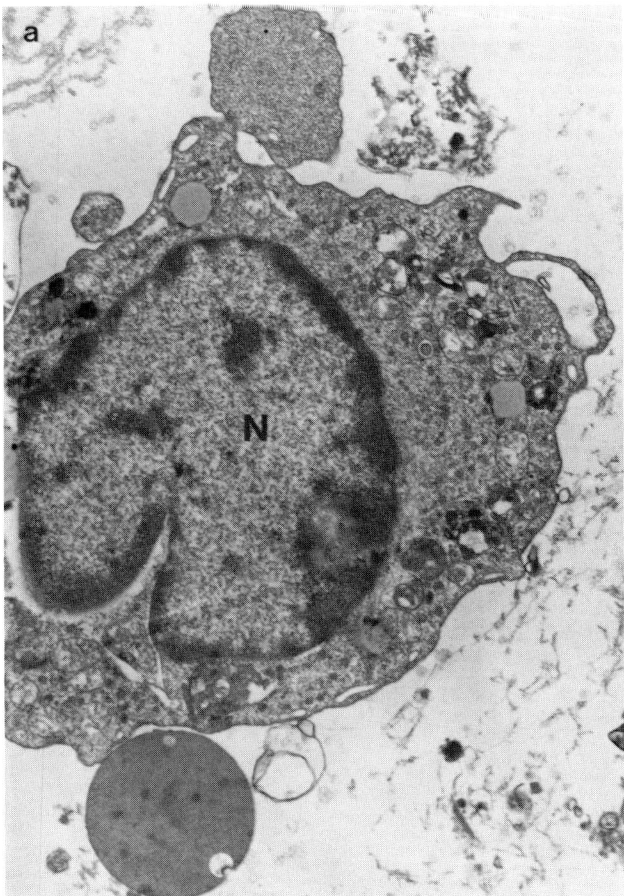

Figure 6-6a. A monocyte, characterized by a notched nucleus (N), can be seen (UA + LC, ×5,000). From *Seminars in Nephrology*, Vol. 6, 1986, with permission.

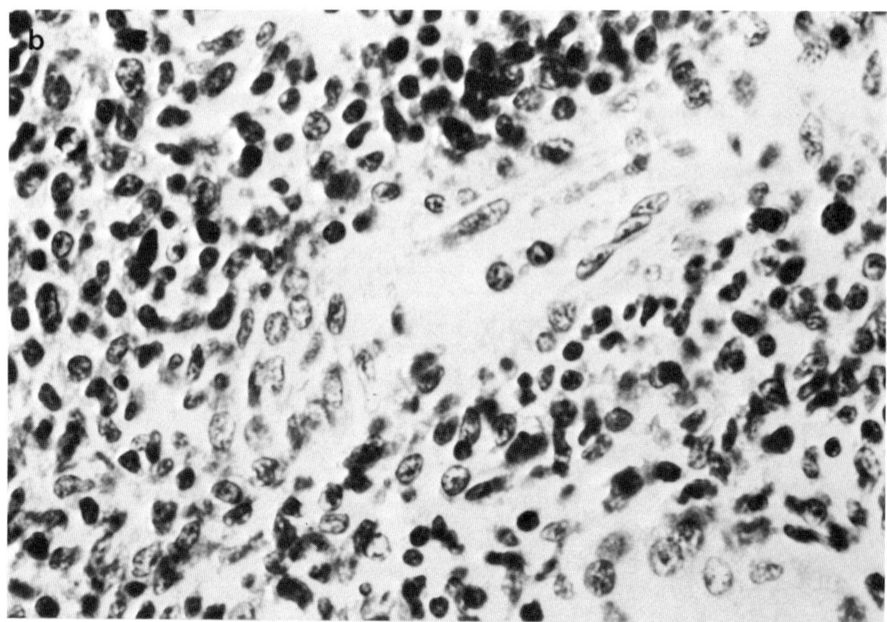

Figure 6-6b.   A light micrograph of a section from a renal biopsy shows mononuclear cellular infiltration (H & E, ×80).

was collected for TEM analysis two weeks posttransplant. The grafted kidney did not function well, and he was treated with cyclosporine, prednisone, and hemodialysis. He was discharged from the hospital on March 17, 1984. His serum creatinine on the day of discharge was 5.8 mg/dl. He was readmitted April 26, 1984, with a complaint of polyuria, his serum creatinine was 2.7 mg/dl and his serum glucose, 584 mg/dl, so treatment with NPH insulin was initiated. His urine output of 5 liters/24 hr decreased to 2,350 ml/24 hr with insulin treatment. He continued to receive cyclosporine and prednisone at reduced dosages.

The TEM study of urinary sediment showed a variety of epithelial cell casts and numerous red blood cells (RBC) (Fig. 6-11 a,b,c). Few necrotic tubule cells and no fibrin or platelet aggregates were found.

Comments: The TEM findings were consistent with ATN, but renal function recovery was considered likely, as confirmed by a slow but continuous improvement.

Patient No. 4, L. H., a 30-yr-old white female, had received a kidney donated by a relative at the Medical College of Georgia Hospital on March 21, 1984. She later developed features of graft rejection and infection and was readmitted to the Medical

College of Georgia Hospital on May 13, 1984, at which time a urine sample was collected for TEM analysis. She was found to have *Pneumocystis carinii* pneumonia. Immunosuppressive drugs included cyclosporine, azathioprine, and antilymphocytic serum. Her admission serum urea nitrogen and serum creatinine were 33 mg/dl and 1.9 mg/dl, respectively. Her renal function rapidly deteriorated; on the 11th hospital day her serum urea nitrogen and serum creatinine were 75 mg/dl and 3.7 mg/dl, respectively. She died on May 24, 1984 from severe hypoxemia, acidosis, and hyperpyrexia.

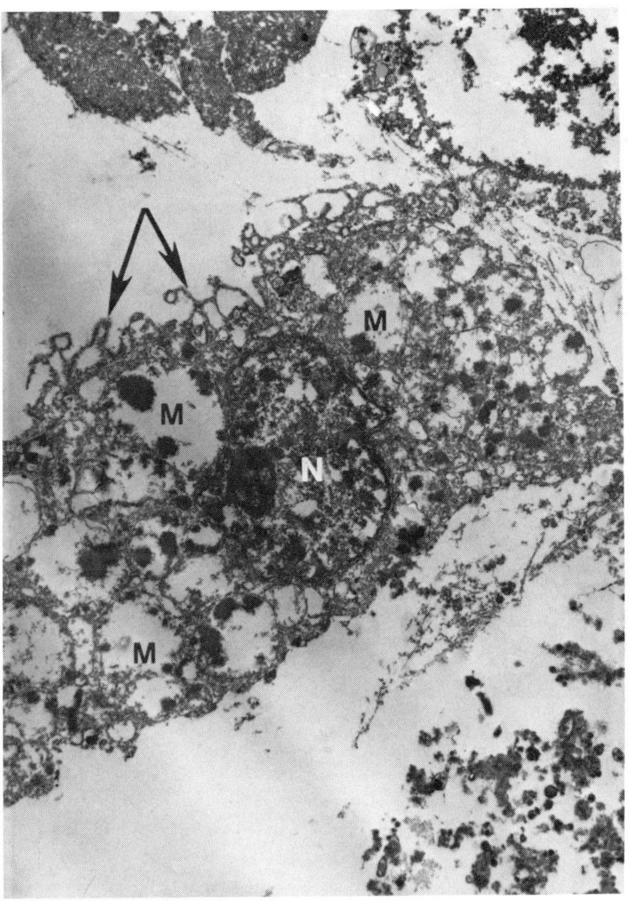

Figure 6-7.   This transmission electron micrograph shows a proximal tubule cell characterized by many mitochondria (M) and remnants of microvill (arrows). The mitochondria are swollen and devoid of cristae; most of them contain amorphous dark bodies (a sign of ischemia). The nucleus (N), though it distinguishes between proximal and distal tubules by its location, often becomes displaced in a necrotic cell and loses this distinguishing feature (UA + LC, ×3,300).

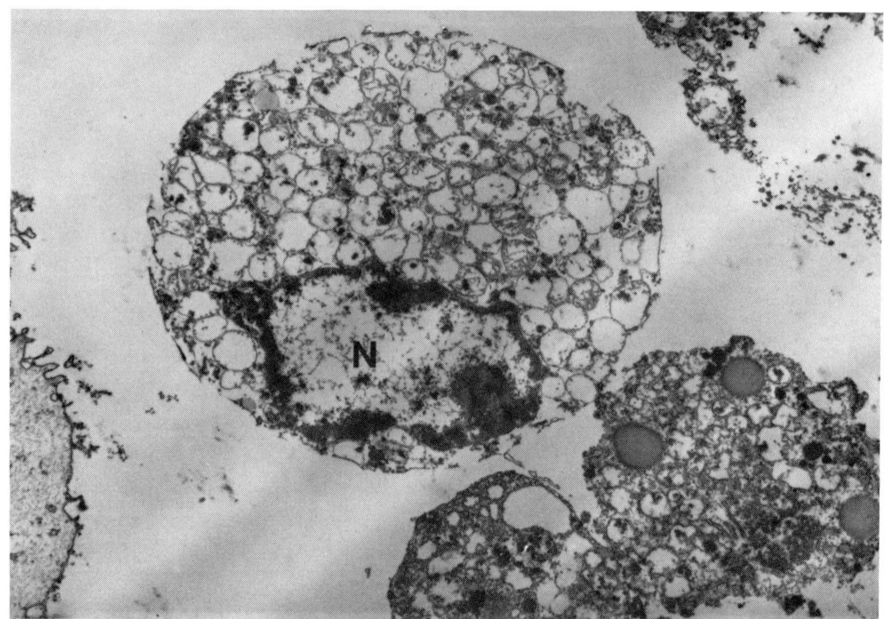

Figure 6-8.   A cross section of a proximal tubule cell shows a large nucleus (N) and numerous mitochondria. There is nuclear condensation of chromatin and all the mitochondria are swollen and devoid of cristae (UA + LC, ×2,600).

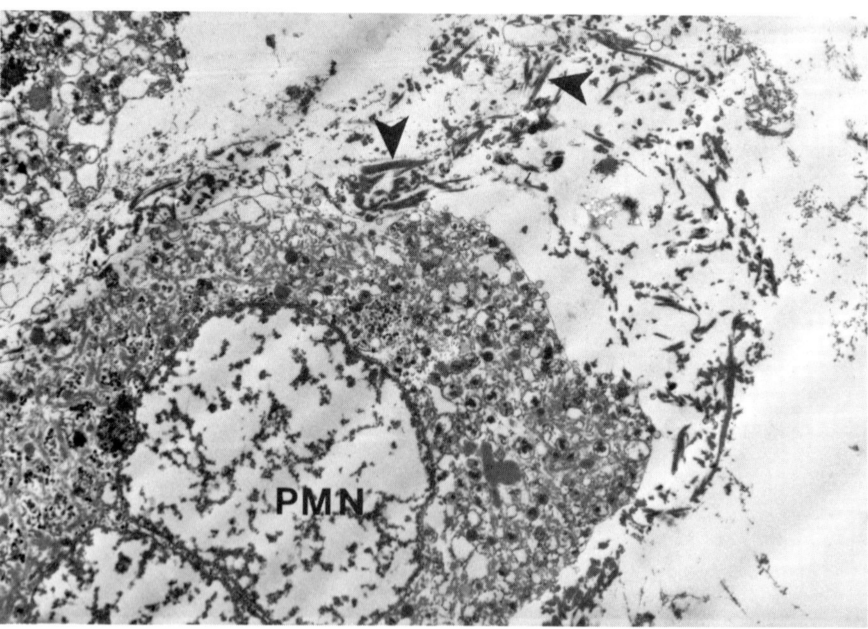

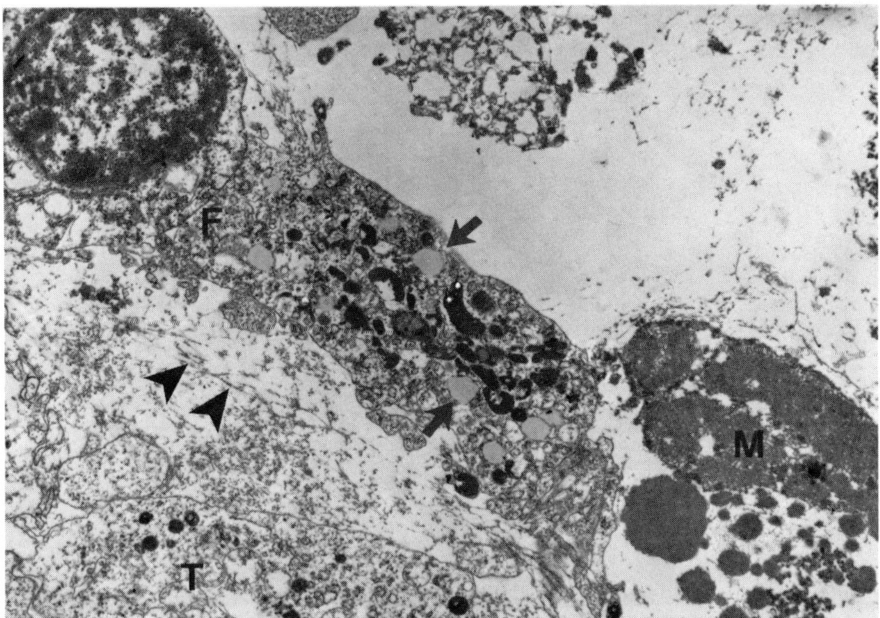

Figure 6-10.   A free fibroblast (F), characterized by a cytoplasmic extension and many lipid droplets (arrows), is seen. There are many collagen fibers (arrowheads), a portion of a tubule cell (T), and a mast cell (M) are seen in the interstitium (UA + LC, ×3,300).

The TEM analysis showed many tubule epithelial cells. The origin of the cells could not be determined, though they appeared to be from proximal tubules. There was marked swelling of the mitochondria with loss of cristae but no dark bodies. Nuclei showed condensation of chromatin material, but the membranes were intact. A large amount of collagen fibers was found (Fig. 6-12), but no fibrin or inflammatory cells.

Comments: The urinary sediment findings were consistent with ATN, which was confirmed clinically by renal function deterioration.

Patient No. 5, R. B., 24-yr-old black male, received a cadaveric renal transplant at the Medical College of Georgia Hospital on January 22, 1984. The graft was functioning well and the patient's serum creatinine was 2.7 mg/dl at the time of discharge. A sample

Figure 6-9.   A neutrophilic leukocyte (PMN) and interstitial infiltration by fibrin (arrowheads) can be seen (UA + LC, ×2,600).

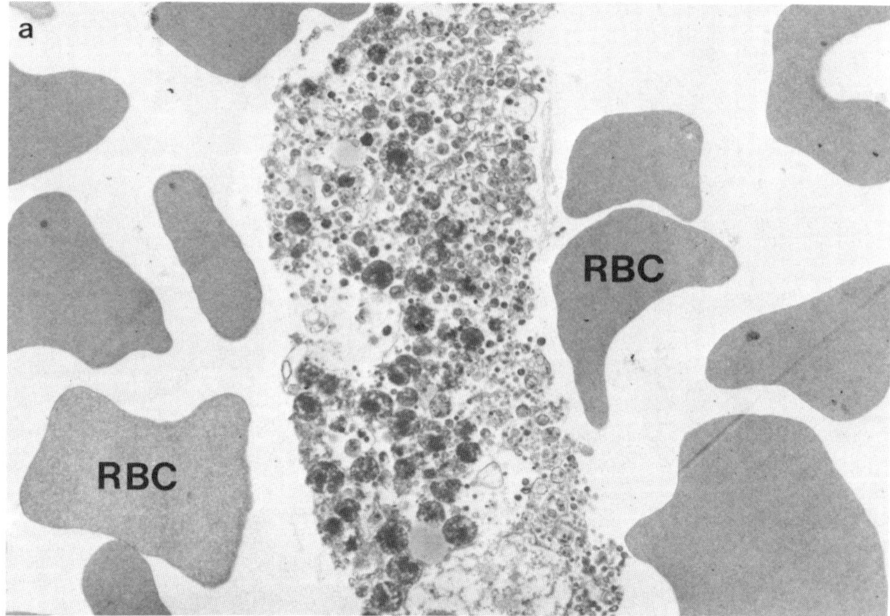

Figure 6-11a.   An epithelial cell cast, consisting of degenerated mitochondria and cellular fragments, is seen. Numerous red blood cells (RBC) are also seen (UA + LC, ×2,600).

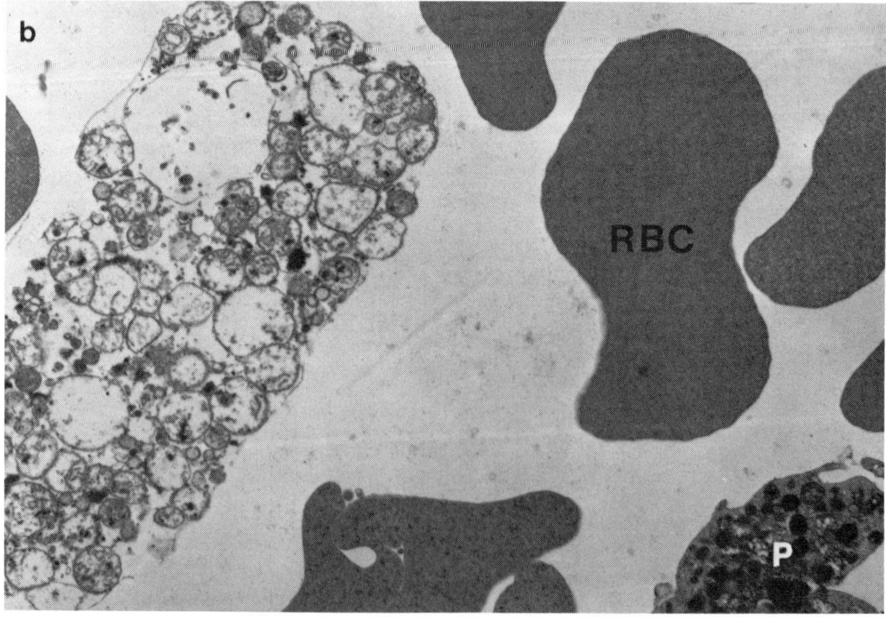

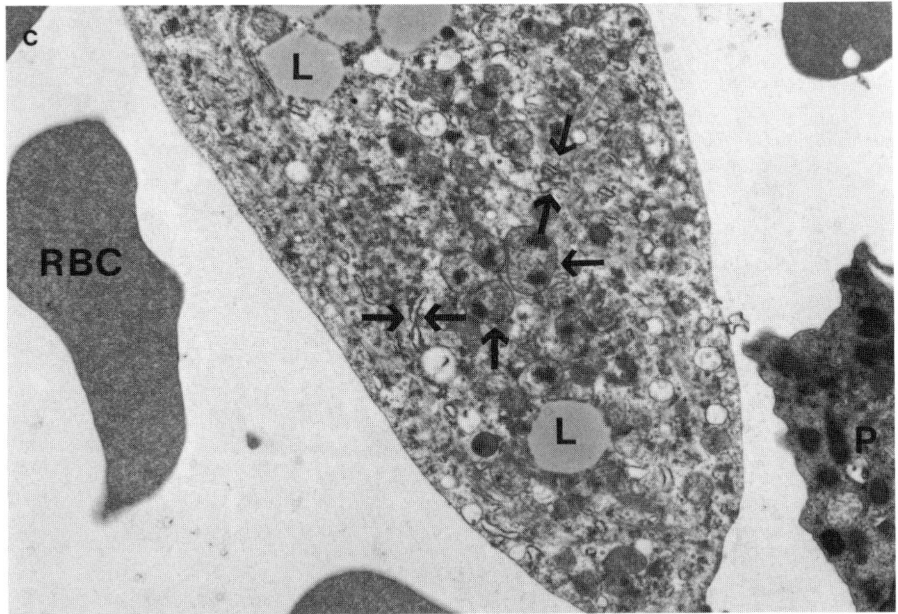

Figure 6-11c. An epithelial cell, in the form of a cast, contains lipid droplets (L), many mitochondria with amorphous dark bodies (arrows), and a large amount of rough-surfaced endoplasmic reticulum (between arrows). A red blood cell (RBC) and a platelet (P) are seen adjacent to the cast (UA + LC, ×3,300).

of urine was collected within a few hours of transplantation, and a second sample was collected seven days after transplantation for TEM analyses.

The TEM study of the first urinary sample showed many tubule epithelial cells (Figs. 6-13–6-15) and numerous neutrophils (Figs. 6-15 and 6-16). Almost all the tubule cells showed such changes as swelling of the mitochondria, amorphous dark bodies in the mitochondria (Fig. 6-14), and large vacuoles in the cells (Fig. 6-15). The TEM study of the second urinary sample showed few tubule cells but excessive numbers of inflammatory cells, including neutrophils, lymphocytes, monocytes, and plasma cells (Figs. 6-17–6-20). These inflammatory cells were found singly or in clumps, and platelets were also found in the clumps (Fig. 6-19). There were few granular casts and RBC (Fig. 6-21). The TEM finding of tubule epithelial and inflammatory cells in the absence of bacteria indicated an ongoing cellular rejection.

Figure 6-11b. A different type of epithelial cell cast, consisting of swollen mitochondria, along with several red blood cells (RBC) and a platelet (P), can be seen (UA + LC, ×3,300).

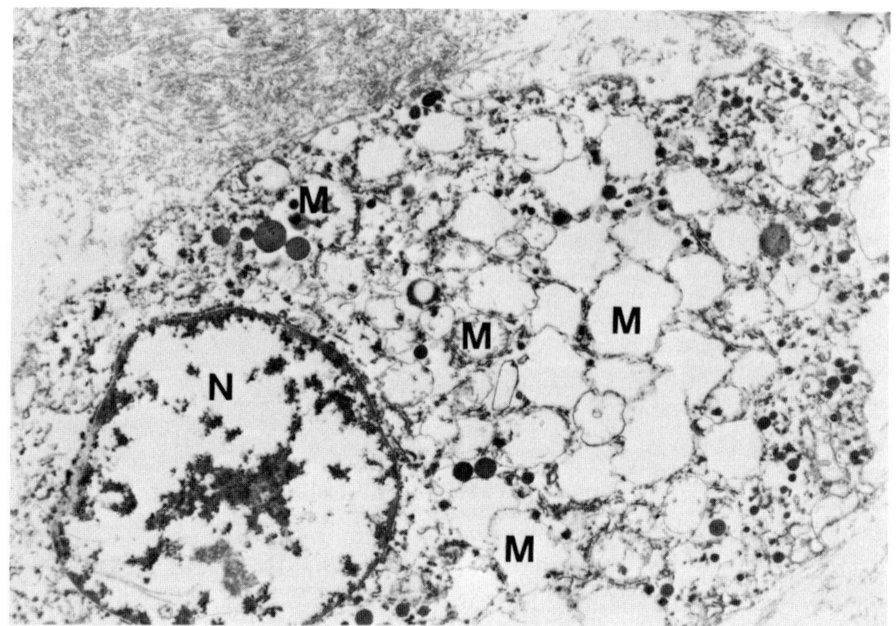

Figure 6-12. In this tubule cell, there is mild to severe swelling of the mitochondria with loss of cristae (M). The nucleus (N) shows condensation of the chromatin and dissolution of the nucleolus (UA + LC, ×3,300).

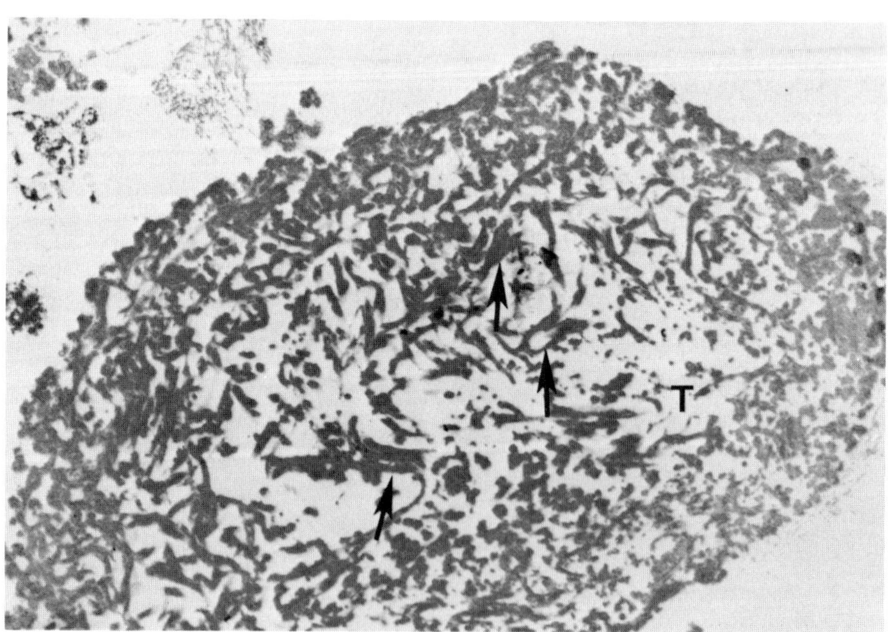

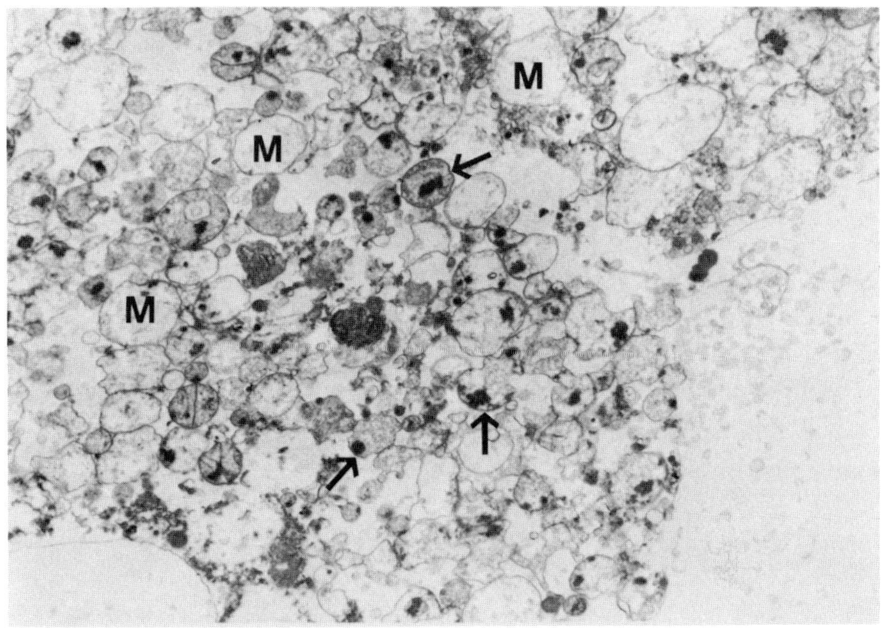

Figure 6-14.   This tubule epithelial cell, of unknown origin, shows mainly dissolution of the mitochondria (M). Some mitochondria contain circular or amorphous dark bodies (arrows) (UA + LC, ×3,300). From *Seminars in Nephrology,* Vol. 6, 1986, with permission.

Comments: The assessment of urinary sediment was confirmed by a percutaneous renal biopsy showing chronic rejection in August, 1984, and by progressive deterioration of renal function as shown below:

Date	Serum urea nitrogen (mg/dl)	Serum creatinine (mg/dl)
September 19, 1984	52	5.0
October 1, 1984	84	5.7
March 26, 1985	61	10.5

The patient was also hypertensive, and was being treated with clonidine and furosemide. Hemodialysis was started May 6, 1985.

Figure 6-13.   This transmission electron micrograph shows bundles of collagen fibers with periodicity (arrows) inside a necrotic tubule. The tubule (T) is totally disorganized (UA + LC, ×3,300).

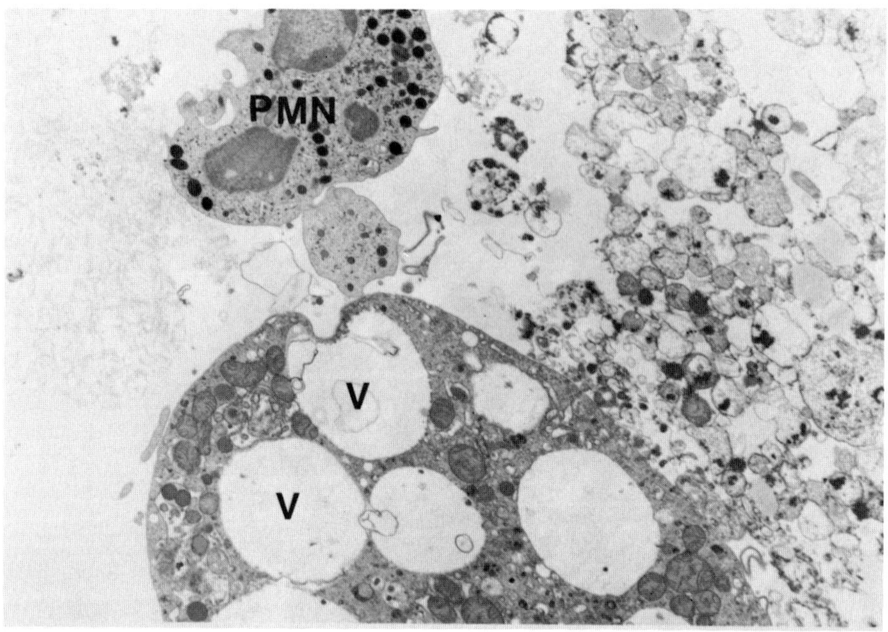

Figure 6-15.   This transmission electron micrograph shows a possible proximal tubule cell characterized by many mitochondria and many large vacuoles (V). A part of the polymorponuclear neutrophil (PMN) is seen (UA + LC, ×2,600).

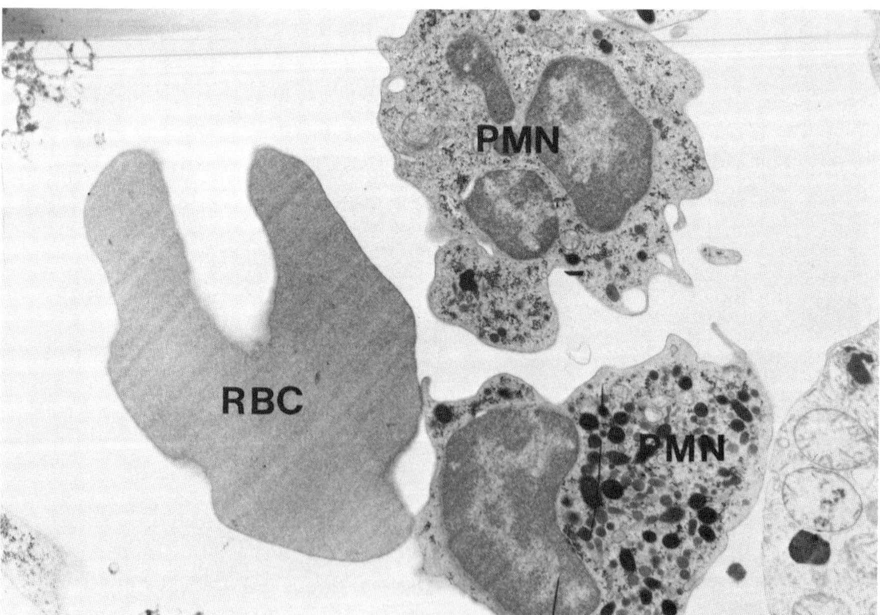

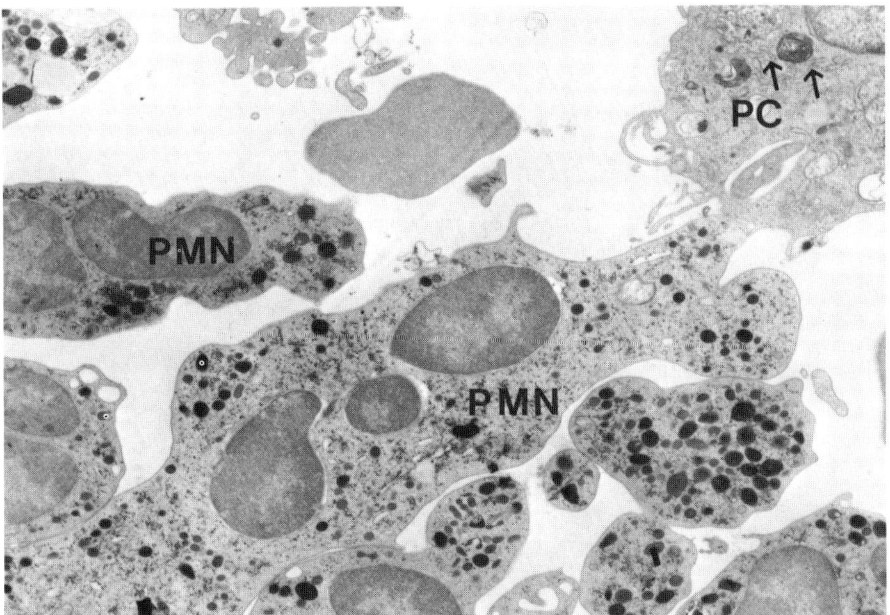

Figure 6-17.   Polymorphonuclear neutrophilic leukocytes (PMN) and a portion of a plasma cell (PC) are shown. The plasma cell contains abundant endoplasmic reticulum (arrows) (UA + LC, ×3,300). From *Seminars in Nephrology,* Vol. 6, 1986, with permission.

Patient No. 6, B. H., a 45-yr-old white male, developed end-stage renal failure secondary to polycystic kidney disease. He received a cadaveric renal transplantation at the Medical College of Georgia Hospital on April 23, 1984. A sample of urine was collected for TEM analysis, on April 25, 1984. The TEM study revealed many bacteria and an occasional tubule epithelial cell.

Comments: The urinary sediment assessment indicated no morphological changes in the grafted kidney. The patient's serum creatinine ranged from 2.3 to 2.8 mg/dl from September 1984, through August 1985.

Patient No. 7, S. E., a 41-yr-old white female, was admitted to the Medical College of Georgia Hospital on April 23, 1984, for renal transplantation. She had developed end-stage renal disease secondary to a suspected childhood glomerulonephritis. She received a renal transplant from her mother on April 25, 1984. She was treated with cyclosporine

Figure 6-16.   Neutrophilic leukocytes (PMN) and a deformed red blood cell (RBC) can be seen (UA + LC, ×3,300).

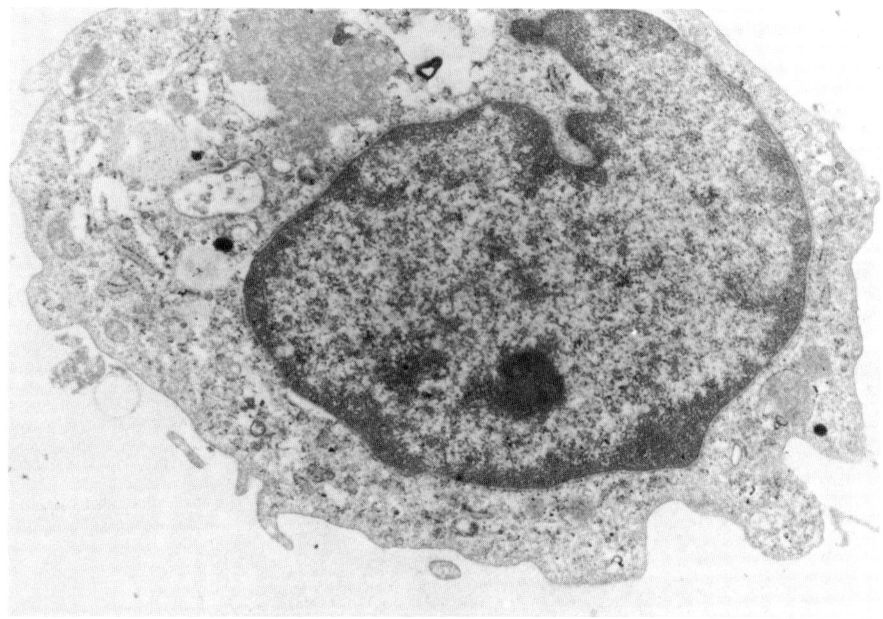

Figure 6-18. A single monocyte, characterized by its notched nucleus, is seen (UA + LC, ×6,600).

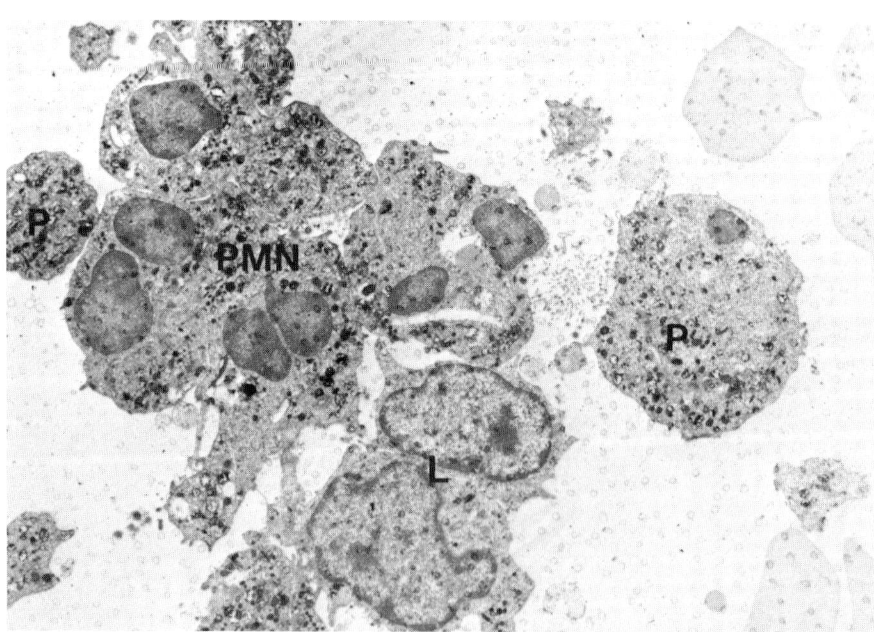

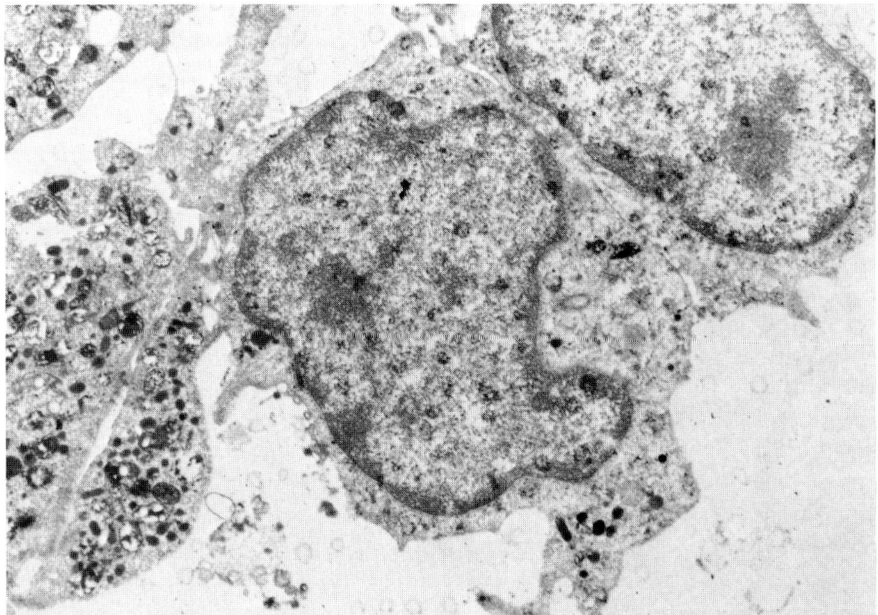

Figure 6-20.   These two lymphocytes are fused together (UA + LC, ×5,000).

(350 mg orally twice daily for five days) before transplantation. From the day of transplantation, 175 mg of cyclosporine was given intravenously twice daily. Her serum creatinine decreased rapidly from the preoperative level of 7.2 mg/dl to 1.3 mg/dl on postoperative day three. A sample of urine was collected on April 26, 1984, for TEM analysis. On postoperative day four, she became febrile and her serum creatinine level increased. A diagnosis of rejection was made, and she was treated with methylprednisolone intravenously, and her treatment regimen was changed to 350 mg of cyclosporine twice daily. She was discharged on May 7, 1984 with instructions to take 350 mg of cyclosporine twice daily and 30 mg of prednisone once daily. Her serum urea nitrogen and serum creatinine levels on the day of discharge were 18 mg/dl and 1.2 mg/dl, respectively. As of April 17, 1985, she was asymptomatic, and her serum urea nitrogen and serum creatinine levels were 21 mg/dl and 2.1 mg/dl, respectively.

The TEM analysis showed few tubule cells; though these cells showed swollen mitochondria, the cristae and membranes were intact. There were no mitochondrial amorphous dark bodies or ischemic tissue changes.

Figure 6-19.   This clump of cells consists of neutrophilic leukocytes (PMN), lymphocytes (L), and platelets (P) (UA + LC, ×2,000). From *Seminars in Nephrology,* Vol. 6, 1986, with permission.

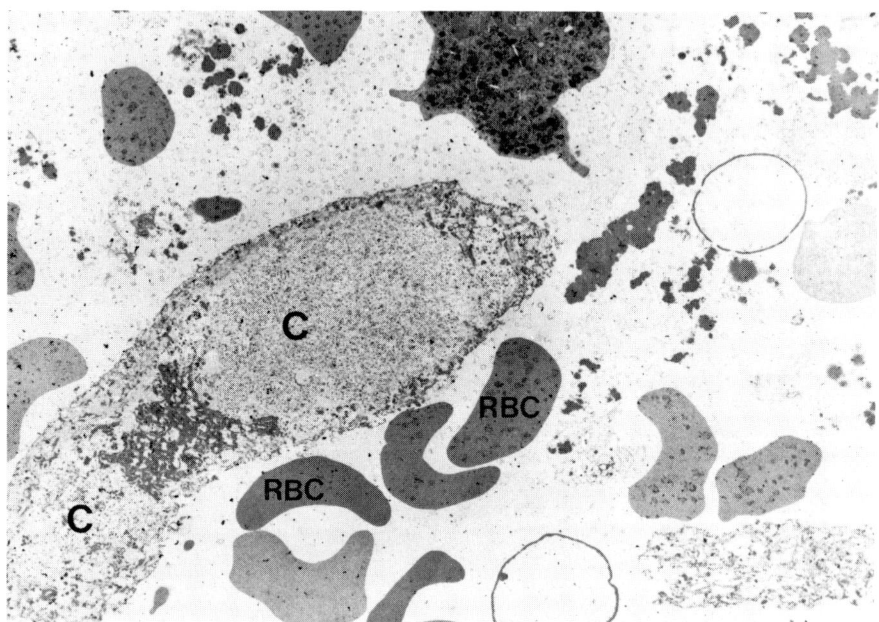

Figure 6-21. A granular cast (C) and many red blood cells (RBC) can be seen. (UA + LC, ×1,300).

Comments: The TEM findings of urinary sediment suggested mild tubule injury, which was confirmed by the normal renal function tests at the time of discharge.

REJECTION OF ALLOGRAFT

Despite careful immunological compatibility studies and the use of potent immunosuppressive drugs, rejection of transplanted organs occurs. Three distinct types of allograft rejection can be distinguished by the types of cellular infiltrate and cellular and humoral responses and the time of onset of these graft abnormalities seen after transplantation.[4]

Hyperacute Rejection

In a presensitized patient, hyperacute rejection may occur as early as 10 min after transplantation. Hyperacute rejection should be considered in patients with anuria in the first 24 to 48 hr after transplantation. A renal biopsy will reveal platelet aggregates and fibrin in the glomerular and peritubular capillaries.

The intrarenal arteries and capillaries are occluded, as a result of thrombosis. If the kidney is left in the recipient for a few days, cortical necrosis occurs. Hyperacute rejection is not reversible by any known therapy and nephrectomy is indicated.

Acute Rejection

Acute rejection can occur in the first three months following transplantation. Acute rejection may show features of both cellular and humoral mechanisms of allograft rejection. Cellular rejection is less common in patients who receive immunosuppressive therapy; it is characterized by widespread interstitial edema and focal interstitial infiltration by lymphocytes and plasma cells; with necrosis of the proximal tubule. Glomeruli and arterial vessesls, however, may show no changes. Conversely, a predominantly humoral rejection is more commonly seen in patients treated with immunosuppressive drugs. Platelet aggregates and thrombi may be found in the glomerular capillaries, arteries, and arterioles and the peritubular capillaries. In addition, arterioles may show fibrinoid necrosis and edema, with infiltration by neutrophilic and mononuclear cells, in both hyper-acute and acute rejection. Acute rejection has been reversed by high doses of corticosteriod or antithymocyte globulin. Recently, monoclonal antibodies have been tried in the treatment of acute rejection. Among these, T lymphocyte antibodies OKT3 monoclonal antibody appears to be highly effective in reversing acute cadaver kidney allograft rejection episodes.[4]

Chronic Rejection

Usually a slow insidious process, chronic rejection leads to a gradual loss of graft function. It may occur as a sequel to repeated bouts of clinically recognizable acute rejection episodes. Chronic rejection is primarily mediated humorally. Histologically, the findings are limited to the arterial vessels, which show subendothelial spaces, thickening of the basement membrane of the smooth muscle cells, and narrowed lumina. Chronic rejection is not amenable to any type of antirejection therapy. For more details about transplant rejection, the reader should consult the chapter "Renal Transplantation" in *Diagnosis and Management of Renal Disease and Hypertension*.[5]

DIAGNOSIS OF REJECTION

Early diagnosis of rejection is essential if irreversible renal damage is to be prevented. In almost all transplant patients, a rise in serum creatinine levels heralds rejection, clinically. It must be remembered, however, that a rise in serum creatinine level may also be the result of dehydration or drug-induced nephrotoxicity, especially from cyclosporine. In the immediate postoperative period following transplantation, continued abnormal renal function might be the result of hyperacute rejection or ATN. Urinalysis, urine enzyme assays, and radionuclide studies are performed to distinguish between rejection and ATN or rejection and cyclosporine nephrotoxicity. None of these tests is sensitive in identifying acute rejection, ATN, and cyclosporine nephrotoxicity precisely.

Percutaneous or open renal biopsy and examination of the renal tissue are considered most useful in distinguishing ATN from acute rejection. Mononuclear cellular infiltrate in the renal biopsy, though regarded by some individuals[6] as an indication that antirejection therapy must be initiated, can be misleading in patients receiving cyclosporine. Mononuclear cellular infiltration can occur in acute tubulointerstitial nephritis, which may be induced by cyclosporine.[7] Therefore, cyclosporine nephrotoxicity may be indistinguishable from cellular acute rejection. Farnsworth *et al.*[8] and Bennett[9] found no difference in the frequency or degree of cellular infiltrates in patients treated with cyclosporine and patients treated by conventional therapy. The renal biopsy study, however, is helpful in distinguishing acute from chronic rejection by the type and degree of vascular changes and the presence or absence of platelet aggregates and thrombi.[6]

The TEM study of urinary sediment by the author has shed some light on the problems of the posttransplant period. The urinary sediment in renal transplant rejection is quite different from that in ATN. The findings of abundant fibrin and inflammatory cells consisting of neutrophilic leukocytes and lymphocytes along with tubule cells in the urinary sediment allow a diagnosis of allograft rejection more than ATN. Urinary sediment findings of rejection were confirmed by renal biopsy findings of rejection in two patients. Urinary sediment findings coincided appropriately with the deterioration or improvement in renal function in other patients. The type of urinary sediment finding in cyclosporine nephrotoxicity has not been determined, however, and it is essential that this information be obtained. Meanwhile, it is prudent to state that urinary sediment TEM can reliably aid in distinguishing ATN from acute cellular and/or humoral rejection. Above all, it is a noninvasive, and cheaper technique and results can be obtained within 24 hr.

REFERENCES

1. Mandal AK, Sklar AH, Hudson JB: Transmission electron microscopy of urinary sediment in human acute renal failure. *Kidney Int* 1985; 28:58–63.
2. Mandal AK, Birnbaum D, Mize GN: Transmission electron microscopy of urinary sediment in aminoglycoside nephrotoxicity, in press.
3. Kahan BD, Van Buren CT, Flechner SM, et al: Clinical and experimental studies with cyclosporine in renal transplantation. *Surgery* 1985; 97:125–140.

 4. Kreis H, Chkoff N, Vigeral PH, et al: Therapeutic use of monoclonal antibodies in kidney transplantation, in Grumfeld JP, Maxwell MH (eds): *Advances in Nephrology*. Chicago, Year Book Medical Publishers, Inc. 1985, pp 389–407.
 5. Mahajan SK: Renal transplantation and its management, in Mandal AK, Jennette JC (eds): *Diagnosis and Management of Renal Disease and Hypertension*. Philadelphia, Lea and Febiger, 1987, in press.
 6. Strom TB: Immunosuppressive agents in renal transplantation. *Kidney Int* 1984; 26:353–365.
 7. Hall BM, Tiller DJ, Duggin GG: Post-transplant acute renal failure in cadaver renal recipients treated with cyclosporine. *Kidney Int* 1985; 28:178–186.
 8. Farnsworth A, Hall BM, Kirwan P, et al: Renal biopsy morphology in renal transplantation: A comparative study of the light microscopic appearance of biopsies from patients treated with cyclosporine A or azathioprine, prednisone and antilymphocyte globulin. *Am J Surg Pathol* 1984; 8:243–252.
 9. Bennett WM: Cyclosporine nephrotoxicity. *Ann Intern Med* 1983: 99:851–854.

7

Hepatorenal Syndrome

The hepatorenal syndrome can be defined as unexplained renal failure in patients with hepatitis or cirrhosis of the liver in the absence of clinical or laboratory evidence of other causes of renal failure. The clinical features of hepatorenal syndrome include severe or advanced liver disease associated with jaundice, ascites, and often encephalopathy and rapid renal failure. This renal failure develops without any apparent precipitating events, such as dehydration or sepsis, and is characterized by a progressive, relentless oliguria. The oliguria and azotemia are not amenable to any known manipulation and thus are usually irreversible. Patients slowly lapse into coma, with hypotension and hypothermia, and die.[1–3]

The pathogenesis of renal failure in decompensated liver disease remains an enigma. In a previous study, acute tubular necrosis (ATN) was suspected in some cases of hepatorenal syndrome on the basis of urinary casts, the low specific gravity of the urine, high urinary sodium, and a low urine/plasma creatinine ratio. A renal histopathological study, however, was not done to confirm the clinical diagnosis of ATN.[2] In light microscopy (LM) studies of kidneys from cases of hepatorenal syndrome, most observers reported inconsistent, mild tubular lesions.[1,4] Further, the findings of an extremely low urinary sodium ($\leq$ 10 mEq/liter) suggesting volume depletion, reversal of renal failure after orthotopic liver transplantation,[5] and recovery of function in kidneys removed from hepatorenal syndrome patients and transplanted into patients with end-stage renal disease[6] tend to argue against ATN as the cause of renal failure in hepatorenal syndrome.

This author has stated that "it is difficult to reconcile with a contradictory situation between progressive and fatal renal failure on one hand and reportedly

165

normal or near normal renal morphology on the other hand." To address this issue further, this author and his colleagues at Oklahoma City, Oklahoma, obtained kidneys at autopsy of five cases of hepatorenal syndrome from 30 to 120 min after death, and studied them extensively by transmission electron microscopy (TEM).[7]

This study was intended to answer the following questions: (1) Is ATN associated with the hepatorenal syndrome? (2) Can TEM study contribute significantly by characterizing the type of renal lesions that may accompany hepatorenal syndrome? and (3) Is a low urinary sodium a reliable criterion in excluding ATN in hepatorenal syndrome?

Our observations indicate that severe acute tubular lesions, or ATN, is a consistent histopathological feature in hepatorenal syndrome. Further, various cellular changes in the proximal tubules suggest the potential for either a reversal or a progression of the ATN. These abnormal ultrastructural findings were not associated with postmortem effects.[7]

Our TEM study was the first report demonstrating cellular necrosis with tubulorrhexis (disruption of basement membrane) in the proximal tubules of cases of hepatorenal syndrome, which suggests an ischemic type of ATN. The study also provided information about the approximate duration of ATN and the potential for recovery from ATN or renal failure.[7] Since then, the author has studied urinary sediments from patients with hepatorenal syndrome by TEM to determine whether the renal morphological changes are similar to those in acute renal failure (ARF).[8,9] The purpose of this chapter is to demonstrate the value of TEM studies of urinary sediment in defining renal morphological changes and to reconfirm our previous findings in hepatorenal syndrome.[7] The findings of urinary sediments from several patients are presented here to demonstrate the clinicopathological correlation between urinary sediment and clinical profile.

Patient No. 1, S. B., an unresponsive, 63-yr-old white male, was admitted to the Veterans Administration Medical Center, Augusta, Georgia, on May 1, 1984, with a history of multiple injuries from an automobile accident. Physical examination revealed a flail chest with a right pneumothorax, a fracture of the left hip, and second- to third-degree burns involving the right chest and hip. He also showed a left lower lobe pneumonia. A chest tube placement was to the right. His temperature was 103° F upon admission; and treatment with ampicillin and gentamicin was started. His past medical history included acute and chronic alcoholism with alcoholic gastritis. A percutaneous liver biopsy study showed moderate fatty changes, a quiescent cirrhosis, and focal mild inflammation.

His serial serum urea nitrogen (SUN), serum creatinine (Scr), serum bilirubin (Bil), serum glutamic oxalacetic transaminase (SGOT), and urine output are shown below.

Dates	SUN (mg/dl)	Scr (mg/dl)	Bil (mg/dl)	SGOT (IU/liter)	Urine output (ml/24 hr)
1983					
July 17	17	1.1	0.5	59	Not available
1984					
May 2	24	2.0	3.7	111	Not available
May 7	30	2.2	13.2	86	Not available
May 14	73	2.8	13.2	72	1353
May 17	96	4.9	Not available	Not available	1425
May 19	108	6.2	Not available	Not available	273
May 21	130	7.7	Not available	Not available	23
May 24	157	9.9	Not available	Not available	15

His serial urinary sodium (UNa), urinary potassium (UK), and urinary osmolality (UOsm) are shown below.

Dates (1984)	UNa (mEq/liter)	UK (mEq/liter)	UOsm (mOsm/kg)
May 14	74	38.2	318
May 17	122	19.5	324
May 19	86	30.9	314
May 21	35	69	325
May 24	122	17	345

The patient died on May 24th. His kidneys were removed at autopsy and studied.

Comments: The patient had progressive oliguria and a severe azotemia in the last week of his life. He was deeply jaundiced and his serum bilirubin was high. On May 21, he showed low urinary sodium, high urinary potassium, and very low sodium/potassium ratios (0.5), but his urine osmolality was consistently low (as were those reported previously). Thus the history of alcoholism, the liver biopsy findings, and the development of oliguric renal failure accompanied by jaundice and encephalopathy satisfy a diagnosis of hepatorenal syndrome. Persistently low urinary osmolality and high urinary sodium are supportive of ATN accompanying hepatorenal syndrome.

Two separate urine samples were collected on May 20 and 21, 1984, for TEM analyses. Kidney tissues were studied by LM and TEM. The urinary samples demonstrated severely damaged tubule cells, with necrotic masses with fibrin and few myeloid bodies (Figs. 7-1 and 7-2). The necrotic masses and the large amounts of fibrin tend to indicate intravascular coagulation associated with severe cellular necrosis. The renal tissue TEM demonstrated necrosis and dis-

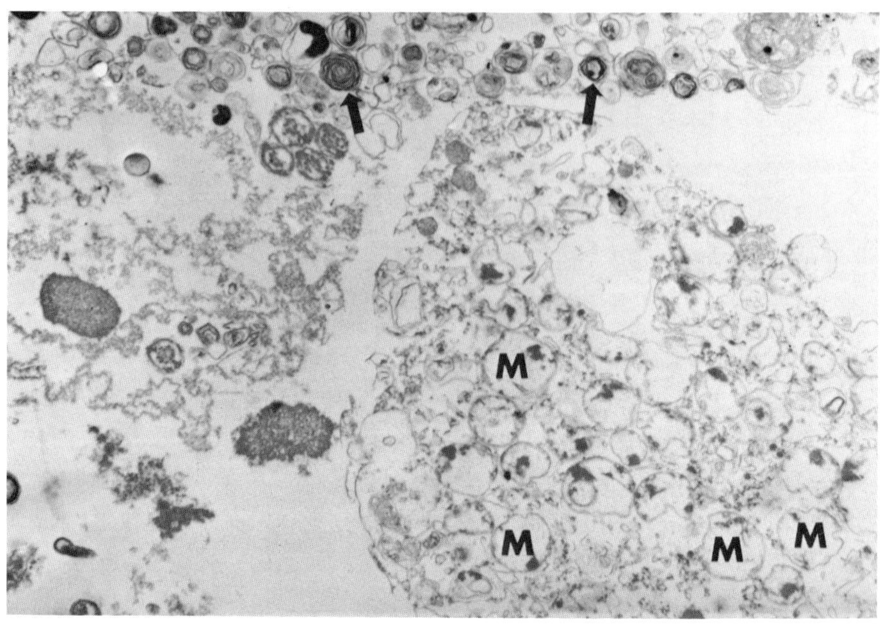

Figure 7-1. A tubule cell characterized by many swollen mitochondria (M), with loss of cristae, is shown. Amorphous dark bodies, a sign of irreversible damage, are present in many mitochondria, though there are few myeloid bodies (arrows) to be found (UA + LC, ×5,000).

ruption of tubules and the presence of many intratubular lysosomes (Figs. 7-3 and 7-4).

Patient No. 2, D. E., a 31-yr-old male American Indian, was admitted to the Veterans Administration Medical Center, Augusta, Georgia, on June 2, 1985, with a history of abdominal swelling and shortness of breath seven days before admission. He was an alcoholic who drank three to six six-packs of beer, as well as unknown amounts of whiskey and wine, a day. Physical examination revealed a temperature of 99.2° F, a pulse of 90/min, regular respiration of 20/min, and a blood pressure of 150/70 mm Hg. His skin was markedly icteric, with several spider angiomas over the anterior chest wall. The liver was percussed to a 13-cm total span with 5 cm below the right costal margin.

Figure 7-3. The intercellular plasma membranes (PM) of this tubule are dilated; individual mitochondria are widely separated by intracellular edema (E). Because the nucleus (N) is basilar in aspect, this is probably a proximal tubule. Many mitochondria demonstrate loss of cristae and contain dark bodies (UA + LC, ×3,300).

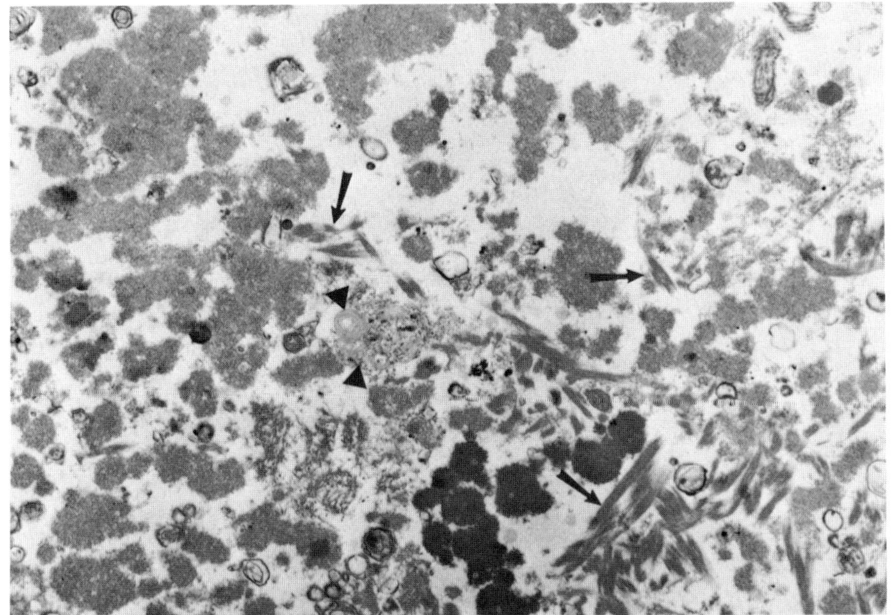

Figure 7-2.   Masses of fibrin fibers (arrows) and myeloid bodies (arrowheads) are seen in this transmission electron micrograph (UA + LC, ×5,000).

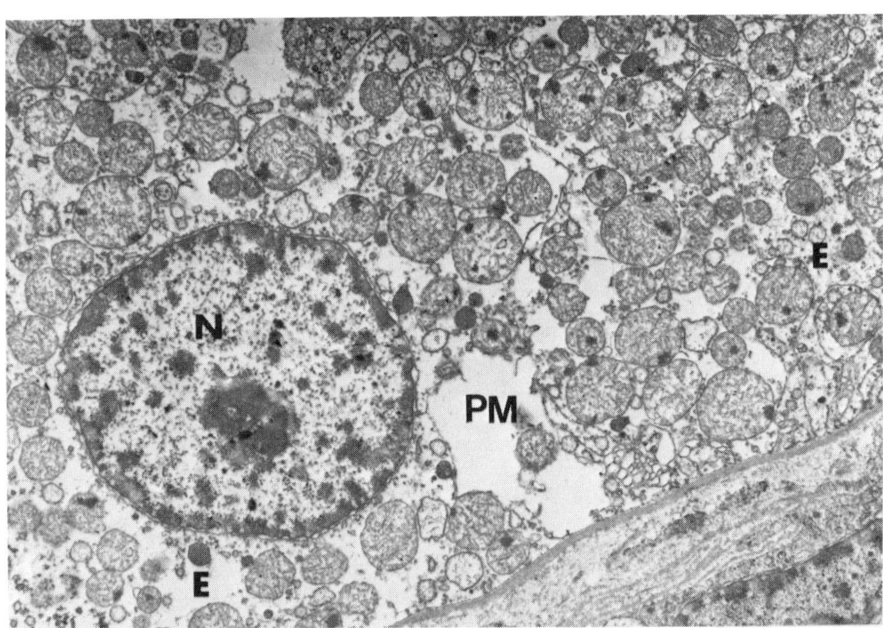

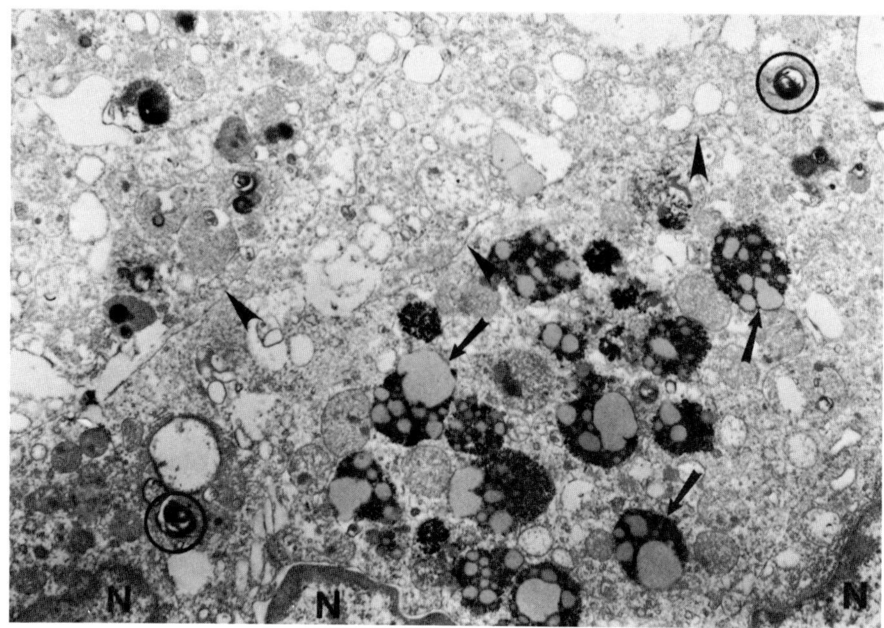

Figure 7-4. Several tubule cells, a portion of the nuclei (N), and intercellular membranes between individual cells can be seen (arrowheads). A striking feature is the many cellular lysosomes (arrows). Occasional myeloid bodies are also observed (circle) (UA + LC, ×5,000).

He had 1^+ pitting edema and moderate ascites. He demonstrated mild asterixis, and his stool occult blood was positive.

Admission laboratory studies showed a serum sodium of 135 mEq/liter; serum potassium, 2.3 mEq/liter; serum chloride, 103 mEq/liter; serum CO_2, 19 mEq/liter; serum glucose, 111 mg/dl; serum urea nitrogen (SUN), 18 mg/dl; and serum creatinine (Scr) 2.1 mg/dl. His prothrombin time was 22.5 sec (C = 11.6 sec), and his partial thromboplastin time was 50.2 sec (C = 25.3 sec). His WBC count was 25×10^3, with a hemoglobin of 9.5 g/dl and a hematocrit of 26.3%. His serial SUN, Scr, serum bilirubin (Bil), alkaline phosphatase (Alk Phos), serum glutamic oxalacetic transaminase (SGOT), and urinary output are shown below.

Date (1985)	SUN (mg/dl)	Scr (mg/dl)	Bil (mg/dl)	Alk Phos (IU/liter)	Urinary output (ml/24 hr)
June 3	17	2.0	36.8	Not available	1200
June 6	40	6.4	36.4	Not available	750
June 10	68	8.5	35.5	204	275

Daily hemodialysis was initiated. His serial urinary sodium (UNa), urinary potassium (UK), and urinary osmolality (UOsm) are shown below.

Date (1985)	UNa (mEq/liter)	UK (mEq/liter)	UNa/UK Ratio	UOsm (mOsm/kg)
June 2	32	28.7	1.11	331
June 3	12	60	0.2	314
June 17	25	85.9	0.29	316
June 24	19	111	0.17	318
July 4	16	105	0.15	

On June 12, a sample of urine was fixed for TEM analysis. Light microscopy of the urinary sediment showed granular casts (Fig. 7-5), a hyaline cast, a red blood cell cast, clusters, and epithelial cell fragments (Fig. 7-6). A red blood cell cast from this patient is shown in Fig. 2-11 (p.35). On June 13, parenteral hyperalimentation was initiated. A urinary sediment study by light microscopy revealed more hyaline, granular, and epithelial cell casts than were present the previous day. From July 1, 1985, his blood pressure

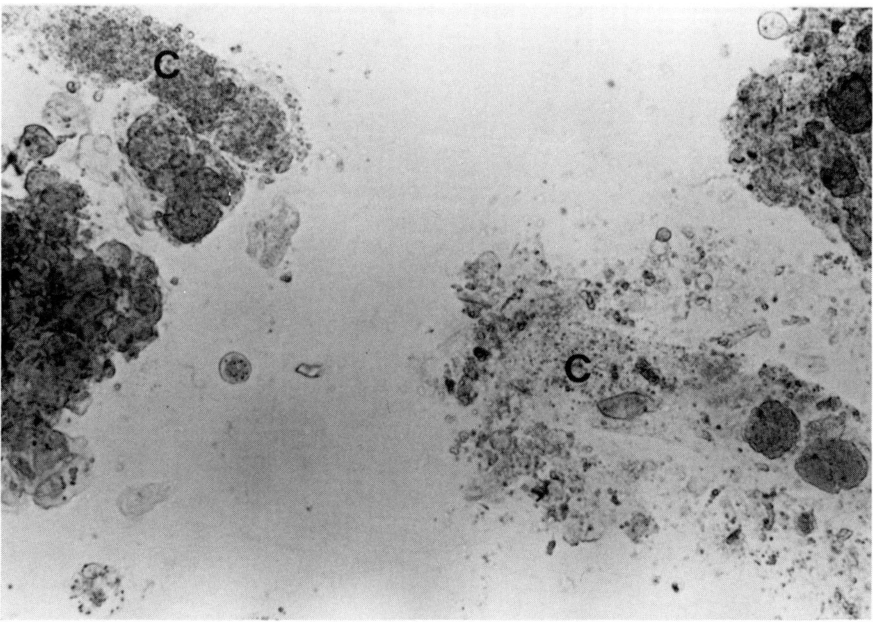

Figure 7-5.   This light micrograph shows two granular casts (C) and an epithelial cell embedded in or adherent to the cast (epoxy tissue stain, × 400).

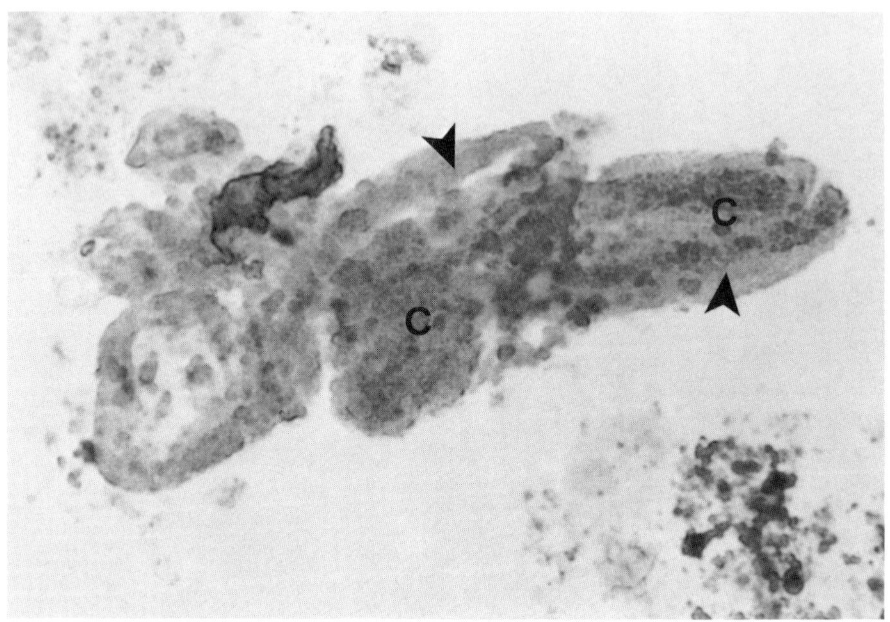

Figure 7-6. This light micrograph reveals what appears to be a segment of a tubule, in which the basement membrane (arrowheads) and several cells (C) are recognizable (epoxy tissue stain, ×400).

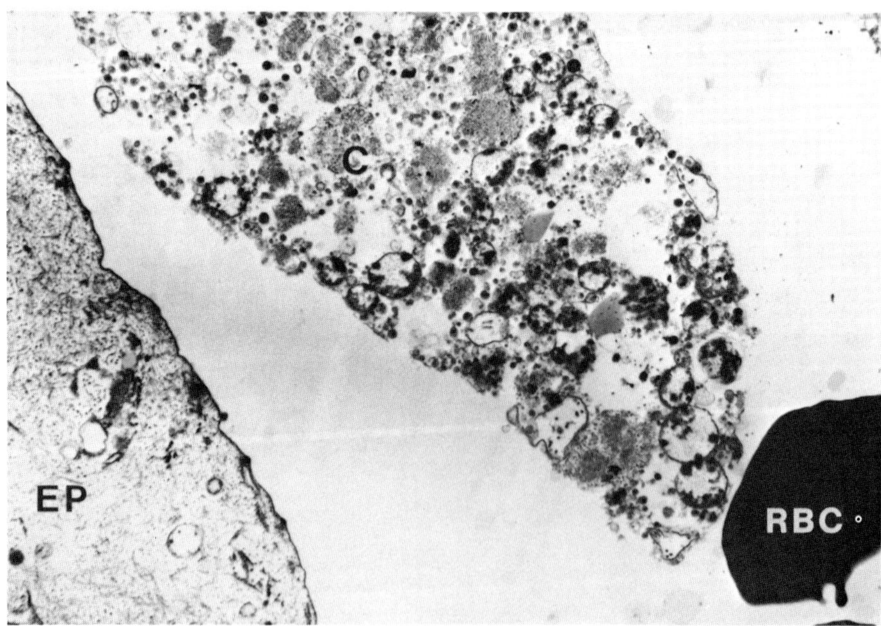

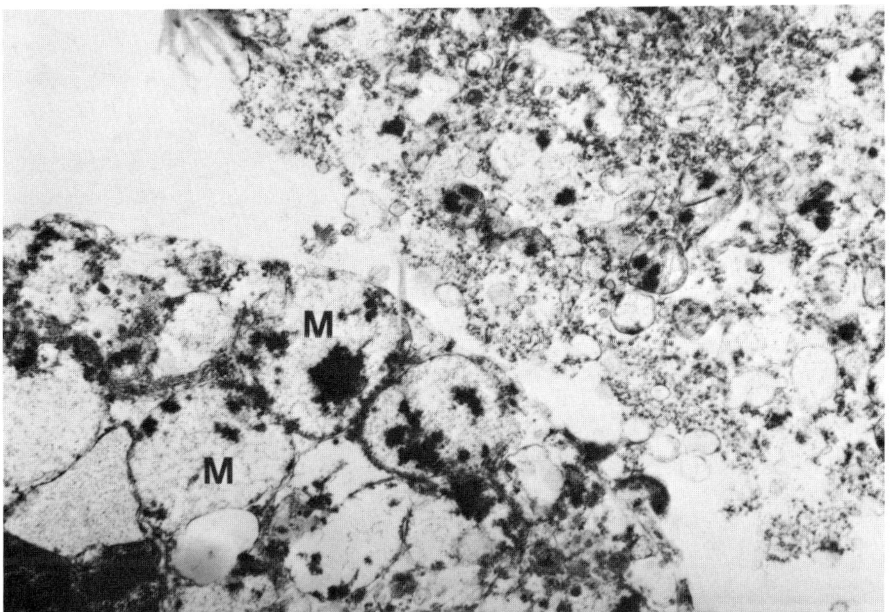

Figure 7-8.   These tubule cells reveal marked swelling of the mitochondria (M); some cells contain large amorphous dark bodies (UA + LC, ×7,500).

began to decrease. From July 1 to July 9, his systolic blood pressure was in the range of 62 to 80 mm Hg; his diastolic pressure, 40 to 50 mm Hg. His urine output decreased to less than 400 ml/24 hr. From July 10, he had no urine output. Despite daily hemodialysis, his SUN and Scr ranged between 90 and 115 mg/dl and 4.4 and 6.1 mg/dl, respectively. He died on July 13, 1985. Autopsy was not permitted.

The TEM analysis of urinary sediment revealed many different types of epithelial casts (Fig. 7-7). (Several epithelial casts from this patient can be seen in Chapter 2.) Many epithelial cells with severe necrotic changes, similar to those described previously,[8] were found (Fig. 7-8).

Comments: The LM urinary sediment findings were consistent with ATN, and the TEM appearance of tubule epithelial cells comply with type 1 sediment or severe ATN. In an earlier study, we showed that renal function recovery is negligible and mortality is very high in patients showing type 1 sediments.[8] Therefore, the urinary sediment findings in this patient shows that hepatorenal

Figure 7-7.   An epithelial cast (C) with many mitochondria, a squamous epithelial cell (EP), and a red blood cell (RBC) can be seen (UA + LC, ×5,000).

syndrome is associated with severe ATN. The urinary sodium and potassium concentrations, urinary Na/K ratios, and the urinary osmolality in this patient are consistent with those in ATN in hepatorenal syndromes reported previously.[7]

Patient No. 3, A. T., a 64-yr-old white male, was admitted to the Veterans Administration Medical Center, Augusta, Georgia, on January 31, 1984, with a possible diagnosis of hepatorenal syndrome. He had a long history of alcohol abuse. He was in his usual state of health until three weeks before admission, when he developed a progressive swelling of his lower extremeties. Laboratory studies during his initial hospital admission one week before his transfer to Augusta showed a serum bilirubin of 1.0 mg/dl and a serum urea nitrogen of 13 mg/dl. His condition rapidly deteriorated and he developed anasarca and became stuporous. His serial serum urea nitrogen (SUN), serum creatinine (Scr), and urine output are shown below.

Date (1984)	SUN (mg/dl)	Scr (mg/dl)	Urine output (ml/24 hr)
January 31	166	3.8	497 (16 hr)
February 1	170	3.5	450
February 3	178	3.4	2,800

His SGOT was 122 IU/liter, and serum bilirubin 3.0 mg/dl, on February 3; also on February 3, a sample of urine was collected for TEM analysis. On February 7, his SUN was 164 mg/dl, his Scr was 3.8 mg/dl, and his urine output was 531 ml/24 hr; his SGOT was 86 IU/liter and his serum bilirubin 3.9 mg/dl. He was treated with continuous infusion of furosemide (20 mg/hr) and low dose dopamine. His serial spot urinary sodium (UNa), urinary potassium (UK), and urinary osmolality (UOsm) are shown below.

Date (1984)	UNa (mEq/liter)	UK (mEq/liter)	UOsm (mOsm/kg)
January 31	11	12.9	326
February 2	10	13.2	770
February 4	82	12.5	Not available
February 5	74	16	Not available

The patient died on February 8, 1984. No autopsy was performed, but the TEM of the urinary sediment revealed severely necrotic tissue, with completely dissolved cell nuclei; the cellular membranes were intact. Some cellular membranes were disrupted. The striking feature was the presence of numerous neutrophilic leukocytes in the absence of bacteria. Within the masses of necrotic cells occasional myeloid bodies and lysosomes were found.

Comments: The urinary sediment findings are commensurate with the rapid deterioration of renal function in this patient. His SUN increased from the normal level of 13 mg/dl to 178 mg/dl within a week. The infiltration by neutrophilic leukocytes in the absence of bacteria may represent an invasion of the necrotic tissue by inflammatory cells.

Patient No. 4, J. B., a 61-yr-old white male, was admitted to the Veterans Administration Medical Center on August 24, 1985, with a history of heavy alcohol intake; he had been drinking one-half gallon of whiskey a day for one month. He had had jaundice for one week and nausea, hematemesis, and melena for five days. Upon admission, he was hypotensive (BP 100 to 112 mm Hg systolic and 40 to 50 mm Hg diastolic). He was jaundiced, edematous, and obtunded. Laboratory studies revealed a serum urea nitrogen (SUN) of 61 mg/dl; serum creatinine (Scr), 5.8 mg/dl; serum sodium, 146 mEq/liter; serum potassium, 3.3 mEq/liter; serum chloride, 101 mEq/liter; serum CO_2 27, mEq/liter; serum alkaline phosphate, 192 IU/liter (normal, 30–115 IU/liter); SGOT, 643 IU/liter (normal, 7–40 IU/liter); CPK, 815 IU/liter (normal 24–195 IU/liter); and serum bilirubin, 24.5 mg/dl. His serial SUN, Scr, and urine output are shown below.

Date (1985)	SUN (mg/dl)	Scr (mg/dl)	Urine output (ml/24hr)
Aug 25	70	7.6	98
	(hemodialysis started)		
Aug 26	93	9.3	29
	(urine sample collected for TEM analysis)		
Aug 27	96	10.6	0

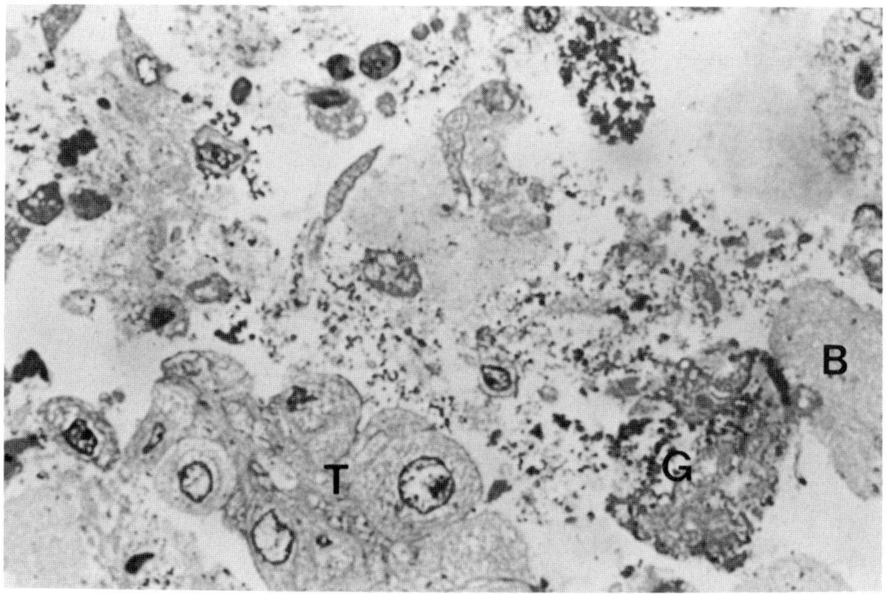

Figure 7-9.   This light micrograph includes a broad cast (B), a granular cast (G), and a portion of the tubule (T) (epoxy tissue stain, × 200).

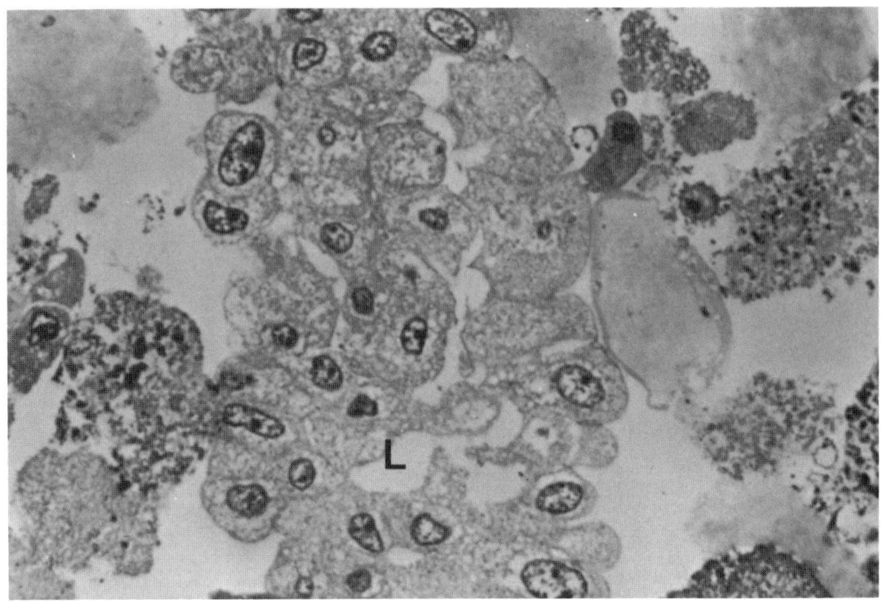

Figure 7-10. The portion of the tubule seen in Fig. 7-9 is shown at higher magnification. The lumen (L) of the segment of the tubule is clearly definable (epoxy tissue stain, ×400). From *Seminars in Nephrology,* Vol. 6, 1986, with permission.

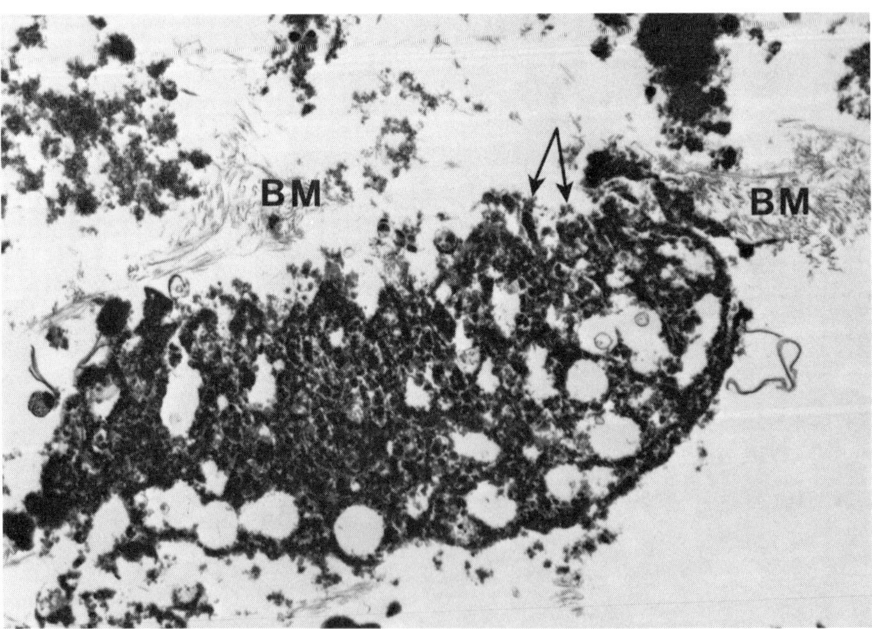

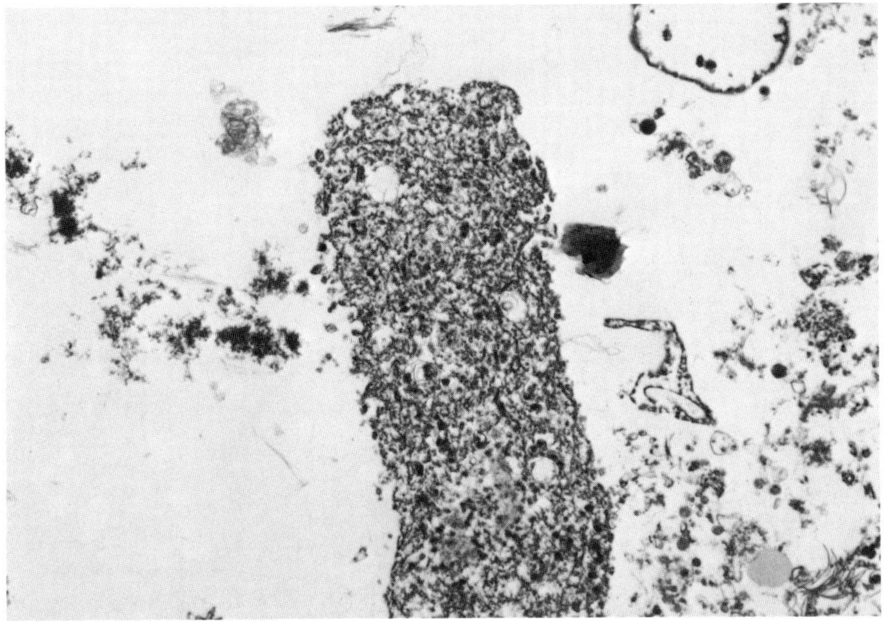

Figure 7-12.   A granular cast is shown (UA + LC, ×5,000).

On this day, his serum uric acid was 26.0 mg/dl; serum potassium, 6.6 mEq/liter; serum phosphate, 13.0 mg/dl; serum calcium, 7.4 mg/dl, SGOT, 10.890 IU/liter; and bilirubin, 20 mg/dl. On August 29, a sample of urine was collected for TEM analysis. On August 30, the patient died.

The thick sections from the first urine specimen on August 26 showed numerous tubule epithelial cells and few hyaline casts. The second specimen, on August 29, showed broad casts and a portion of the tubule (Figs. 7-9 and 7-10).

The TEM study of the first urinary sediment showed many necrotic epithelial cells. Some tubule cells appeared to be of proximal origin (Fig. 7-11); in other tubule cells, the anatomy could not be defined. The basement membranes of the tubules were completely disrupted and appeared to be fibrillar, and the number of cellular lysosomes had increased. The TEM study of the second urinary sediment showed a large number of casts, which included granular casts (Fig. 7-12), an epithelial cast (Fig. 7-13), segments of tubules (Figs. 7-14–7-16), and many isolated and clusters of tubule epithelial cells (Figs. 7-17 and 7-18). The granular casts contained large amounts of coarse granular

Figure 7-11.   This necrotic cell, apparently of proximal tubule origin, contains recognizable remnants of microvilli (arrows) and basement membranes of the tubules (BM) (UA + LC, ×7,500). From *Seminars in Nephrology,* Vol. 6, 1986, with permission.

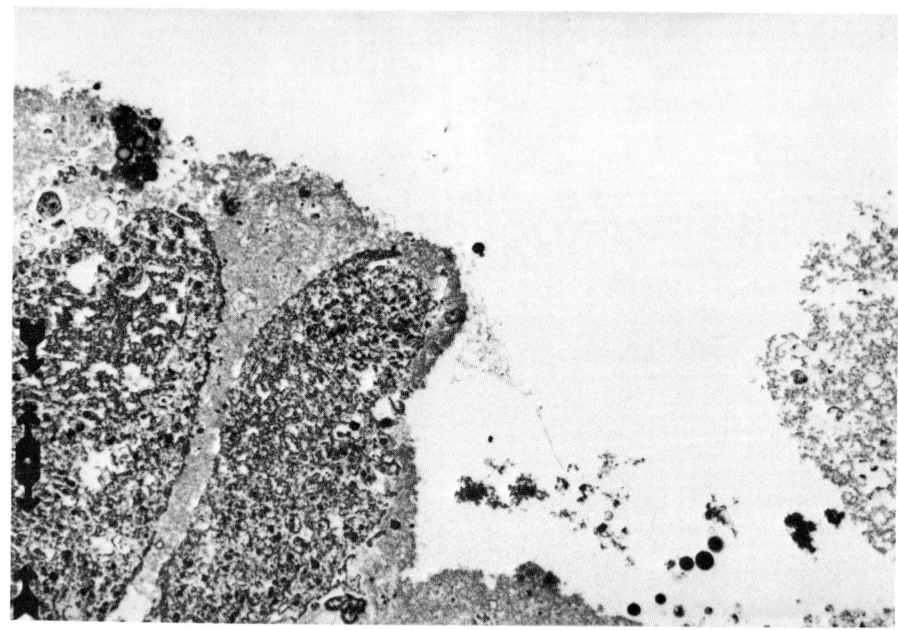

Figure 7-13. This epithelial cast contains a possible proximal tubule cell as shown by remnants of microvilli (between arrows) seen embedded in the cast matrix (UA + LC, ×4,000).

matcrial that appeared to be cellular cytoplasm. Many degenerated epithelial cells were seen adjacent to the granular casts. This latter finding is indirect evidence for the origin of granular casts from degenerated epithelial cells. Segments of tubules consisting of multiple cells, separated by intercellular spaces, were found, but the cellular structure was totally disorganized. These cells appeared to have come from the proximal tubule because of their narrow apexes and the location of the nuclei toward the basilar aspect of the cells. The basement membranes in these necrotic tubules were totally disrupted and fibrillar. Many tubule cells, although severly damaged, contained lysosomes.

Comments: The TEM studies of the first and second urinary sediments demonstrated the presence of numerous epithelial cells, epithelial casts, and granular casts, findings, which are consistent with ATN. Though the cellular changes were severe, the presence of nuclei and lysosomes in many cells might be evidence of a potential for regeneration.

In summary, TEM urinary sediment study has uniformly found most severe changes in the tubule cells in patients with hepatorenal syndrome. The sediment findings confirm our previous renal histopathologic findings and indicate that

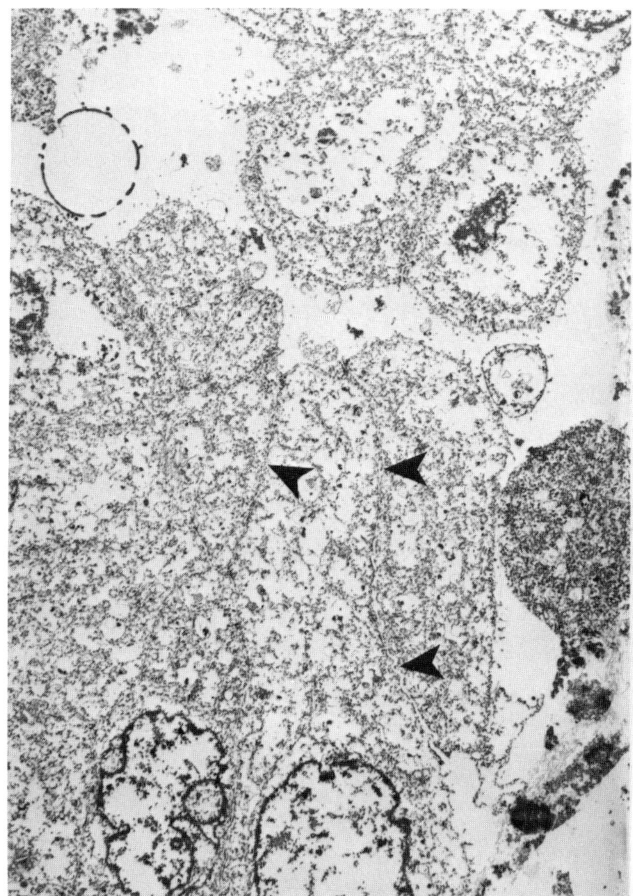

Figure 7-14.   In this segment of the tubule, the cells, which are very necrotic, are in parallel rows. The intercellular membrane separating the cells (arrowheads) can be identified (UA + LC, ×2,000). From *Seminars in Nephrology,* Vol. 6, 1986, with permission.

progressive renal failure in hepatorenal syndrome is due to ATN. Furthermore, the worst sediment findings are consistent with the dismal prognosis of this disorder.[9]

PATHOGENESIS

The pathology of the kidneys in hepatorenal syndrome has been demonstrated to a point, though the pathogenesis of renal failure, or ATN, is not

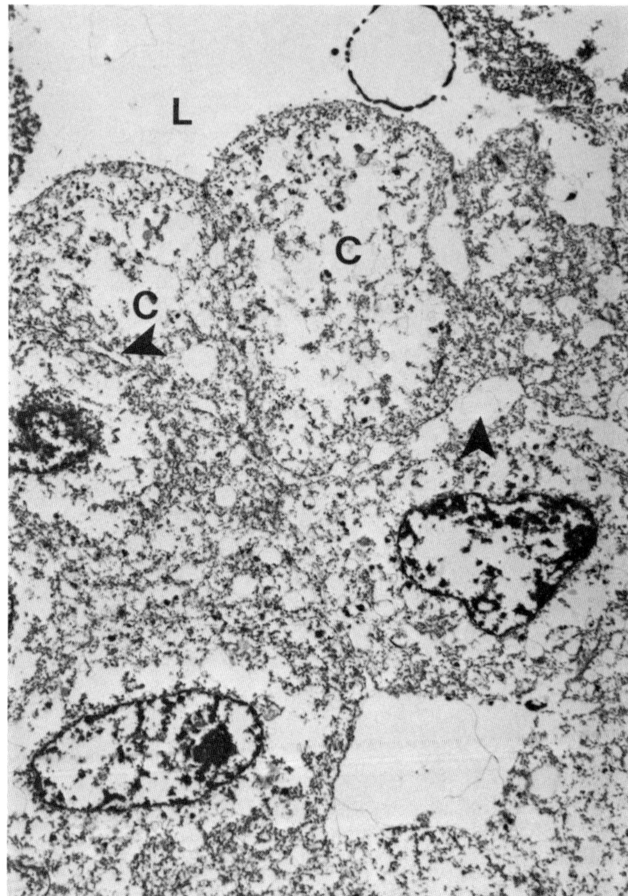

Figure 7-15. This segment of a tubule shows a parallel arrangement of cells (C), which are very necrotic. They are separated by intercellular membranes (arrowheads). The apical aspect of the cells toward the lumen (L) of the tubule is shown (UA + LC, ×2,500).

known. Various theories have been proposed; they include a decrease in effective circulating volume with an underperfused kidney; an increase in renin–angiotensin activity; alterations in vasodilator prostaglandin (PGE_2) and vasoconstrictor thromboxane (TXB_2) activities; a decrease in renal kallikrein activity; and the presence of endotoxins and a hepatic factor, *glomerulopressin*.

The pathogenesis of hepatorenal syndrome, cannot be discussed here, but it should be stated that a decrease in the effective volume of the renal circulation

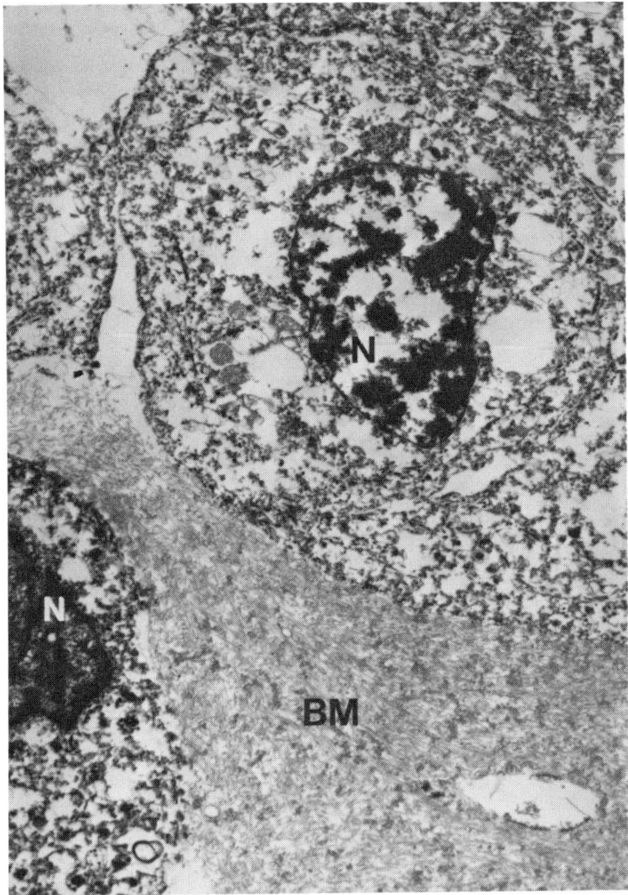

Figure 7-16.   A portion of the tubule with a widened, fibrillar basement membrane (BM) is shown. Though the cells appear to be necrotic, nuclei (N) are still present (UA + LC, ×5,000).

for a prolonged period seems to be the most important factor in the development of ATN. Cirrhotic patients have episodes of vomiting and gastrointestinal bleeding that lead to an intermittent circulatory insufficiency. In addition, a low serum albumin, which almost always occurs, contributes to the low circulatory volume. Another factor is the nephropathy of hypokalemia, which was not addressed. Hypokalemia has also been linked to hepatic encephalopathy. It is probable that the excessive number of vacuoles and lysosomes found in the proximal tubules in hypokalemia could potentiate cellular necrosis during ischemia induced by

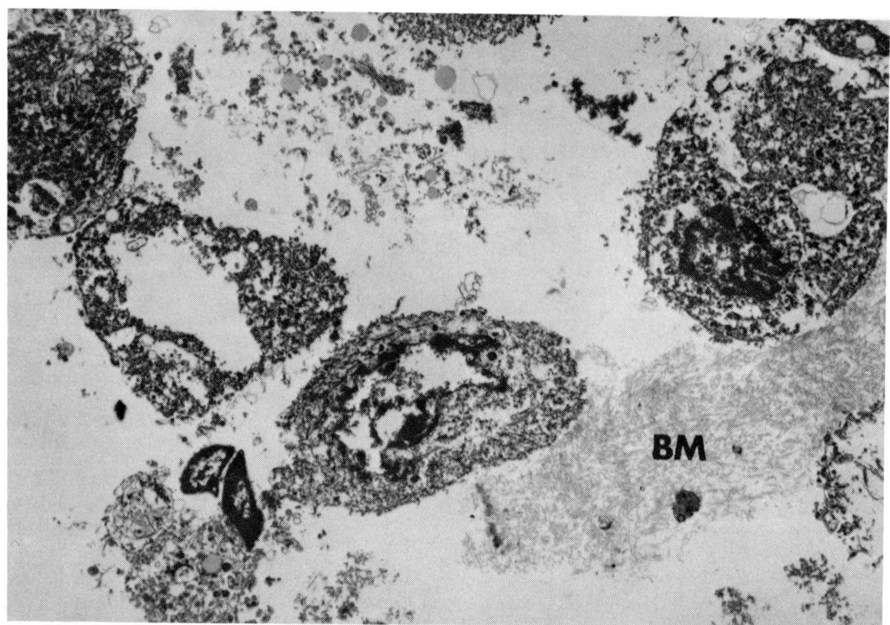

Figure 7-17.   A cluster of epithelial cells that appear to be remnants of a tubule is shown. The cells demonstrate variable changes. The fibrillar basement membrane (BM) of the tubule is still discernible (UA + LC, ×2,500).

circulatory insufficiency. Although a decrease in the circulating vasodilator PGE_2 or an increase in the circulating vasoconstrictor TXB_2 may not exert major effects, separately,[10] the two together could lead to a profound tubule ischemia. An experimental model of hepatorenal syndrome that would allow us to study the pathophysiology of this type of renal failure would be useful.

MANAGEMENT

As stated earlier, this syndrome is irreversible and is almost always fatal. No therapeutic manipulation known can reverse this progressive disorder. Nevertheless, in any patient with hepatorenal syndrome, as with any patient with ATN, attempts must be made to identify and treat reversible conditions. These reversible conditions include volume depletion (fluid, blood, plasma, or albumin IV); hypokalemia (potassium supplements orally or intravenously); urinary tract obstruction; and finally, cautious use of potentially nephrotoxic antibiotics.

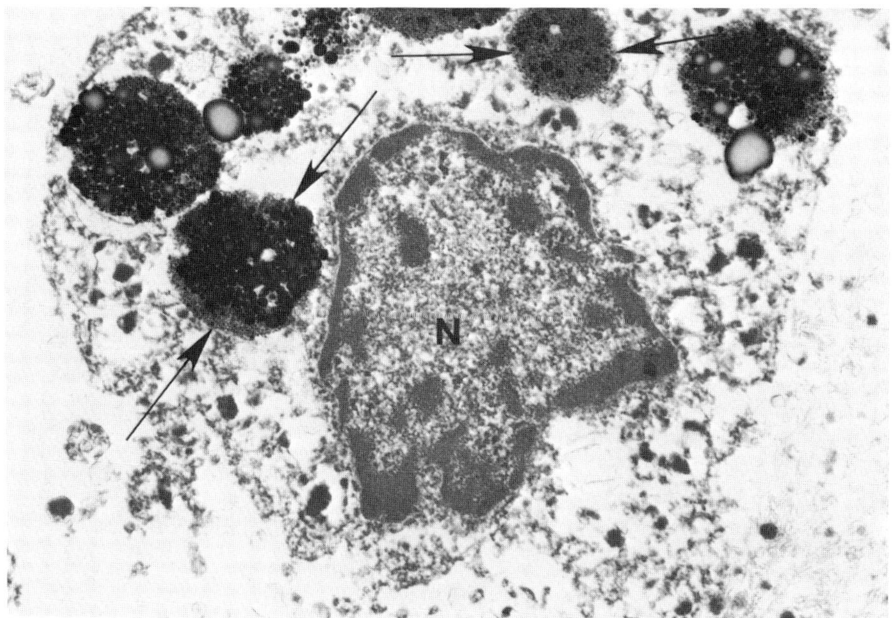

Figure 7-18.   In this cell, though the mitochondria have undergone complete dissolution, the nucleus (N) is intact and there are many lysosomes (between arrows) (UA + LC, ×10,000).

REFERENCES

1. Vaamonde CA, Papper S: The kidney in liver disease, in Strauss and Welt's *Diseases of the Kidney*, ed 3. Boston, Little, Brown and Company, 1979, pp 1289–1317.
2. Shear L, Kleinerman J, Gabuzda GJ: Renal failure in patients with cirrhosis of the liver. 1. Clinical and pathologic characteristics. *Am J Med* 1965; 39:184–198.
3. Wong PY, McCoy GC, Spielberg A, *et al:* The hepatorenal syndrome. *Gastroenterology* 1979; 77:1326–1334.
4. Goresky CA, Kumar G: Renal failure in cirrhosis of the liver. *Canad Med Assoc J* 1964; 90:353–356.
5. Iwatsuki S, Popvtzer MM, Corman JL, *et al:* Recovery from "hepatorenal" syndrome after orthotopic liver transplantation. *N Engl J Med* 1973; 289:1155–1159.
6. Koppel MH, Coburn JW, Mims MM, *et al:* Transplantation of cadaveric kidneys from patients with hepatorenal syndrome. *N Engl J Med* 1969; 280:1367–1371.
7. Mandal AK, Lasing M, Fahmy A: Acute tubular necrosis in hepatorenal syndrome: An electron microscopy study. *Am J Kid Dis* 1982; 2:363–373.
8. Mandal AK, Sklar AH, Hudson JB: Transmission electron microscopy of urinary sediment in human acute renal failure. *Kidney Int* 1985; 28:58–63.

9. Mandal AK: Transmission electron microscopy of urinary sediment in renal disease. *Sem Nephrol* 1986; 6:346–370.
10. Zipser RD, Radvan GH, Kronborg IJ: Urinary thromboxane B and prostaglandin E in the hepatorenal syndrome: Evidence for increased vasoconstrictor and decreased vasodilator factors. *Gastroenterology* 1983; 84:697–703.

8

Neoplasms and the Kidney

Renal manifestations in neoplasm vary and depend on whether the neoplasm is primary or secondary. Manifestations generally are florid with secondary involvement of the kidneys, especially in acute leukemia, lymphoma, and myeloma. Clinically, there is microscopic or gross hematuria, mild to heavy proteinuria, renal tubular acidosis, and acute or chronic renal failure. These overt characteristics may be the result of renal interstitium infiltration by abnormal white blood cells (WBC); deposition of uric acid, calcium, or myeloma protein(s) in the tubules or interstitium; and/or chemotherapeutic agent toxicity. Some of the renal complications in malignancy are transient and cause slight concern, whereas others are persistent and of major importance. Among the renal complications, the most frequent nephrological consultation is done for progressive renal failure in patients with multiple myeloma. Twenty-five or thirty years ago, tumor lysis syndrome and acute uric acid nephropathy were common. Since the advent and use of allopurinol, acute urate nephropathy is rare, but acute renal failure (ARF) from sepsis or the effect of newer chemotherapeutic agents [cisplatinum, gallium, m-AMSA or amsacrine (acridinyl anisidide)] still occurs. The use of amsacrine tends to be a common reason for nephrological consultation.

Irrespective of the type of renal disease and the malignancy that produced it, renal biopsy is infrequently performed to document renal histopathological changes. Many patients with acute leukemia or lymphoma are seriously ill, often with bleeding abnormalities, which make renal biopsy extremely hazardous.

The urinary sediment can be examined by light microscopy (LM) to assess the type and severity of renal changes, but because of low resolution, findings are not generally rewarding. We have observed that transmission electron microscopy (TEM) of urinary sediments from patients with ARF is highly informational about the renal changes and that changes found in the tubules in urinary sediment correlate well with the recovery of renal function and the clinical outcome.[1]

Urinary sediments from several patients with malignancy have been examined by TEM. The purpose of this chapter is to demonstrate that such TEM studies can aid in delineating the renal changes in malignancy.

Patient No. 1, E.H., a 73-yr-old black male, was admitted to the Veterans Administration Medical Center, Augusta, Georgia, on November 9, 1983, complaining of lower back pain. Other significant complaints at the time of admission included an approximately 45-lb weight loss over the past several years. His past medical history included a total prostatectomy in 1971. Admitting laboratory studies showed a normochromic, normocytic anemia, a hemoglobin of 9.6 g/dl, and a hematocrit of 28.1%. Initial urinalysis revealed 4$^+$ protein. The diagnosis of multiple myeloma was suspected because of the elevated serum total protein and a monoclonal spike in a serum protein electrophoresis. No Bence Jones proteinuria was noted in the initial work-up. Immunoelectrophoresis of serum proteins showed IgG and kappa light chain and urine immunoelectrophoresis showed free kappa light chain only. The diagnosis of myeloma was confirmed by the finding of 40 to 50% plasma cells in the bone marrow aspirate. The patient was treated with prednisone, melphalan, and vincristine and discharged to be followed up by the Hematology/Oncology Clinic. He was readmitted to the Veterans Administration Medical Center on January 3, 1984, after suffering a cardiac arrest in the elevator while on the way to the Dental Clinic for routine outpatient work; he was successfully resuscitated. It was felt that his arrest was due to cardiac dysrrhythmia. The patient then developed an oliguric ARF that was attributed to his ischemic acute tubular necrosis (ATN) secondary to hypoperfusion. A Tenchkhoff peritoneal catheter was placed on January 10, 1984, for peritoneal dialysis. Hemodialysis was undertaken later. A sample of urine collected 10 days after the onset of ARF was processed for TEM study. On February 2, 1984, the patient was found in acute respiratory distress and a chest X ray revealed acute pulmonary edema and a left upper lobe infiltrate. He was started on broad spectrum antibiotics. On February 4, 1984, he developed a cardiopulmonary arrest. Resuscitation was attempted, but it was unsuccessful. At autopsy, renal tissue was fixed for conventional LM and TEM studies.

The TEM study of urinary sediment showed a segment of a glomerular capillary (Fig. 8-1), many plasma cells (Figs. 8-2 and 8-3), polymorphonuclear neutrophils, tubule cells, and moderate numbers of red blood cells (RBC). The characteristic finding, however, was the presence of nonperiodic fibrils (Figs. 8-3 and 8-4), with dark granules at the periphery. They were found inside the tubule cells and were thought to be consistent with light chain fibers. Conventional LM studies of the renal tissue showed many tubules with fractured or lamellated casts (Figs. 8-5 and 8-6), and some tubules with casts that showed cellular reactions (Fig. 8-7). Necrotic changes were found in an occasional glomerulus (Fig. 8-8), and plasma cells were found in the lumen of a few tubules. The TEM study of the renal tissue showed tubules changes consistent with ATN (Fig. 8-9).

Figure 8-2.   Many cells that appear to be plasma cells are seen. The eccentric position of the nucleus (arrows), the cartwheel appearance of the nuclear chromatin, the clear halo around the nucleus, the large amount of cytoplasm, and the multivesicular bodies (arrowheads) indicate that these are plasma cells. Many red blood cells (RBC) and platelets (P) are seen among the plasma cells. The striking feature of these cells is the presence of nonperiodic fibrils that may be light chain fibers (double arrows) (UA + LC, ×2,000).

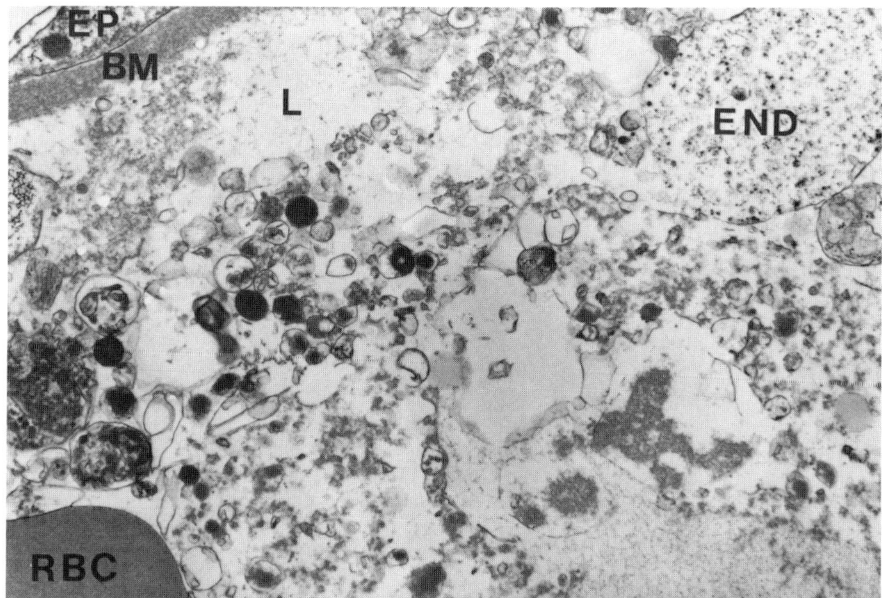

Figure 8-1.   This transmission electron micrograph shows a segment of a glomerular capillary characterized by the basement membrane (BM) and a portion of an epithelial cell (EP). Inside the capillary lumen (L), a swollen endothelial cell (END); fragments of inflammatory cell, as shown by granules; and a portion of a red blood cell (RBC) are seen (UA + LC, ×6,600).

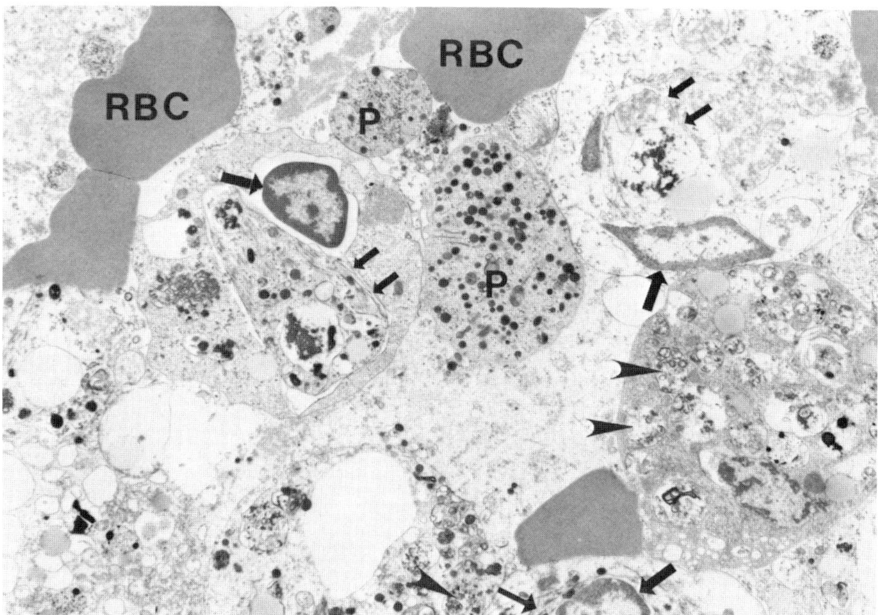

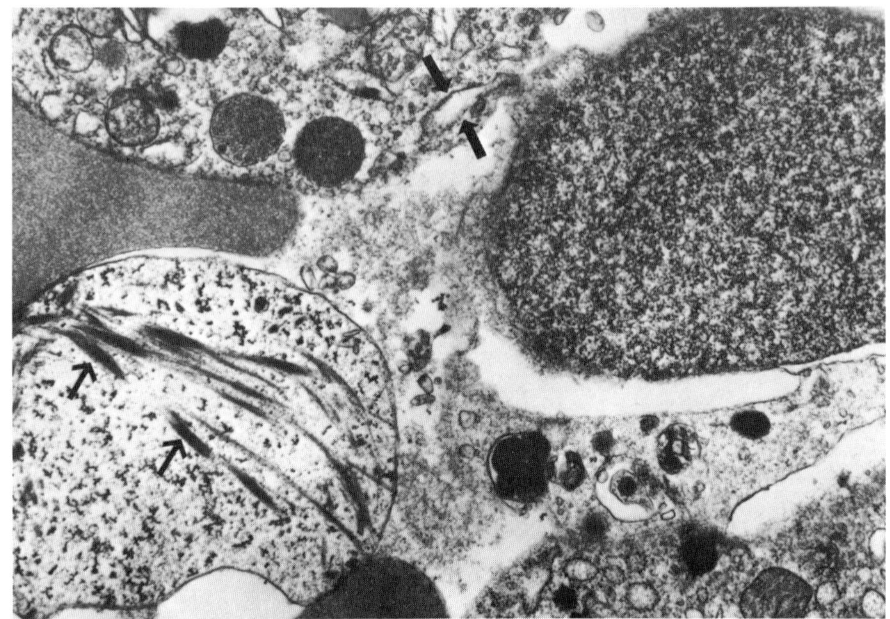

Figure 8-3. In this transmission electron micrograph, a portion of a plasma cell, characterized by dilated endoplasmic reticulum (between thick arrows), is seen. In the tubule cell are nonperiodic fibrils that may be light chain fibers (thin arrows) (UA + LC, ×8,300).

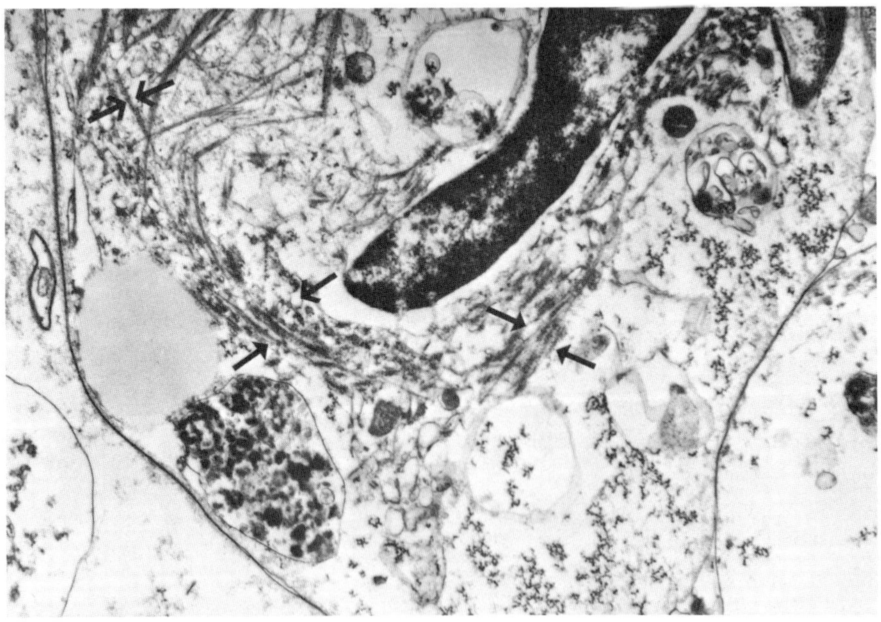

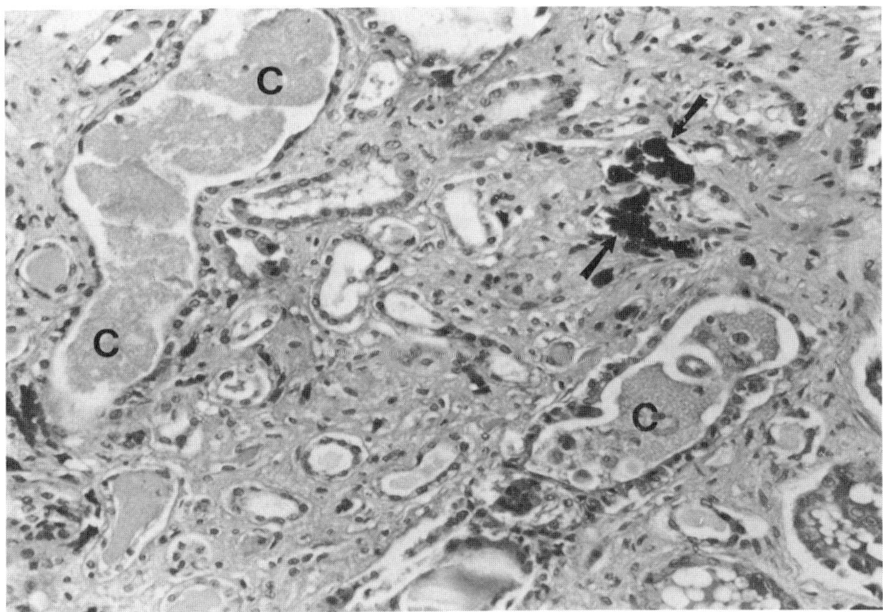

Figure 8-5.   This conventional light micrograph of renal tissue shows collecting tubules filled with fractured casts (C). The tubule epithelium is atrophic and flattened. There is a separation of the epithelium from the basement membranes in some Henle's loops; otherwise the tubules are intact. A large calcium deposit in the necrotic tubules is seen (between arrows) (H & E, ×200).

Comments: The presence of many tubule epithelial cells in the urinary sediment is consistent with ATN, as confirmed by the concomitant presence of ATN in the renal tissue examined by conventional LM and by TEM. The presence of many plasma cells in the urine suggests that circulating plasma cells were filtered and reaching the tubules. This was supported by the histological finding of plasma cells inside the tubules.

The significance of the plasmacyturia, whether as evidence of an advanced state of myeloma or as a diffuse involvement of the kidneys by myeloma, is unknown.

Until serial studies of urinary sediments from patients with multiple myeloma are done, the relationship of plasmacyturia to renal function cannot be determined. Similarly, the significance of nonbranching, nonperiodic fibrils,

Figure 8-4.   An unidentified cell contains nonperiodic fibrils, suggestive of light chain fibers, with granular material surrounding the fibrils (between arrows) (UA + LC, ×6,600).

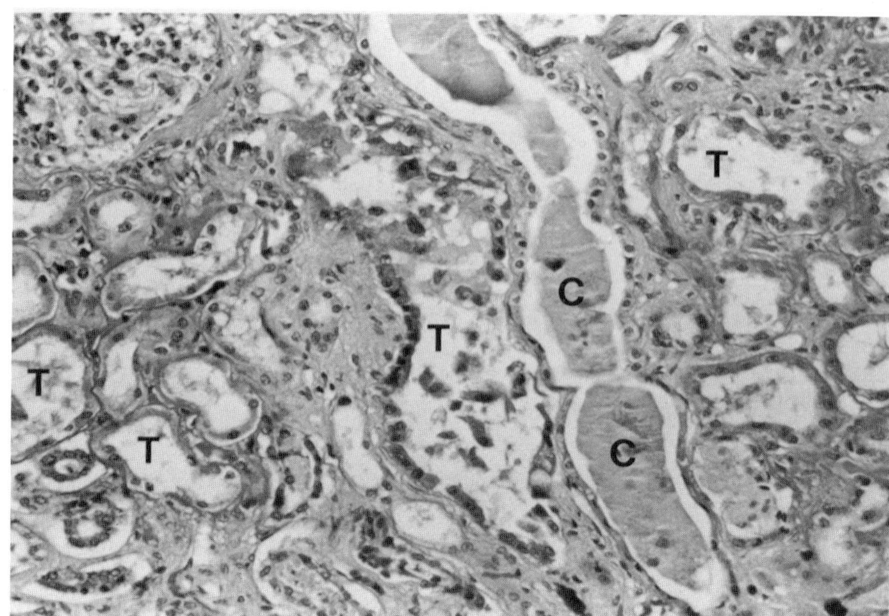

Figure 8-6.   In this light micrograph, a long dilated collecting tubule is filled with fractured cast (C). Most of the tubule lumina are dilated and the epithelium is somewhat flattened. Some tubules (T) appear to be necrotic (H & E, ×200).

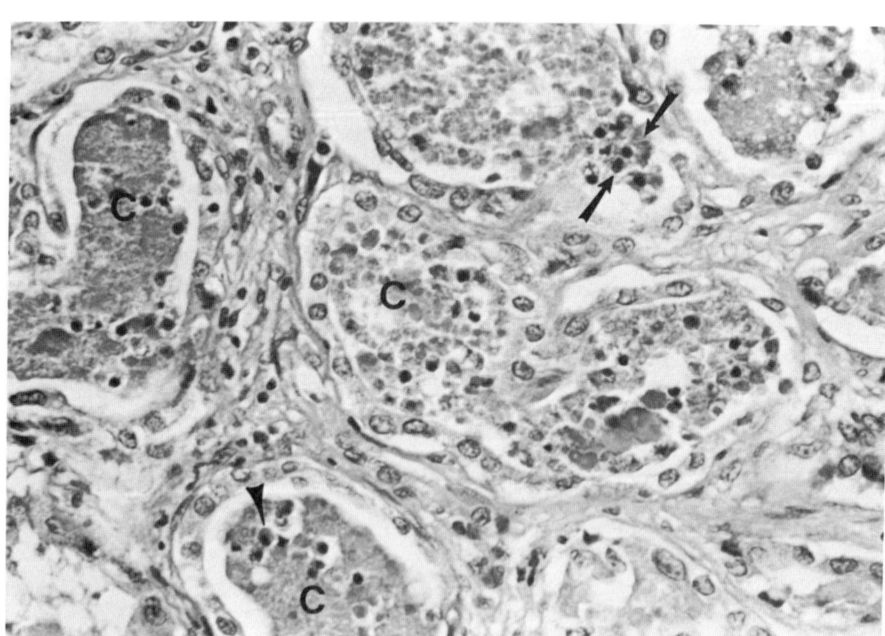

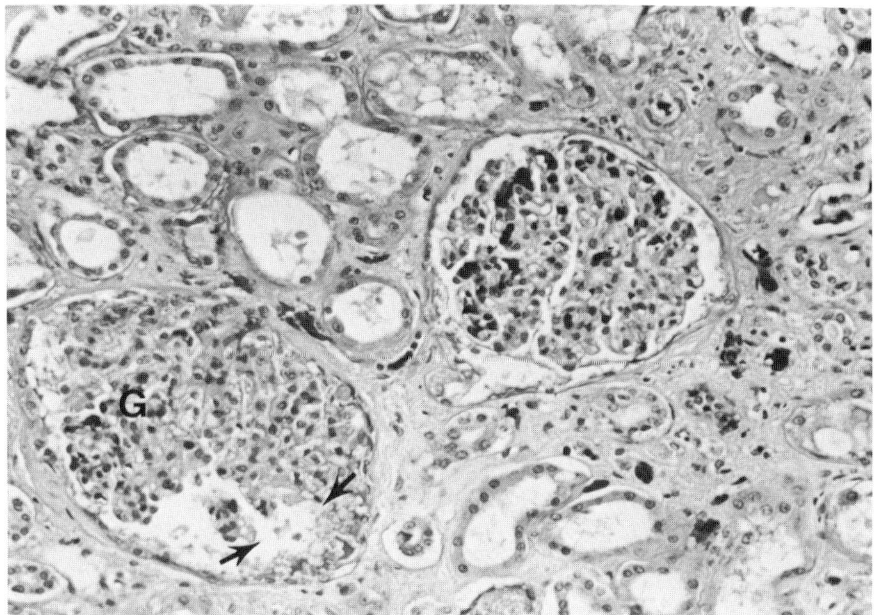

Figure 8-8. A glomerulus (G) shows adhesion with the Bowman's capsule, and partial necrosis (between arrows). The neighboring glomeruli appear to be intact (H & E, ×200).

which appear to be light chain fibers, inside tubule epithelial cells or neutrophilic leukocytes, is not known. It is prudent to mention that these fibrils may be precursors of amyloid fibrils.

The next patient is very interesting in that there were light chain fibers in his urinary sediment without evidence of overt myeloma.

Patient No. 2, J. B., a 62-yr-old black male with a long history of hypertension and gout, presented to his local physician with symptoms of dysuria in November 1984. Urinalysis showed pyuria. He was given a 10-day course of trimethoprim–sulfamethoxazole (Bactrim), with rapid resolution of the symptoms and pyuria, though he complained of a skin rash associated with the antibiotic. He next saw his local physician for a routine physical examination and was found to have 2^+ proteinuria and hematuria. In January 1985, he was admitted to the Urology Service of the Veterans Administration Medical Center, Augusta, Georgia, for evaluation of hematuria and benign prostatic hypertrophy. Physical examination was essentially normal, except for a blood pressure

Figure 8-7. In this section, the cast (C) shows a cellular reaction including a giant cell reaction (between arrows). Occasional plasma cells (arrowheads) are seen (H & E, ×200).

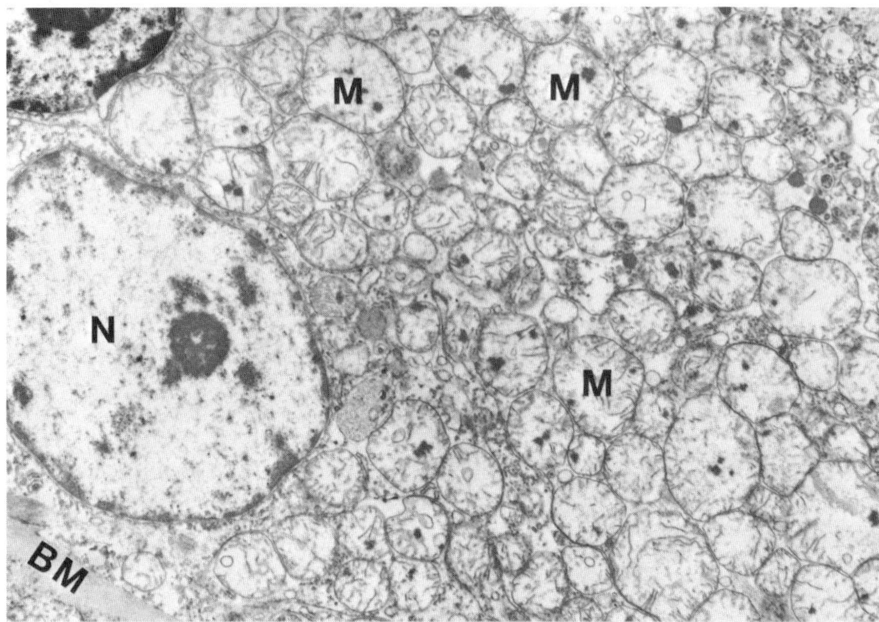

Figure 8-9. This transmission electron micrograph of a proximal tubule shows marked swelling, with loss of cristae in the majority of mitochondria (M). Many mitochondria contain amorphous dark bodies, though the location of the nucleus (N) is unaffected. The nucleus shows dissolution of chromatin material, but the nuclear membrane and the nucleolus appear intact, as does the basement membrane (BM) (UA + I C, ×3,300).

of 150/90 mm Hg. Renal evaluation at the that time included a serum urea nitrogen (SUN) of 35 mg/dl, a serum creatinine (Scr) of 2.9 mg/dl, and a 24-hr urinary study that showed a creatinine clearance of 48 cc/min and 2.0 g of protein (there was no history of prior renal disease). A renal sonogram, a bilateral retrograde pyelogram, and a cystogram, as well as serum protein electrophoresis and urine protein electrophoresis, were all normal. The patient underwent a transurethral prostatic resection (TURP) with only 1 of 35 "chips" positive for adenocarcinoma. The patient was discharged soon after the procedure and given the "usual" post-TURP three-day course of Bactrim orally. He came to the Renal Clinic at the Veterans Administration Medical Center for a routine follow-up approximately two weeks after discharge. Laboratory studies indicated further renal function deterioration, with a SUN of 64 mg/dl and a Scr of 4.1 mg/dl. He was admitted to the hospital with the presumptive diagnosis of acute interstitial nephritis secondary to Bactrim. No fever, skin rash, peripheral eosinophilia, or eosinophiluria was noted. A percutaneous renal biopsy attempt was unsuccessful. He was given a trial of corticosteroid (60 mg prednisone every morning) for four weeks. No appreciable change was noted in his renal function after therapy. An immunoelectrophoresis of urine was reported to be positive for free kappa and lambda light chains. He was readmitted to the VA Medical Center on

May 17, 1985, from the Renal Clinic for further evaluation of the original diagnosis and treatment of a metabolic acidosis. Admitting laboratory studies included SUN, 87 mg/dl; Scr, 4.4 mg/dl; serum sodium, 139 mEq/dl; serum potassium, 5.3 mEq/dl; serum chloride, 112 mEq/dl; and serum bicarbonate, 15 mEq/dl. Other studies included a serum uric acid, 10.8 mg/dl; serum phosphate, 5.1 mg/dl; and total serum protein, 5.6 g/dl. The complete blood count included a WBC of 14,000, with 82% segmented forms, 3% bands, 10% lymphocytes, and 5% monocytes. No eosinophils were noted. He had a hemoglobin of 12.2 g/dl and a hematocrit of 35.8%. The platelet count was 243×10^3. An electrocardiogram and a chest X ray were normal. The admission urinalysis showed a pH of 6.0, a specific gravity of 1.010, 2^+ protein, occasional WBC, and occasional granular casts. No eosinophils were found with Wright staining of the urine sediment. A sample of urine was collected for TEM study. No appreciable change in the patient's renal function was noted, and a repeat 24-hr urinary study showed a creatinine clearance of 20 cc/min and 0.5 g of protein; a repeat urine protein immunoelectrophoresis showed free kappa and lambda light chains, and a bone marrow biopsy showed less than 10% plasma cells. A percutaneous renal biopsy was performed and the tissue was fixed for LM, immunofluorescence (IFM), and TEM studies. The urine sample was processed for TEM study, as described in Chapters 1 and 2. The TEM study of urinary sediment showed many epithelial cells that appeared to be glomerular or parietal epithelial cells (Fig. 8-10), many multinucleated giant cells (Fig. 8-11), and nonbranching, nonperiodic fibrils

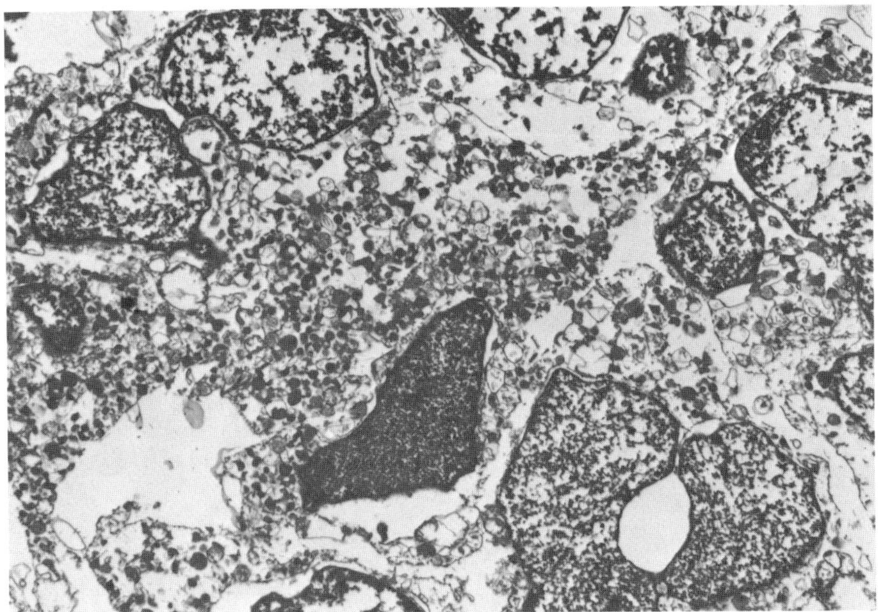

Figure 8-10. In this transmission electron micrograph of urinary sediment, the epithelial cells with large nuclei appear to be parietal epithelial cells of Bowman's membrane (UA + LC, ×5,000).

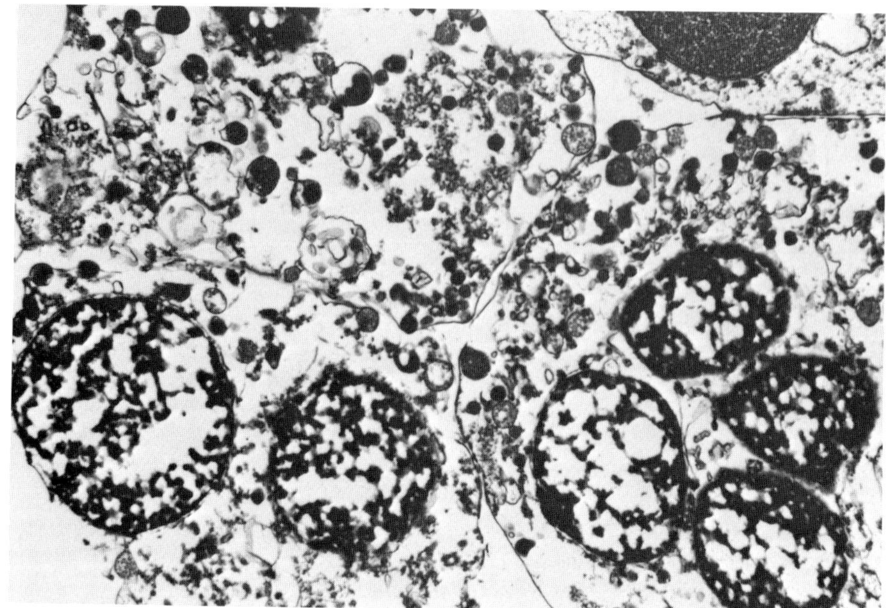

Figure 8-11. Many multinucleated giant cells are seen in this transmission electron micrograph. These cells may be derived from tubules as a reaction to light chain deposition in the tubules (UA + LC, ×7,500).

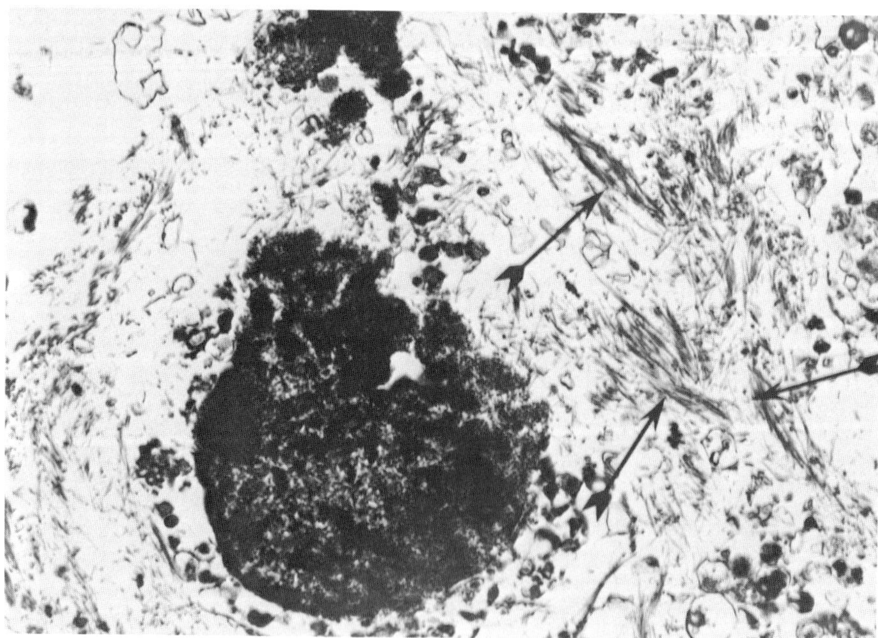

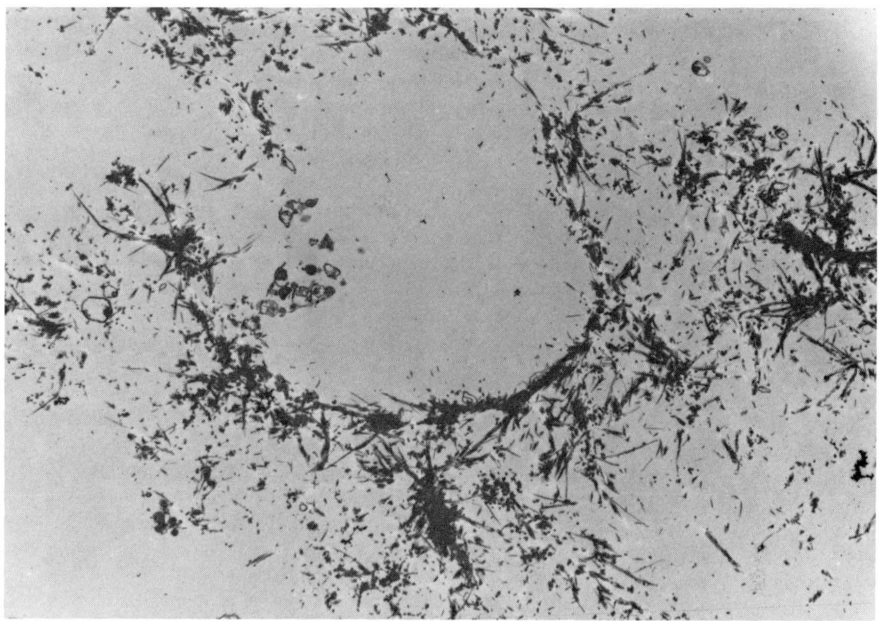

Figure 8-13.   The granular appearances of these bunches of nonperiodic fibrils suggests that they may be light chain fibers (UA + LC, ×5,000).

(Fig. 8-12). These fibrils appeared granular at the periphery and at the end and were thought to be light chain fibers (Fig. 8-13).

The LM study of the biopsied kidney showed nodular sclerotic changes in the glomeruli that resembled nodular diabetic glomerulosclerosis (Fig. 8-14). Staining with Congo red demonstrated dichroism (green birefringence) under polarized light in sclerotic nodule areas and in the arteriole walls. Many tubules contained casts that stained positively with Congo red and showed dichroism under polarized light.

The IFM study of the biopsied kidney demonstrated brilliant (4$^+$) positive staining for kappa light chain (Fig. 8-15) and faintly positive staining for lambda light chain in the mesangium and arteriolar walls. The TEM study of glomerular nodules showed a granular appearance at low magnification (Fig. 8-16) but a nonbranching fibrillar appearance at higher magnification. The basement membrane of the glomerular capillaries adjacent to the sclerotic nodules appeared darker than usual; however, discrete electron-dense deposits were not observed. The tubules uniformly revealed marked thickening and splitting of the basement membranes (Fig. 8-17). The most conspicuous change was found

Figure 8-12.   These nonperiodic, nonbranching fibrils (arrows) appear to be light chain fibers (UA + LC, ×10,000).

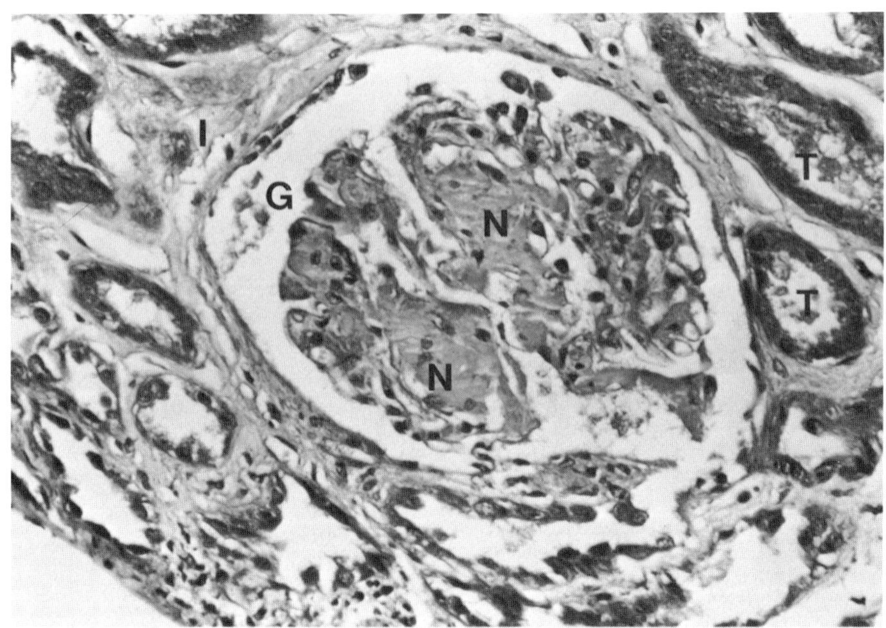

Figure 8-14. This light micrograph of a biopsy specimen shows a glomerulus (G) with mesangial nodules (N). The tubules (T) appear to be normal, though they are separated by conspicuous interstitium (I) (H & E, ×200).

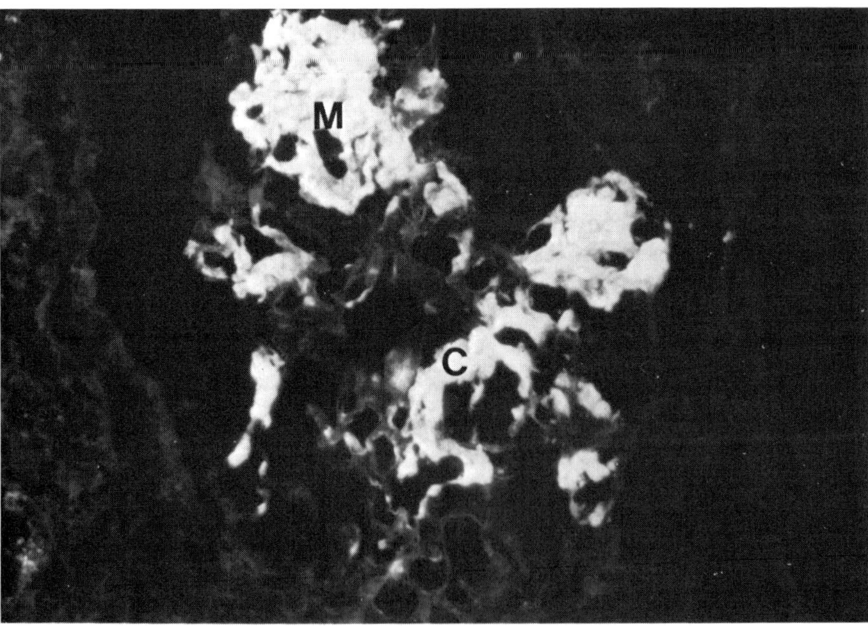

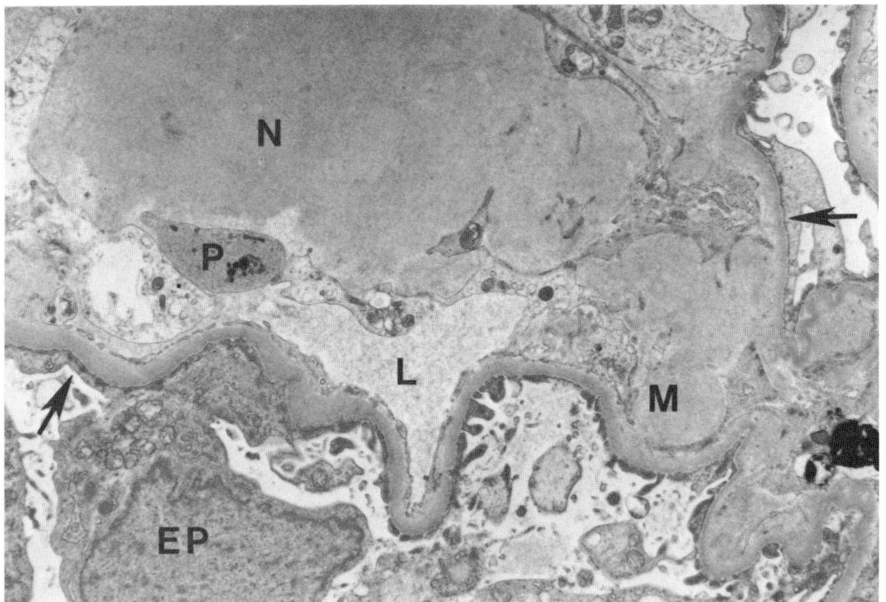

Figure 8-16.   A mesangial sclerotic nodule (N), in the mesangial area, occupies a large area of the capillary and almost obliterates the lumen (L). On close inspection and at higher magnification, nonbranching fibrils are seen. There is a moderate increase in the mesangial (M) matrix. Also seen is a segmental fusion of foot processes (arrows), but the epithelial cell (EP) appears to be normal (UA + LC, ×4,000).

in the interstitium, in which large amounts of collagen fibers, many fibroblasts, and few neutrophilic leukocytes were seen (Fig. 8-18).

Comments: The unexplained renal failure, proteinuria, and hyperchloremic nonanion gap metabolic acidosis led to a presumptive, diagnosis of myeloma for this patient. This was further supported by the presence of free light chains (kappa and lambda) in the urine and the finding of light chainlike fibers in the urinary sediment. The diagnosis of light chain nephropathy accompanied by amyloidosis was confirmed by the positive immunofluorescence for kappa and lambda light chains in the glomeruli and by the TEM finding of nonbranching fibrils in the glomeruli. The presence in the urinary sediment of many epithelial cells, with abundant mitochondria and large nuclei, that appeared to be parietal

Figure 8-15.   This immunofluorescent micrograph shows brilliantly positive (4⁺) kappa light chains in the mesangium (M) and in the peripheral capillary loops (C) (×400).

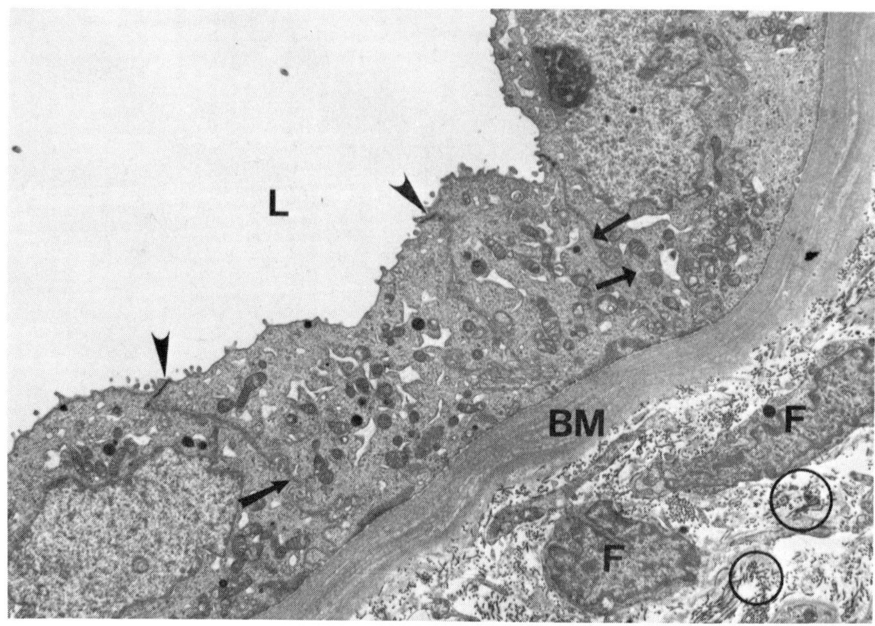

Figure 8-17.   This transmission electron micrograph shows a collecting tubule cell with rudimentary microvilli and fewer mitochondria. The cells, cuboidal in shape, are separated by irregularly shaped intercellular spaces (arrows) except at the most luminal part, where the lumen (L) is sealed off from the intercellular space by a tight junction (arrowheads). The striking feature is the marked thickening and splitting of the tubule basement membrane (BM). The interstitium shows two fibroblasts (F) and many collagen fibers (circles) (UA + LC, ×3,000).

or proximal tubule epithelial cells and many multinucleated giant cells was indirect evidence of proximal tubule injury. The latter possibility was clinically evident as hyperchloremic nonanion gap metabolic acidosis.

The distinctive feature in this patient was the presence of both kappa and lambda light chains in the urine and the presence of amyloid in the glomeruli and vessels in the absence of overt myeloma. Light chain nephropathy (LCN) has been associated with the deposition of one subclass of light chain, kappa light chain, in most cases.[2] Thus far, there is only one report of LCN in which both kappa and lambda light chains were demonstrated.[3] The significance of the positive staining for amyloid in the patient presented here, as well as in a patient reported in the literature,[3] is not clear. Whether the presence of both kappa and lambda light chains involves a different pathogenesis and course than of kappa light chain alone in LCN also remains to be determined. The type of light chain in the fibrils in the urinary sediment could not be determined. This finding, however, suggests that further investigation, such as immunoelectron microscopy of urinary sediments from patients with myeloma, be undertaken to elucidate the presence of kappa and/or lambda fibers in the urine (see also Chapter 9).

Patient No. 3, J.R., a 66-year-old black male, was admitted to the Veterans Administration Medical Center, Augusta, Georgia, on May 4, 1985, with the complaint of spiking fever of 104–105°F. Six days before this admission, he was admitted to the Self Memorial Hospital, Greenwood, South Carolina, with a history of bleeding from the nose and hemoptysis. A complete blood count there showed total WBC, 1,000/mm^3, with 16% segmented neutrophils, 2% bands, 78% lymphocytes, and 2% monocytes. A bone marrow biopsy revealed increased cellularity, with the majority of cells in the myelocytic series and prominent maturation arrest at the promyelocytic stage. Urinalysis showed 1$^+$ blood. Upon admission to the Veterans Administration Medical Center, his a complete blood count showed hemoglobin, 10.9 g/dl; hematocrit, 31.8%; total WBC, 1100/mm^3; segmented neutrophil, 12%; bands, 2%; lymphocytes, 77%; monocytes, 8%; and eosinophils, 1%. The platelet count was 84,000/mm^3. Urinalysis showed pH 6.0, protein trace, blood 1$^+$, and an occasional WBC.

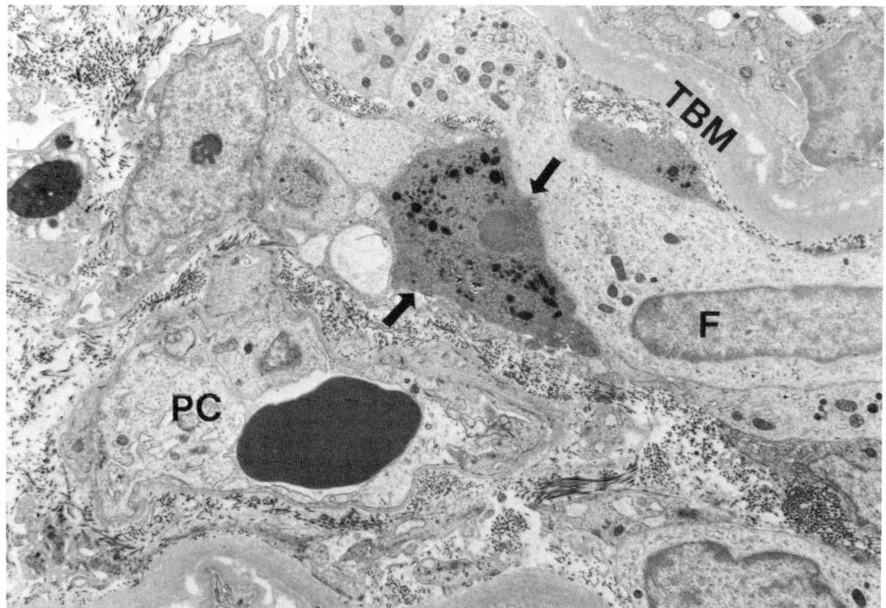

Figure 8-18.   A very conspicuous interstitium containing a fibroblast (F), a neutrophilic leukocyte (between arrows), abundant collagen fibers, and a peritubular capillary (PC) can be seen. Again, there is a marked thickening of the tubule basement membrane (TBM) (UA + LC, ×3,000).

The patient had been treated with Dyazide (hydrochlorothiazide 25 mg and triamterene 50 mg), one tablet daily, from April 1983. For a possible but undocumented diagnosis of septicemia, he was treated with numerous antibiotics from May 5 through May 28, 1985. Some of these antibiotics include gentamicin (May 5 through May 13), clindamycin (May 5 through May 21), amikacin (May 8 through May 13), and carbenicillin (one dose, May 25). His serial serum potassium (K), serum urea nitrogen (SUN), and serum creatinine (Scr) are shown below.

Date (1985)	Serum K(mEq/liter)	SUN (mg/dl)	Scr (mg/dl)
May 4	4.1	14	1.4
May 16	5.3	22	2.5
May 18	5.3	35	3.4
(urine sample collected for TEM analysis)			
May 20	4.4	48	4.3
May 22	3.7	39	3.6
May 24	3.9	30	2.9
May 27	3.9	26	2.7

The patient died on May 28th. The final diagnosis was acute promyelocytic leukemia.

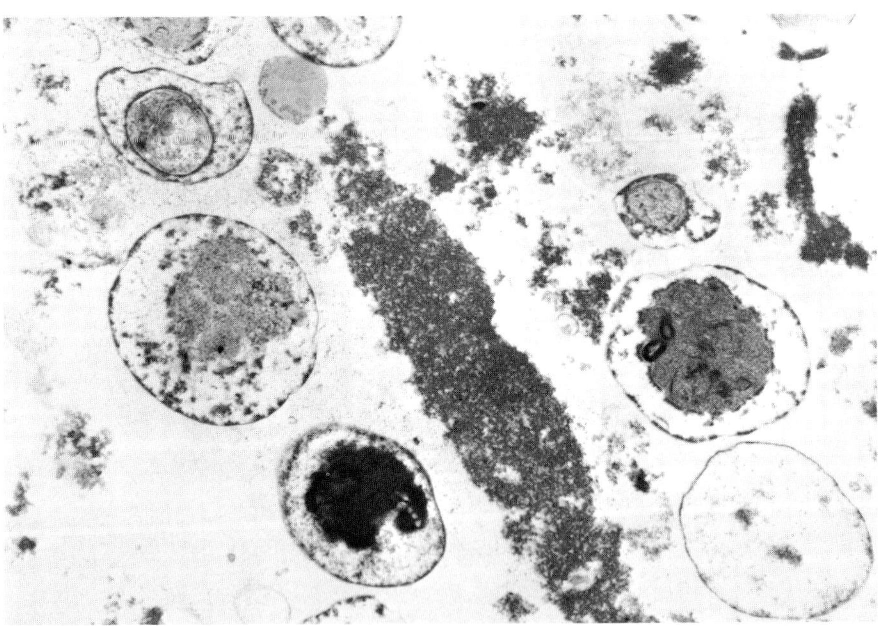

Figure 8-19.   This transmission micrograph shows a hyaline cast consisting of a smooth homogeneous matrix. Also shown are numerous secondary lysosomes (UA + LC, ×10,000).

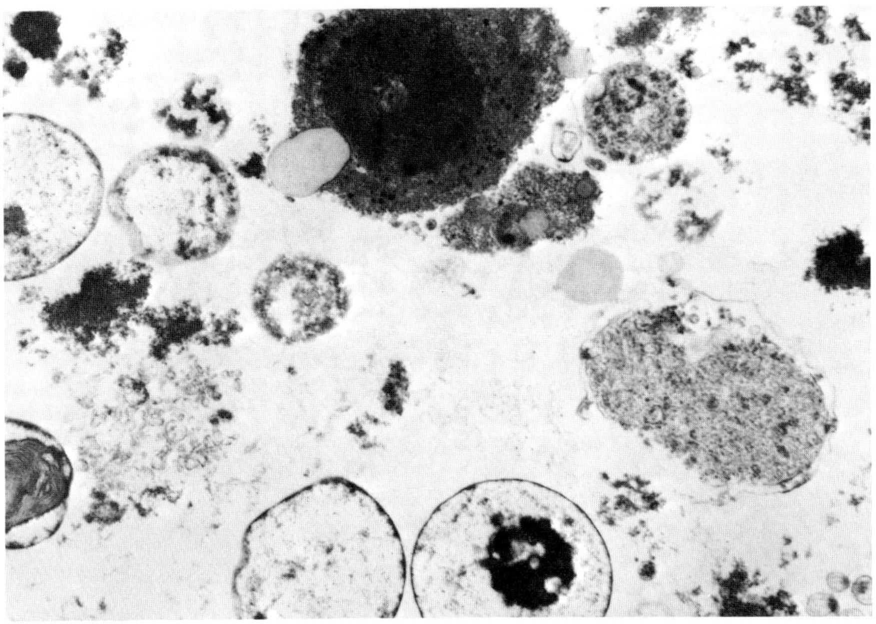

Figure 8-20.   An electron micrograph of a secondary lysosome (UA + LC, × 10,000).

Comments: The TEM study of urinary sediment showed a hyaline cast (Fig. 8-19), an epithelial cast, and numerous lysosomes of different sizes and shapes. A lysosome is a membrane-bounded particle containing a number of hydrolytic enzymes. It is difficult to describe the typical morphology of this organelle because of the structural heterogeneity of the cytoplasmic bodies. Some morphologists separate them into primary and secondary lysosomes, whereby fusion of a primary lysosome with a particle brought into the cell from outside produces a secondary lysosome. The secondary lysosome is a pleomorphic and is shown in Figs. 8-20–8-24. Some of the lysosomes had membranes, and some of the lysosomes were intermediate between lysosomes and lipofuscin pigments (the latter are large lobulated structures that contain vacuoles, membranous lamellae, and possibly, protein droplets). The patient had many abnormal leukocytes with abundant lysosomes (Figs. 8-25–8-27).

Patient No. 4, C. C., a 76-year-old white male, was admitted to the Veterans Administration Medical Center, Augusta, Georgia, on August 9, 1985, with the complaints of nausea, vomiting and weakness. One month before admission, he was found to have acute myelogenous leukemia, with leukocytosis. He had been put on allopurinol (300 mg daily) to block purine biosynthesis and to protect against uric acid nephropathy. Upon admission to the hospital, he showed evidence of a mild renal dysfunction, but

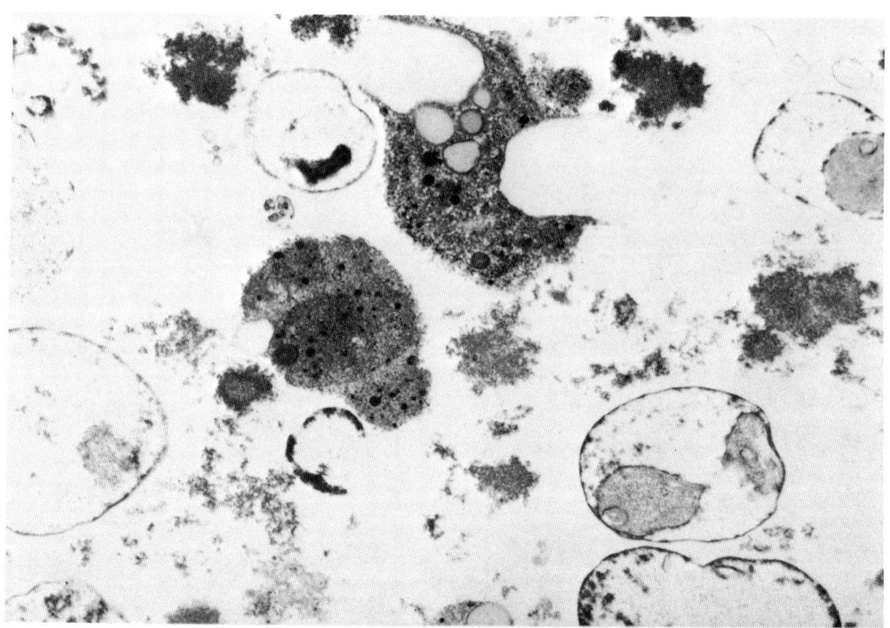

Figure 8-21.   An electron micrograph of a secondary lysosome (UA + LC, ×10,000).

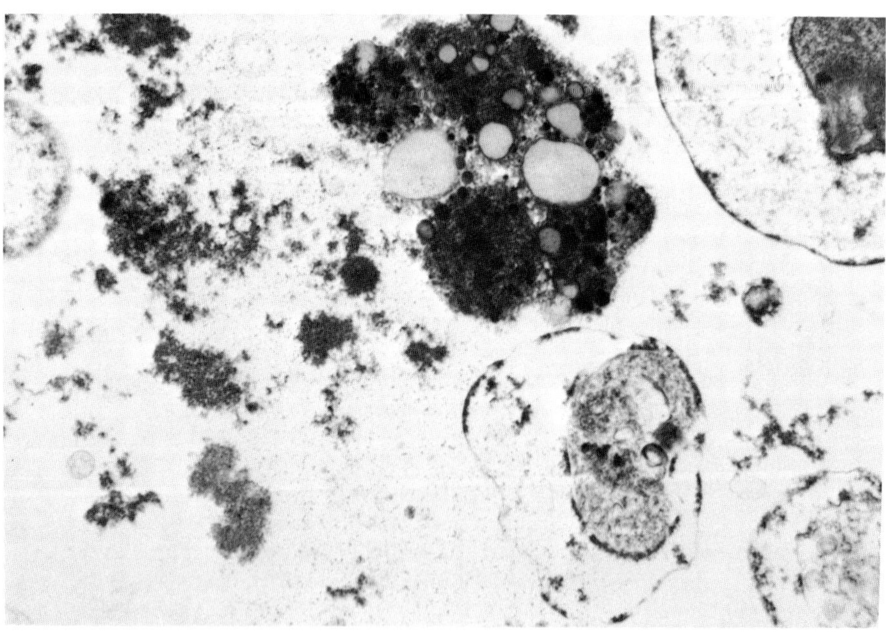

Figure 8-22.   An electron micrograph of a secondary lysosome (UA + LC, ×13,000).

following chemotherapy with arabinoside C and m-AMSA, his renal function deteriorated further. It returned to baseline levels after treatment with fluids, bicarbonate, and furosemide. He also manifested gross hematuria, however, which gradually cleared with the above treatment.

Terminally, he showed progressive deterioration of renal function, which did not respond to therapy. His serial serum potassium (serum K^+), serum urea nitrogen (SUN), and serum creatinine (Scr) levels are shown below.

Date (1985)	Serum K^+	SUN (mg/dl)	Scr (mg/dl)
August 9	3.4	18	2.3
August 12	4.3	Not available	2.7
August 13	3.3	13	3.1
August 17	3.5	44	3.2
August 19	3.5	32	2.4
August 22	3.7	43	2.6
August 26	3.9	30	2.2
	(urine sample collected for TEM analysis)		
August 29	5.4	60	3.3
August 30	4.2	91	5.1

The patient developed acute respiratory distress. A bronchoscopy on August 30, 1985, revealed a mucus plug secondary to *Candida* infection. He became obtunded and died on August 30, 1985.

The urinary sediment TEM study showed proximal and distal tubule cells. The tubule cells showed mitochondrial swelling, with loss of cristae, and some mitochondria that contained amorphous dark bodies (Fig. 8-28). The most striking feature of the study was the presence of excessive numbers of cellular lysosomes (Figs. 8-29 and 8-30).

Comments: The urinary sediment findings are consistent with ATN. The excessive number of lysosomes in tubule cells might have been caused by the aminoglycosides used to treat the unconfirmed sepsis. It is interesting that this patient, like patient No. 3, showed low normal or below normal serum potassium despite azotemia.

FEATURES OF THESE CASES

Two features are of interest in the two cases presented. These are hypokalemia and renal failure. Serum potassium levels were low normal or below normal, despite renal dysfunction in both cases. Patient No. 3 was given triamterene (Dyazide: hydrochlorothiazide and triamterene), which is known to cause hyperkale-

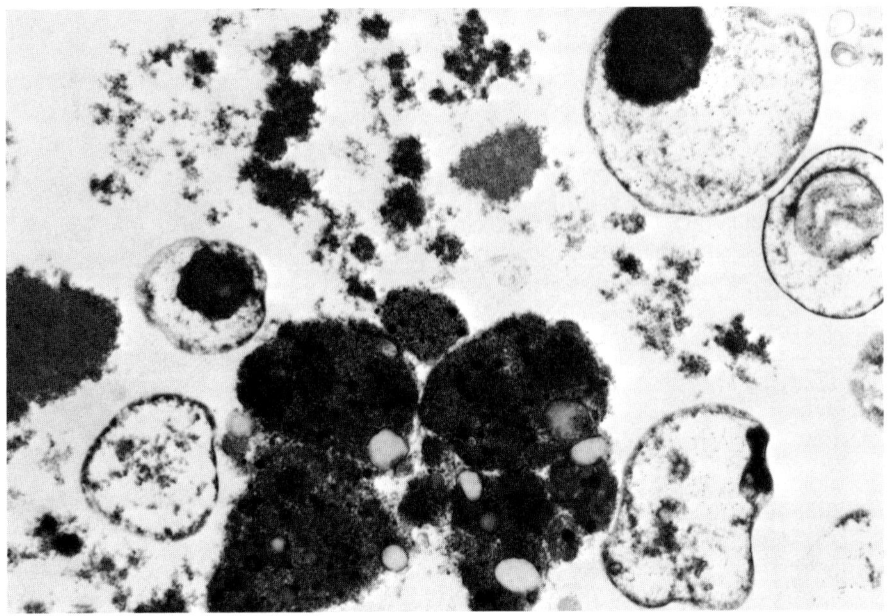

Figure 8-23. An electron micrograph of a secondary lysosome (UA + LC, ×10,000).

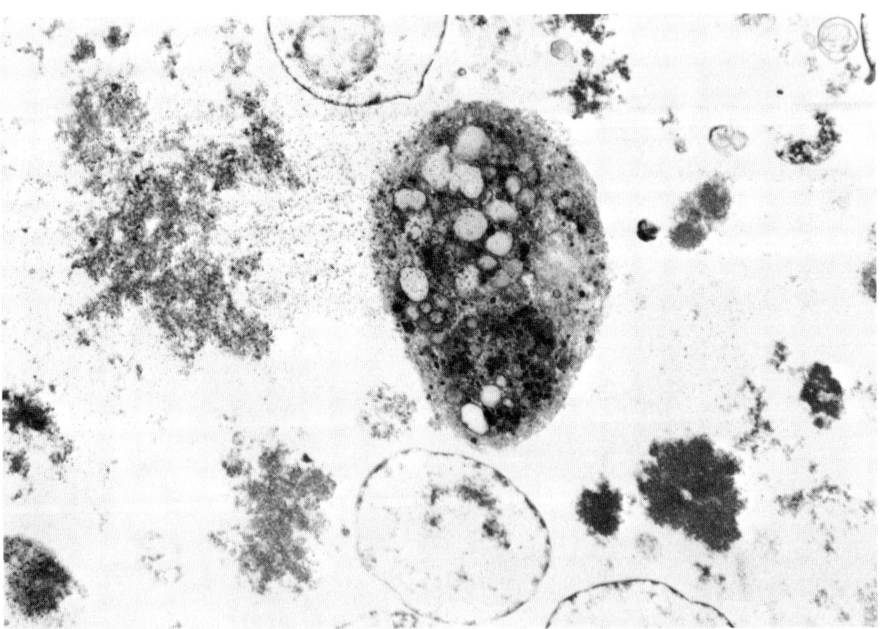

Figure 8-24. An electron micrograph of a secondary lysosome (UA + LC, ×10,000).

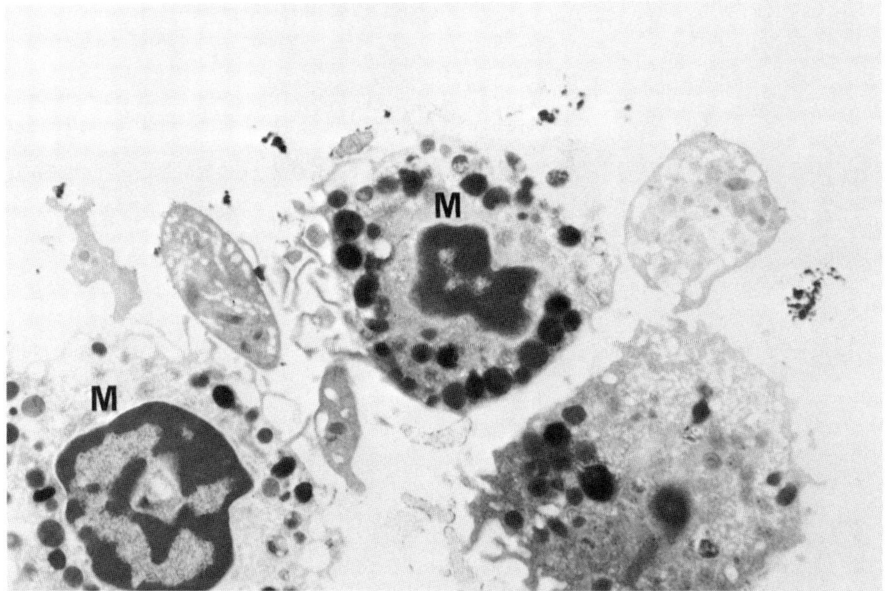

Figure 8-25. This transmission electron micrograph shows two myelocytes (M) with conspicuous lysosome granules (UA + LC, ×7,500).

mia, especially in the presence of renal failure. His urinary sediment showed granular and epithelial casts and tubule epithelial cells, which are consistent with ATN. The excessive numbers of free lysosomes in the urinary sediment and in the tubule epithelial cells was striking. This finding could be significant in (1) the relationship of urinary lysosomes to hypokalemia, (2) the relationship of lysosomes to lysozymuria, and (3) the relationship of lysosomes to ARF.

The Relationship of Urinary Lysosome to Hypokalemia

It has been proposed by several investigators that lysozymuria in acute myeloid leukemia accounts for the kaluresis and the hypokalemia.[4-7] Lysozyme, a low molecular weight protein, is excreted in excessive amounts in the urine in patients with acute myeloid leukemia. However, the serum lysozyme level is also elevated. A study in chloroleukemic rats has shown that prolonged elevation in serum lysozyme levels only can produce detectable lysozymuria accompanied by kaluresis.[6] Furthermore, once lysozymuria has begun, renal loss of lysozyme and potassium often persist after the serum lysozyme level has returned to normal. This animal experiment also may explain the high incidence of lysozymuria and

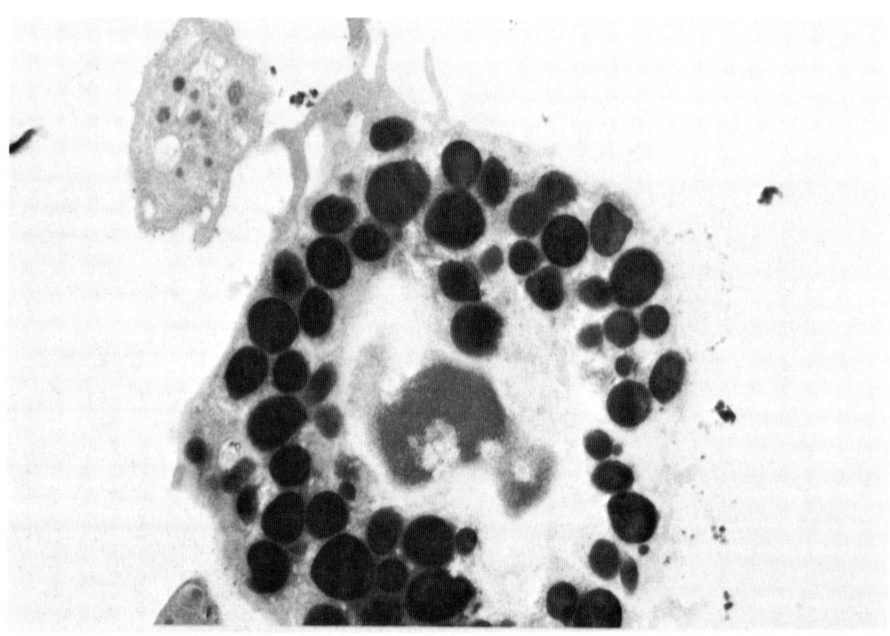

Figure 8-26.   A magnified view of a myelocyte. This immature neutrophil, with its content of lysosomal granules, is very conspicuous (UA + LC, ×10,000).

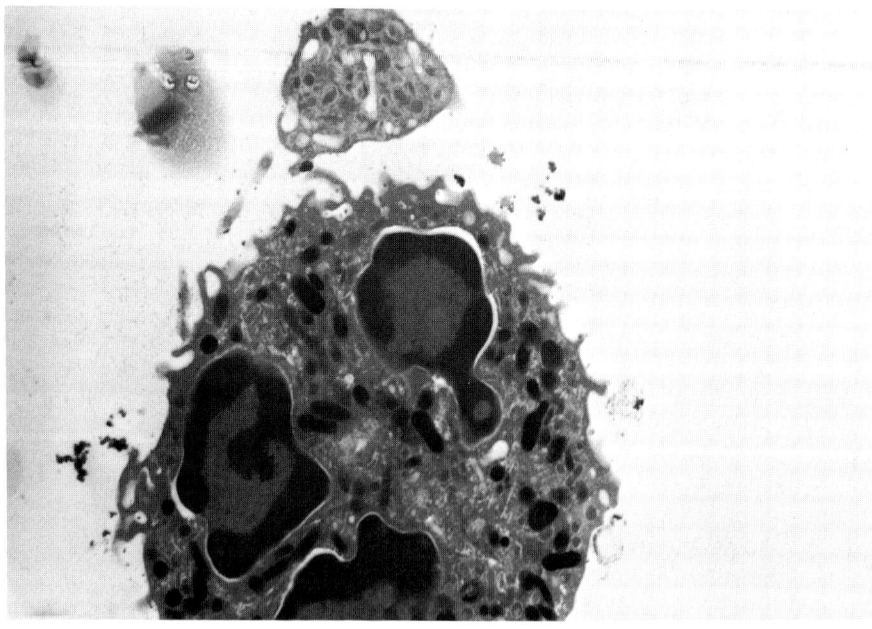

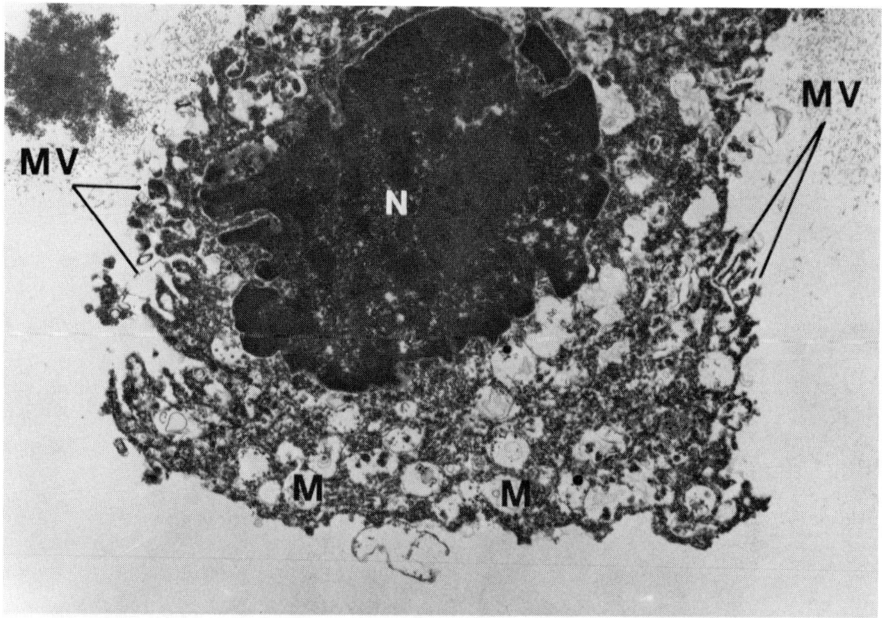

Figure 8-28. This transmission electron micrograph shows a proximal tubule cell with microvilli (MV) and many mitochondria. All mitochondria (M) are swollen and devoid of cristae, but the nucleus (N) is intact (UA + LC, ×7,500).

hypokalemia in patients with myeloproliferative disorders terminating in acute leukemia.

Although it is generally agreed that lysozymuria causes hypokalemia in acute myelocytic leukemia, the reason for renal loss of potassium is not known. In an experiment using isolated rat kidney,[7] purified human muramidase (lysozyme) was added after a control 40-min perfusion. The glomerular filtration rate (^{14}C-inulin), urinary sodium, and urinary potassium were determined in successive 10-min periods. At increasing concentrations of muramidase, muramidase excretion increased linearly as the filtered load increased. When muramidase was added to the perfusion medium, there was an immediate increase in urinary potassium excretion in the first 10-min collection period, which persisted for the remaining 30 to 60 min of perfusion. This increase in potassium excretion was observed at all concentrations of muramidase, but the highest

Figure 8-27. In this neutrophilic leukocyte, the lysosome granules appear normal (UA + LC, ×7,500).

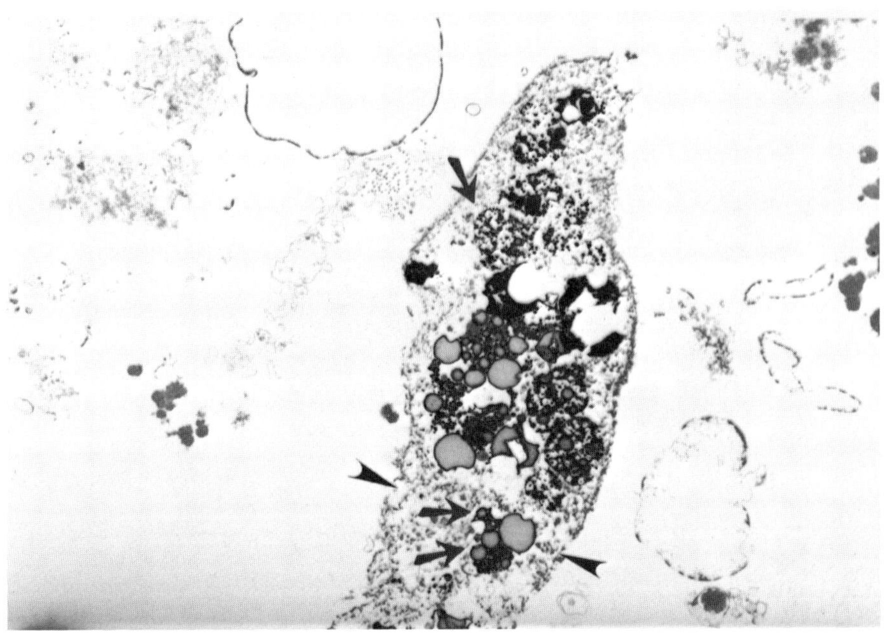

Figure 8-29.   This tubule epithelial cell is rich in both primary (single arrow) and secondary (double arrows) lysosomes. Disruptions (arrowheads) of the cellular membrane can be seen (UA + LC, ×4,000).

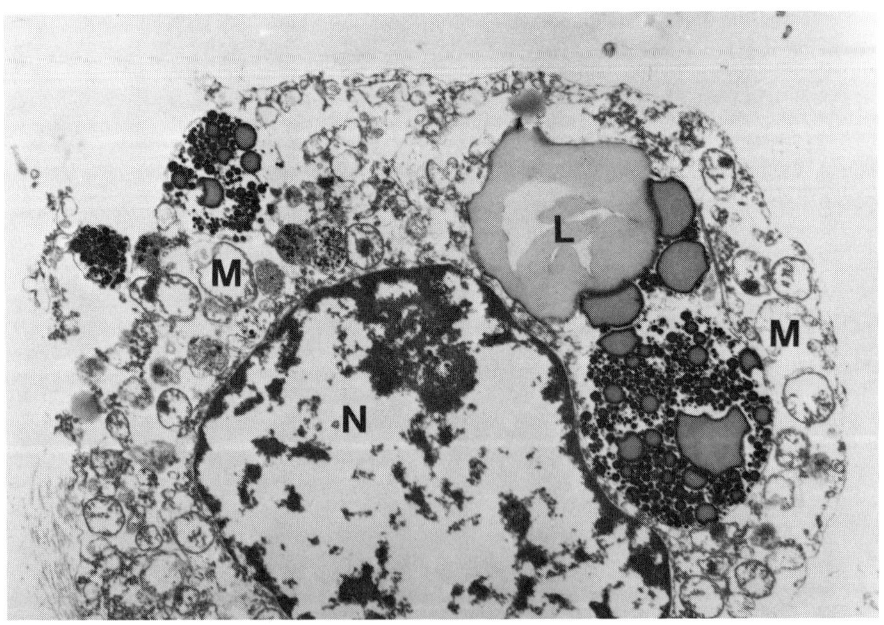

doses of muramidase did not further enhance excretion of potassium, so that the urinary/plasma potassium/urinary/plasma inulin ratio did not exceed one. Histochemically, there was intense lysozyme staining in the lining of the proximal tubule cells. The glomeruli or distal tubule cells, took up little or no stain, but some positively staining material was found in the collecting tubule lumina. This experiment thus provides evidence that lysozyme accumulates in the proximal tubules and that an increase in filtered lysozyme is associated with an increase in urinary potassium excretion. It does not, however, provide evidence that the enhanced secretion of potassium produces kaluresis. More importantly, the lysozyme-rich proximal tubule is not the potassium secretion site.

Other mechanism(s) to explain kaluresis and hypokalemia were investigated. That potassium wasting is the result of an antibiotic-induced renal dysfunction is unlikely, since it seems to depend on alterations in renin–aldosterone secretion.[8]

The Relationship of Urinary Lysosome to Lysozymuria

A review of the literature reveals that lysosome is the source of lysozyme, as shown in the following brief summary of the study in rats by Ottosen, Bode, and Madsen.[9]

After a single IV injection of ^{125}I-labeled lysozyme, the blood concentration of the protein was followed under experimental conditions that simulated an increased or a decreased transtubular transport of protein, which rapidly increased the blood level of ^{125}I-lysozyme in recipient rats. Determination of radioactivity in subcellular fractions isolated from the kidney cortex was by differential centrifugation 30 min after injection and revealed an accumulation of ^{125}I-lysozyme in the lysosomal fraction. The labeled lysozyme was found to be enriched 4.1 times, and acid phosphatase was enriched 3.3 times, in the lysosomal fraction compared to the homogenate. In the control experiments in which ^{125}I-lysozyme was added to kidney cortical homogenates from noninjected animals, ^{125}I-lysozyme was not enriched in the lysosomal fraction. Electron-microscope autoradiography of proximal tubules revealed that most grains were located over lysosomes or endocytic vacuoles. Of a total 911 grains, 80.1% were located over the lysosomes and L-cytoplasm (cytoplasm within 0.5 μ from the lysosomes), and 14.9% were located over endocytic vacuoles and EV-cytoplasm

Figure 8-30. This tubule epithelial cell, like the preceding one, is rich in lysosomes. A membrane-bound primary lysosome (L) shows the attachment of membrane-bound bodies. The cell is necrotic, as evidenced by the dissolution of the nuclear (N) chromatin and the swelling of the mitochondria (M), with loss of cristae (UA + LC, ×7,500).

(cytoplasm within 0.5 μ from the endocytic vacuoles). This study confirms and extends the view that lysozyme filtered in the glomeruli is reabsorbed in the proximal tubule by endocytosis and is transferred to the lysosomes, where it can be catabolized. In our study, we found excessive numbers of lysosomes in the distal and collecting tubule cells of patient No. 4. That these tubule cells secrete potassium implies an association among lysosomes, lysozymuria, and kaluresis.

The Relationship of Urinary Lysosome to Renal Failure

Again, the two cases presented here demonstrate renal dysfunction and an excessive number of free lysosomes in the urine or of lysosomes in the distal tubule cells. As in hypokalemia, it can be asked whether the lysosomes in the urine or tubule cells contributed to the development of ARF in these cases, as well as in other patients, with acute myelocytic leukemia and ARF.

In another experiment, an intravenous infusion of egg white lysozyme into male Wistar and Wistar/Furth rats for different periods of time achieved plasma levels of lysozyme in the range of 30 to 8,000 mg/ml. A plasma lysozyme level of 700 to 3,000 mg/ml significantly increased the fractional excretion of sodium and potassium, though the glomerular filtration rate (GFR) did not change. Lysozyme infusion for over 30 min led to oliguria and a subsequent anuria. After 60 minutes of lysozyme infusion, the observed morphological changes appeared to be related to the plasma lysozyme level; these included alteration of glomerular podocytes and cast obliteration of most of the tubules. At a plasma lysozyme level of 6,700 mg/ml, precipitated protein blocked the lumina of almost all tubular segments. At a plasma lysozyme level of 8,200 mg/ml, the urinary space was filled with a solid mass of precipitated protein and all the tubules were obstructed by vacuolized casts.[10] Tubular obstruction by the lysozyme-induced casts, obviously, would lead to oliguria and azotemia. From these experiments, one may infer that urinary excretion of excessive numbers of lysosomes and the consequent lysozymuria are in some way related to hypokalemia and ARF, though the exact mechanisms are not known.

Patient No. 5, S. A., a 59-year-old white male, was admitted to the Veterans Administration Medical Center, Augusta, Georgia, on May 1, 1984, with the complaints of shortness of breath, cough productive of yellowish sputum, fever, and poor appetite. Multiple myeloma had been diagnosed in 1977. Physical examination revealed a blood pressure of 130/80 mm Hg; pulse, 88/min; regular respiration, 28/min and labored; and a temperature of 100.7°F. Upon examination of the lungs, bilateral rales and rhonchi were heard over the lower lungs fields. Laboratory studies showed serum urea nitrogen (SUN) 62 mg/dl, serum creatinine (Scr) 9.0 mg/dl, serum sodium 132 mEq/liter, serum potassium 4.8 mEq/liter, serum chloride 100 mEq/liter, serum CO_2 22 mEq/liter, serum phosphate 7.4 mg/dl, and serum calcium 8.3 mg/dl. Urinalysis showed 4^+ protein, 2^+ blood, 0–3 WBC in a high power field, and 4^+ bacteria. Gram stain of the sputum showed many neutrophilic leukocytes and a moderate number of gram-positive diplococci. A chest X ray revealed bilateral infiltration of the lower lobes. Serum immunoelectrophoresis showed IgG-lambda type with IgG level of 7000 mg/dl. Subsequent chemotherapy consisted of vincristine, prednisone, and melphalan. The patient's SUN and Scr continued to increase. On May 10th, his SUN and Scr were 92 mg/dl and 17.6 mg/dl, respectively. Another urinalysis showed 18–19 WBC in a high power field. A sample of urine was collected for TEM analysis, and hemodialysis was started.

The TEM study of urinary sediment showed numerous plasma cells and neutrophilic leukocytes (Figs. 8-31–8-34). No bacteria, no casts, and no tubule epithelial cells were observed.

Comments: The absence of casts or renal tubule cells argue against ATN as the cause of renal failure in this patient. The presence of few neutrophilic leukocytes in the absence of bacteria does not suggest urinary tract infection. The plasmacyturia, with some plasma cells showing degenerative changes, implies tubule infiltration by plasma cells, as in patient No. 1.

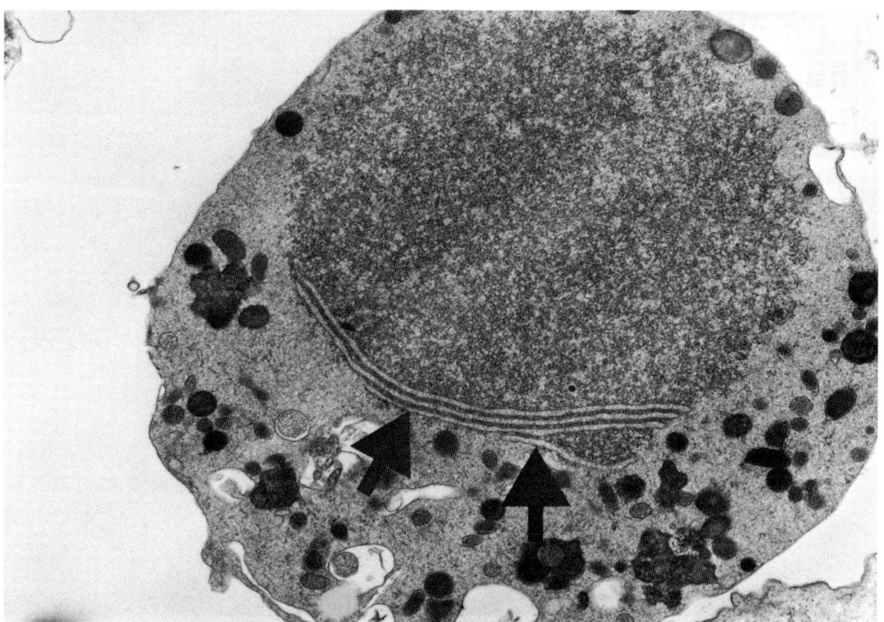

Figure 8-31. The endoplasmic reticulum (arrows) of this plasma cell is highly developed (UA + LC, ×6,600).

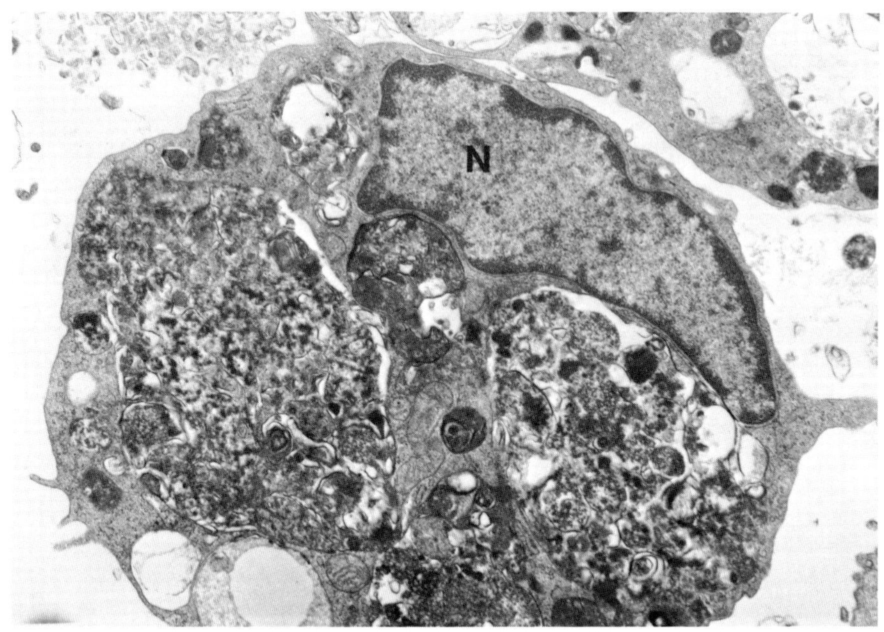

Figure 8-32.   Shown is a plasma cell with an eccentric nucleus (N) (UA + LC, ×5,000).

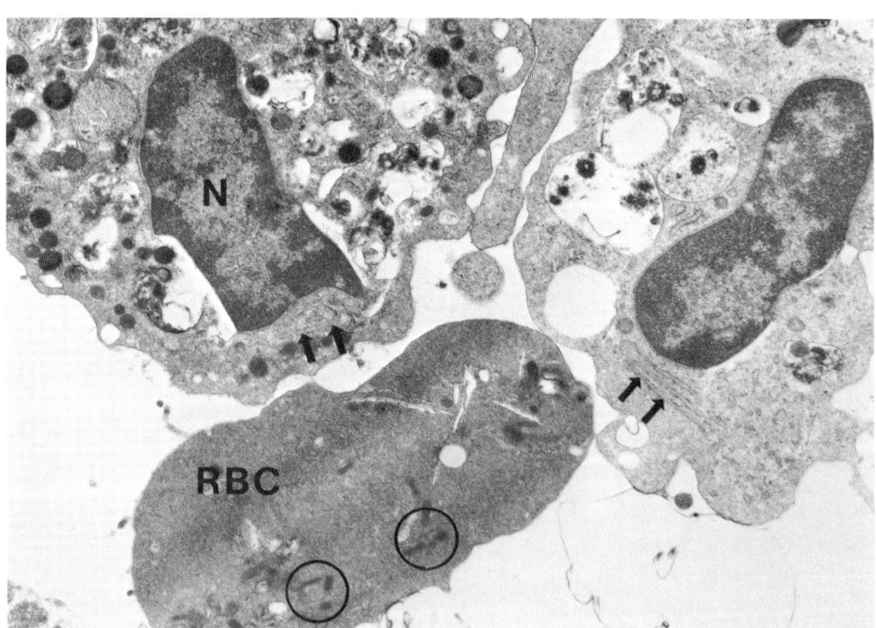

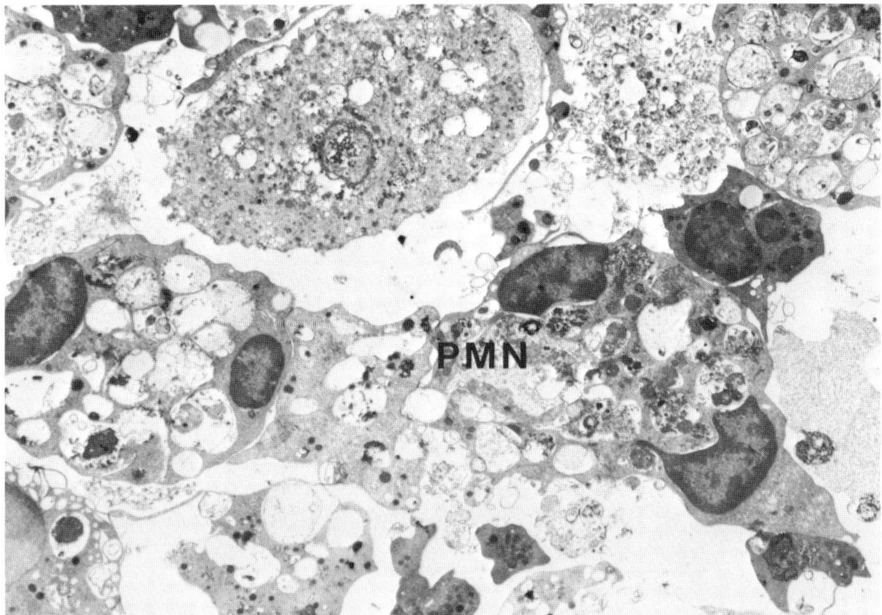

Figure 8-34.   This transmission electron micrograph shows a neutrophilic leukocyte (PMN), almost in the form of a macrophage. Several other neutrophilic leukocytes can be seen (UA + LC, ×2,000).

URINARY SEDIMENT TEM IN PATIENTS WITH MALIGNANCY

Acute or chronic renal failure is a common event in patients with malignancy, and TEM can be used to demonstrate findings that are consistent with ATN. Since urinary tract obstruction often leads to ARF, a TEM study of urinary sediment that revealed ATN would save unnecessary investigations. In myeloma patients, TEM seems to be unique in revealing the presence of plasma cells in urinary sediment. Whereas, plasmacyturia has been found to be associated with advanced myeloma, its absence may rule out a diagnosis of overt myeloma. Thus, urinary sediment TEM can be used to distinguish light chain nephropathy from kidney disease in overt myeloma.

←————————————————————————————————

Figure 8-33.   In this transmission electron micrograph, two plasma cells, one with an eccentric nucleus (N), are seen. Both have a prominent endoplasmic reticulum (arrows). Also seen is a red blood cell (RBC), with mitochondria (circles), which appear to be fibrillar. The latter signify hemolysis (UA + LC, ×5,000).

REFERENCES

1. Mandal AK, Sklar AH, Hudson JB: Transmission electron microscopy of urinary sediment in human acute renal failure. *Kidney Int* 1985; 28:58–63.
2. Geneval D, Noel LD, PreudHomme JL, Droz D, Grunfeld JP: Light chain deposition disease: Its relation with AL-type amyloidosis. *Kidney Int* 1984; 26:1–9.
3. Alpers CE, Hopper J, Biava CG: Light chain glomerulopathy with amyloid-like deposits. *Hum Pathol* 1984; 15:444–448.
4. Mir MA: Lysozyme: A brief review. *Postgrad Med J* 1977; 53:257.
5. Mir MA, Brabin B, Tang OT, *et al:* Hypokalemia in acute myeloid leukemia. *Ann Intern Med* 1975; 82:54–7.
6. Greenberger JS, Rosenthal DS, Moloney WC: Hypokalemia in leukemia (Letter) *Ann Intern Med* 1975; 82:854.
7. Mason DY, Howes DT, Taylor CR: Effect of human lysozyme (muramidase) on potassium handling by the perfused rat kidney. *J Clin Pathol* 1975; 28:722–727.
8. Perry MC, Bauer JH, Farhangi M: Hypokalemia in acute myelogenous leukemia. *South Med J* 1983; 76:958–61.
9. Ottosen PD, Bode F, Madsen KM: Renal handling of lysozyme in the rat. *Kidney Int* 1979; 15:246–54.
10. Cojocel C, Docie N, Baumann K: Early nephrotoxicity at high plasma concentrations of lysozyme in the rat. *Lab Invest* 1982; 46:149–157.

9

Glomerular Disease

Diverse types of glomerulonephritis (acute and chronic) are manifested by proteinuria, cylindriuria, and decreased renal function. In the past, much emphasis was placed upon cylindriuria in assessing the severity of glomerulonephritis. The presence of red blood cell casts was once considered a characteristic of acute glomerulonephritis but no longer is. Red blood cell casts have been and can be found in acute tubular necrosis (ATN) (see Chapter 2).

Very little or no sediment is observed in patients with glomerular disease. Urinary samples collected at different times and on repeated occasions from an unspecified number of patients with biopsy-proven glomerular disease, produced no sediment or so little sediment that sometimes it was not possible to do transmission electron microscopy (TEM) studies. Urinary sediments in patients with glomerular disease are soft and fluffy and often do not form stable pellets; also, such pellets may break down during the lengthy processing for TEM study. Therefore, there have been very few TEM studies of urinary sediment in glomerular disease, compared to ATN or acute tubulointerstitial nephritis.

Urinary sediment TEM studies from several patients will be presented here to demonstrate the importance of this study in the diagnosis of glomerular disease.

Patient No. 1, C.B., a 22-year-old white female, developed a urticarial rash in May 1981. This recurred intermittently over the next three years, though some improvement was noted with prednisone therapy. She also experienced recurrent facial swelling and arthralgias. During 1983, she was found to have persistent hematuria and proteinuria, despite 20 mg of prednisone daily. Her creatinine clearance in December of 1983 was 95 ml/min.

In February of 1984, she was admitted to North Carolina Memorial Hospital for renal biopsy. At that time, she had a blood pressure of 150/95 mm Hg, no fever, multiple

215

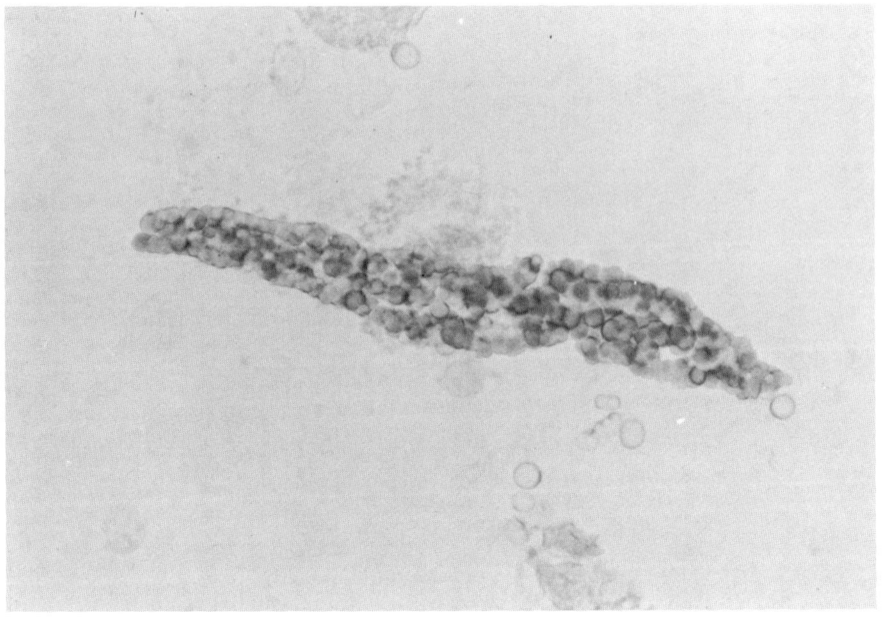

Figure 9-1. Discrete RBC are discernible in this red blood cell cast (unstained wet preparation, ×400).

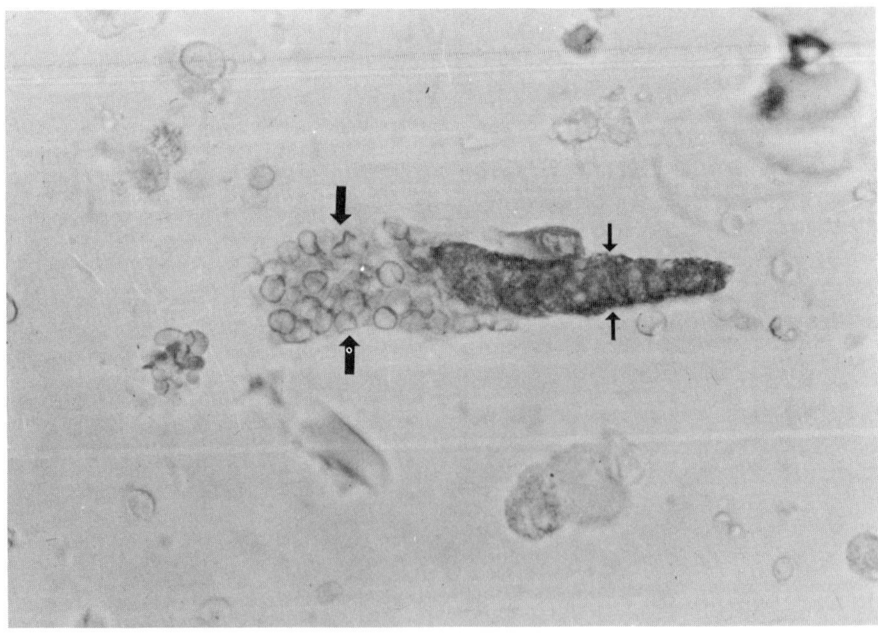

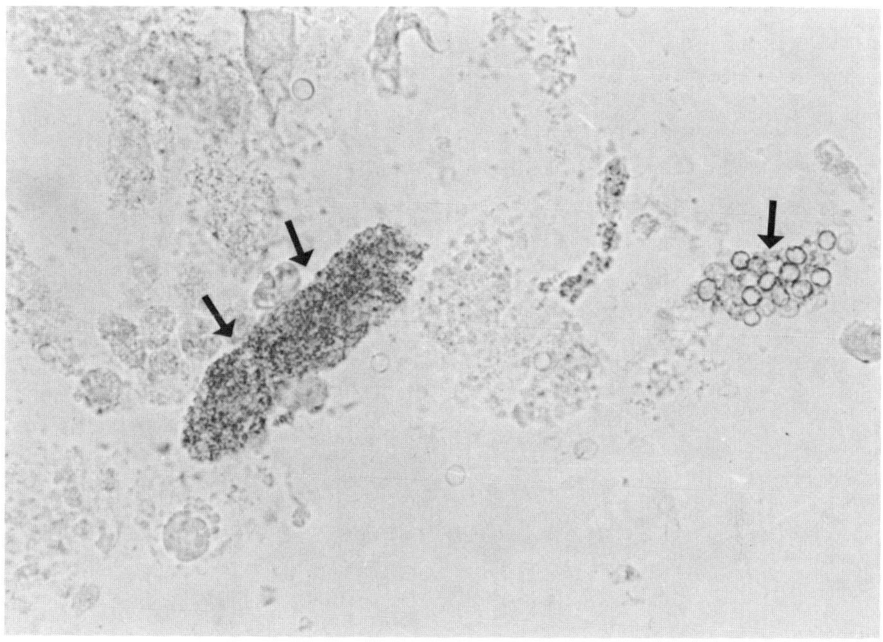

Figure 9-3.   A red blood cell cast (single arrow), a pigmented cast (double arrows), and many WBC are seen (unstained wet preparation, ×400).

urticarial lesions, and trace pitting edema of the lower extremities. Laboratory data included serum creatinine, 1.6 mg/dl; creatinine clearance, 65 ml/min, a 4.8-g 24-hr proteinuria, and a high power field of 25–50 red blood cells (RBC) in the urine. Urinary sediment examined by light microscopy revealed red blood cell casts (Figs. 9-1–9-3), a pigmented cast (Figs. 9-2 and 9-3), and granular casts (Fig. 9-4). The patient had low serum complement (C3 84, C4 5, CH50 less than 10). Collagen vascular disease studies were negative, and serum cryoglobulins were present.

A renal biopsy specimen revealed a diffuse proliferative glomerulonephritis with 60% crescents (Fig. 9-5). There was an extensive glomerular capillary wall and mesangial granular localization of IgG, IgA, IgM, C3, and Clq and lesser degrees of tubular basement membrane and extraglomerular vascular localization. Glomerular subendothelial, subepithelial, and mesangial electrons dense deposits (Fig. 9-6), as well as

Figure 9-2.   A red blood cell cast (between thick arrows) and a pigmented granular cast (between thin arrows) are seen in apposition. In this cast, as well as in the cast in Fig. 9-1, though red cell aggregation is conspicuous, the matrix is not evident (unstained wet preparation, ×400).

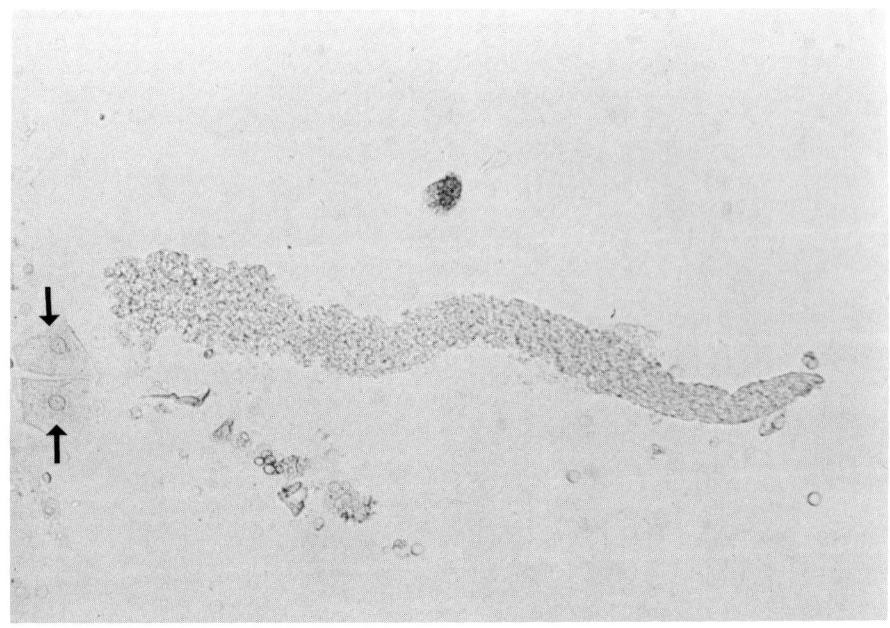

Figure 9-4. A long slender granular cast and two squamous type epithelial cells (between arrows) can be seen (unstained wet preparation, ×400).

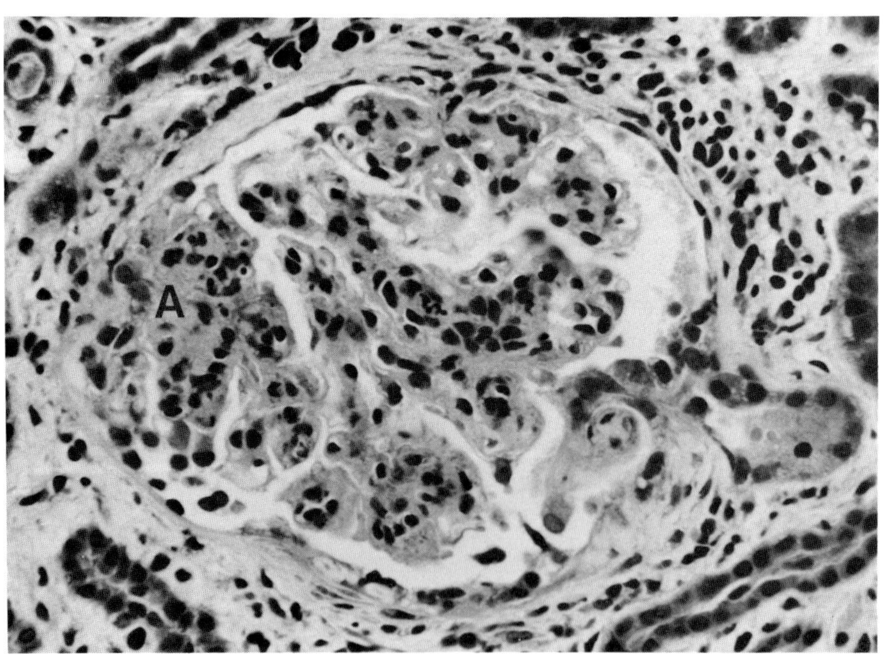

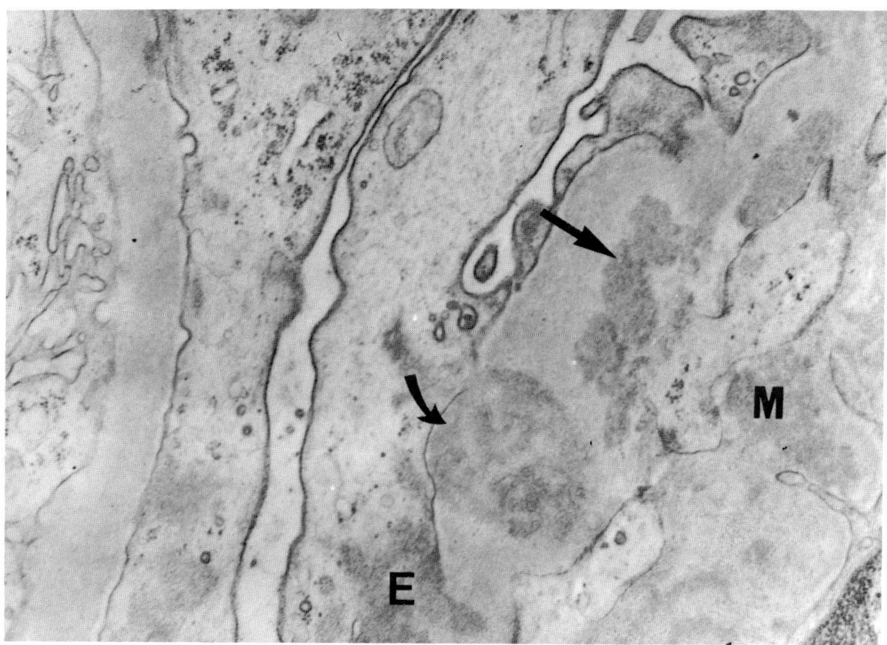

Figure 9-6. This transmission electron micrograph of a glomerular capillary loop shows electron-dense deposits in the subendothelial area (straight arrow), the basement membrane (curved arrow), epimembranous (or extramembranous) area (E), and the mesangial area (M) (UA + LC, ×11,000).

tubular basement membrane and extraglomerular vascular electron-dense deposits, were seen by TEM.

A skin biopsy specimen showed a leukocytoclastic angiitis (Fig. 9-7) and immunoglobulin and complement localization at the dermoepidermal junction and in vessels.

The patient was diagnosed as having hypocomplementemic urticarial vasculitis with active glomerulonephritis. (The clinical summary and the photographs of the urinary sediment study were kindly provided by J. Charles Jennette, M.D., Department of Pathology, University of North Carolina at Chapel Hill.)

Patient No. 2, L.H., a 3-year-old white female, was admitted to the Medical College of Georgia Hospital, Augusta, Georgia, on August 25, 1985, with a chief complaint of colored urine of one week's duration. Approximately three weeks before admission, sores had appeared on the patient's legs, and impetigo was diagnosed. Two weeks before

Figure 9-5. This glomerulus shows proliferative and exudative changes with occlusion of most of the capillary lumina and adhesion (A) of the capillary loops to Bowman's capsule (H & E, ×400).

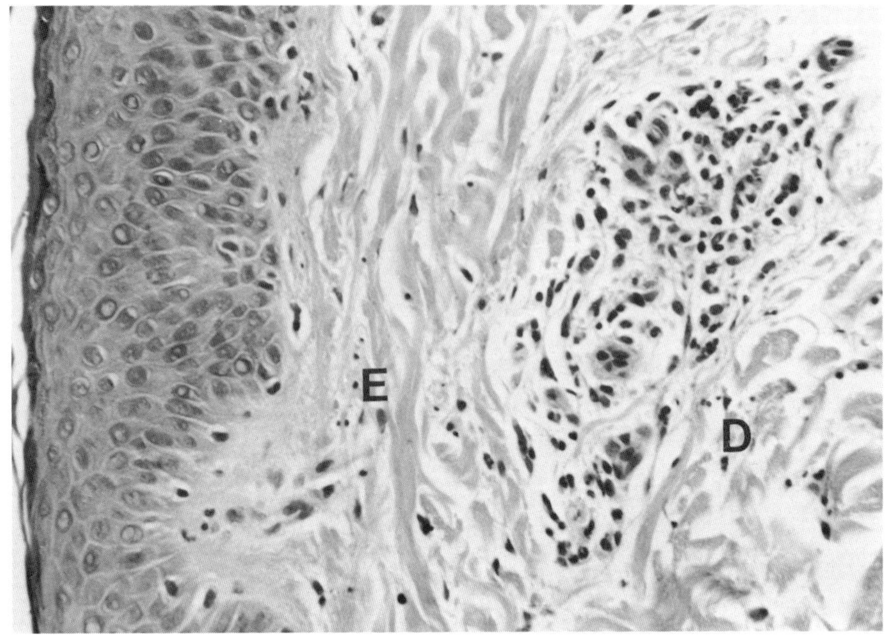

Figure 9-7.   This skin biopsy specimen demonstrates a collection of inflammatory infiltrates between the epidermis (E) and the dermis (D) (H & E, ×400).

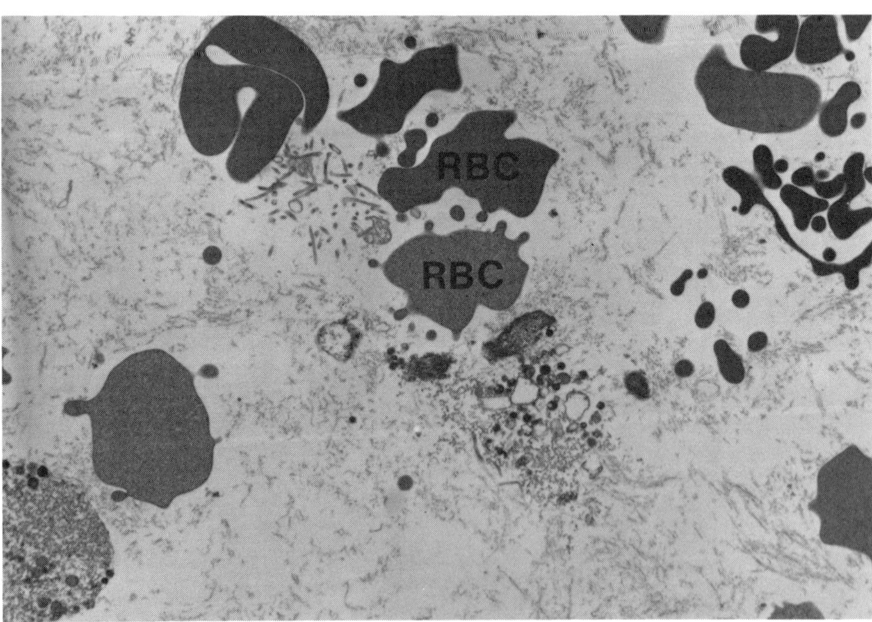

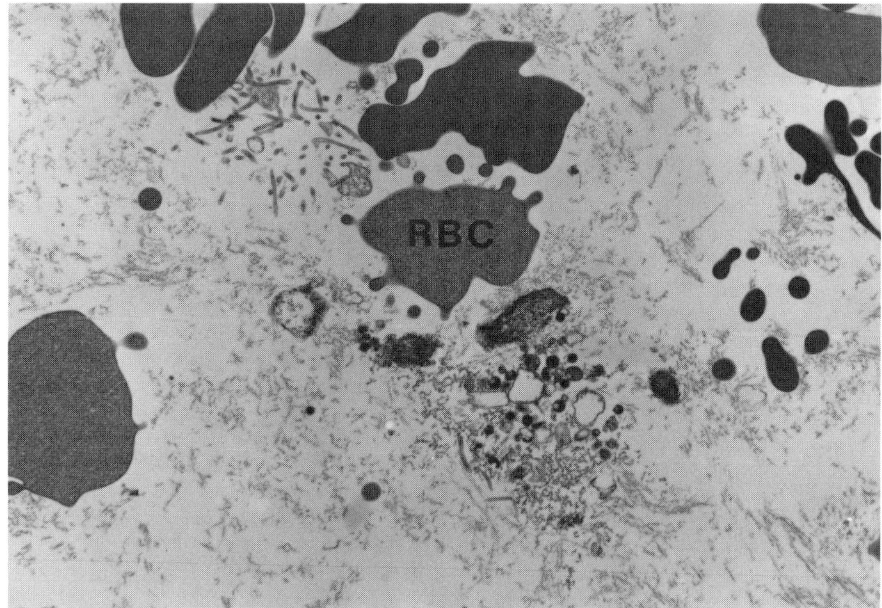

Figure 9-9.   In this magnified view of the red blood cell cast shown in Fig. 9-8, the aggregate of RBC, surrounded by the protein matrix, is evident (UA + LC, ×5,000).

admission, the patient had complained of abdominal pain, headache, and earache and was treated for otitis media with ampicillin for 1 week. One week before admission, the patient began to pass Coca-Cola-colored urine; two days later, the urine was bloody. One day before admission, the patient was found to have high blood pressure. The caretaker also noticed a puffiness of the patient's face, hands, and feet, though physical examination showed no edema. The liver and spleen were palpable below the right and left costal margins, respectively. Her blood pressure then was 113/72 mm Hg. Also, several healing skin lesions were seen on her upper and lower extremities.

A urinalysis showed a 3^+ protein, 20–50 white blood cells (WBC), occasionally hyaline casts, and rare white blood cell casts. Red blood cells were too numerous to count. The serum chemistry showed urea nitrogen, 14 mg/dl; creatinine, 0.5 mg/dl; total protein, 6.2 g/dl; and albumin, 3.4 g/dl. A sample of urine was collected for TEM analysis on August 26, 1985.

The TEM study of urinary sediment showed many free RBC, occasional tubule epithelial cells, and a structure that could be described as red blood cell cast (Figs. 9-8

←──

Figure 9-8.   A similitude of a red blood cell cast shown in Fig. 9-1. The RBC are in close apposition, surrounded by the protein matrix material (UA + LC, ×4,000).

and 9-9). (This urinary sample was provided by Dr. Sharon Pearlman, Pediatric Nephrologist, Medical College of Georgia, Augusta, Georgia.)

Comments: Though with TEM, red blood cell casts may not be found as an aggregate of RBC, as they are seen by light microscopy (LM) (Figs. 9-1, 9-2), a close apposition of many RBC within a proteinous matrix indicates that red blood cell casts are present. An explanation is that the exact aggregate of RBC seen by LM (Fig. 9-1) may have been disrupted, at least in part, by the lengthy processing of the sediment, and especially, during thin sectioning for TEM study.

Patient No. 1 had an acute diffuse proliferative glomerulonephritis as shown by renal biopsy; in patient No. 2, though renal biopsy was not done, the history and urinalysis were very suggestive of acute glomerulonephritis. In patient No. 1, florid red blood cell casts were found in the urinary sediment by LM; in patient No. 2, no red blood cell casts were noted with LM of the urinary sediment. This does not mean that these casts were not present, especially since there was severe microscopic hematuria. In this patient, the TEM finding of urinary sediment was suggestive of red blood cell casts. Most nephrologists would agree that red cell casts are a characteristic urinary sediment finding in acute glomerulonephritis of diverse etiology, though it is not known how they are formed. Similarly, the significance of red blood cell casts relative to the severity of clinical manifestations or renal function abnormalities is not known.

Patient No. 3, W. N., a 63-year-old black male, was admitted to the Medical College of Georgia Hospital from Americus Sumter County Hospital, Americus, Georgia, on April 6, 1984. The patient was in good health up to three weeks before admission at which time he developed malaise, anorexia, and intermittent nausea. He denied such urinary symptoms as dysuria, frequency, or nocturia.

At the Americus Sumter County Hospital, the admission serum creatinine concentration was 6 mg/dl and urine output was 600 ml/24 hr. A sonogram of the kidneys showed no evidence of obstruction. Peritoneal dialysis was initiated, and a bovine graft was placed in the left forearm to institute hemodialysis. Also, the left kidney was biopsied percutaneously.

Upon admission to the Medical College of Georgia Hospital, a urinalysis showed a specific gravity of 1.020, 2^+ protein, and large amount of blood and, reportedly, several red blood cell casts, granular casts, and a few white blood cell casts. The renal biopsy findings were consistent with a rapidly progressive (acute) glomerulonephritis. On April 8th, the patient had a creatinine clearance of 2 ml/min and a 24-hr proteinuria of 325 mg/dl (total volume of urine, 330 ml). On April 9, 1984, a sample of urine was collected for TEM analysis. Treatment was with corticosteroids and immunosuppressive drugs.

The TEM analysis of the urinary sediment showed a hyaline cast and cellular casts. There were also some structures that might be interpreted as viral-like particles (Fig. 9-10), and necrotic glomerular segments. An occasional tubule cell was found. The viral-like particles had a central electron-dense core and a less electron-dense, wide peripheral

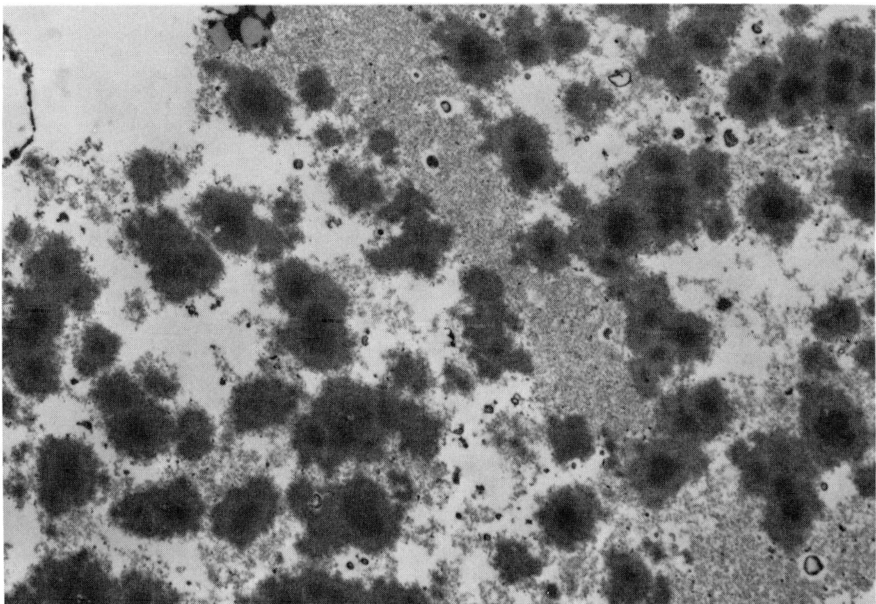

Figure 9-10.   The discrete spherical structures consisting of a central electron-dense core surrounded by less electron-dense peripheral material are consistent with viral particles (UA + LC, ×3,300).

rim. The diameter of the peripheral rim ranged from 61.06 to 78.51μ, with an average diameter of 67.17μ. The ultrastructural features and diameter of these urinary particles are consistent with such myxoviruses as influenza, mumps, and measles.[1] On April 16th, the patients serum urea nitrogen and serum creatinine were elevated to 98 mg/dl and 6.4 mg/dl, respectively. He was treated symptomatically and returned to his private physician for tapering of immunosuppressive therapy and consideration of maintenance hemodialysis.

Comments: The sediment findings provided subtle evidence for glomerular necrosis and a severe pathological condition. Viruses have been implicated in the pathogenesis of rapidly progressive glomerulonephritis, but none has been isolated. Therefore, the finding of viral-like particles in the urinary sediment in this study should stimulate further investigations to determine the role, if any, of these types of viruses in the pathogenesis of rapidly progressive glomerulonephritis.

Patient No. 4, L. D., a 59-year-old black male, developed polyarthritis and was found to have a rheumatoid factor titer of 1:10,240 and a nephrotic syndrome. At the

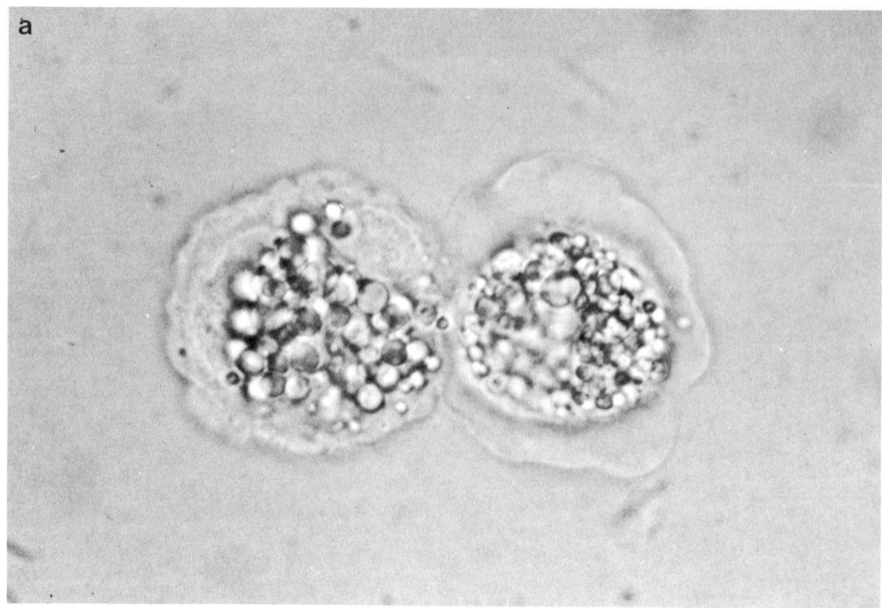

Figure 9-11a.   Two oval fat bodies containing many lipid droplets engulfed within a tubule epithelial cell are shown. The peripheral parts of the tubule cells are also evident (unstained wet preparation, ×400).

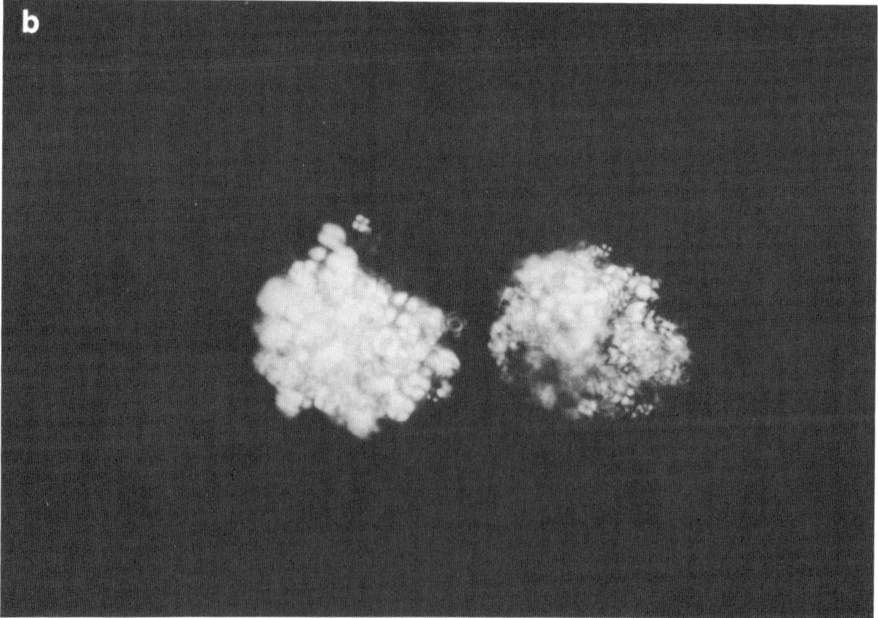

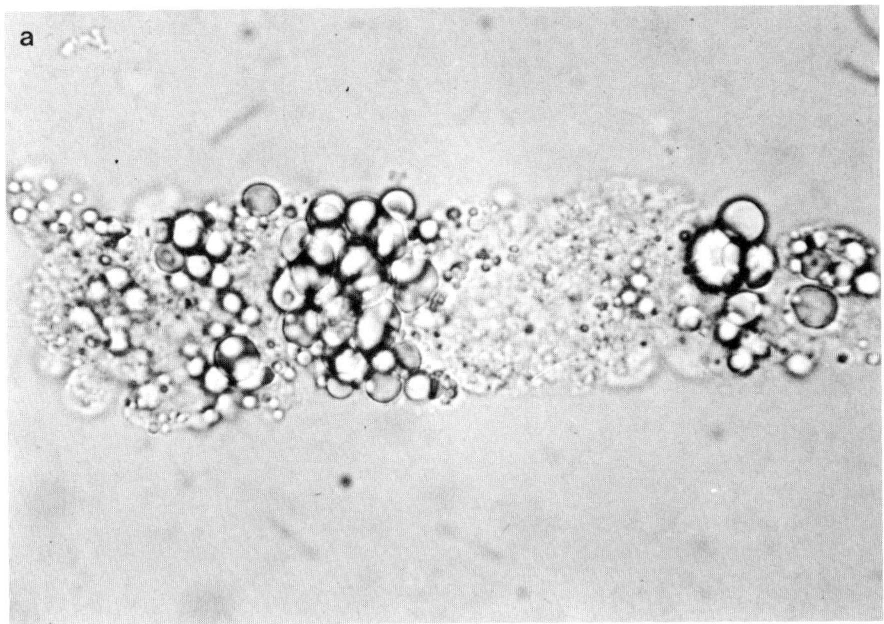

Figure 9-12a.   Lipid droplets are embedded within a matrix in this fatty cast (unstained wet preparation, ×400).

time of renal biopsy, the laboratory studies showed a 6.75 g/24-hr proteinuria; serum creatinine, 1.3 mg/dl; serum urea nitrogen, 18 mg/dl; serum cholesterol, 250 mg/dl; serum albumin, 2.5 g/dl; and normal C3, normal C4, and CH50. The antinuclear antibody determination was negative. The urine contained 5–10 WBC, 5–10 RBC, oval fat bodies (Fig. 9-11a,b), and fatty casts (Fig. 9-12a,b).

A renal biopsy specimen studied by LM showed a uniform, slight thickening of peripheral capillary loops, which is consistent with an early stage of membranous glomerulonephritis. Transmission electron microscopy revealed numerous, regularly distributed, subepithelial electron-dense deposits with adjacent projections of basement membrane material or stage II membranous glomerulonephritis (Fig. 9-13b). (The clinical summary and the photographs of the urinary sediment study were kindly provided by J. Charles Jennette, M.D., Department of Pathology, University of North Carolina at Chapel Hill.)

Patient No. 5, B. P., a 28-year-old black male, was admitted to the Veterans Administration Medical Center, Augusta, Georgia, on October 5, 1984, with a history

Figure 9-11b.   The same oval fat bodies, examined under polarized light, have a characteristic Maltese cross appearance (×400).

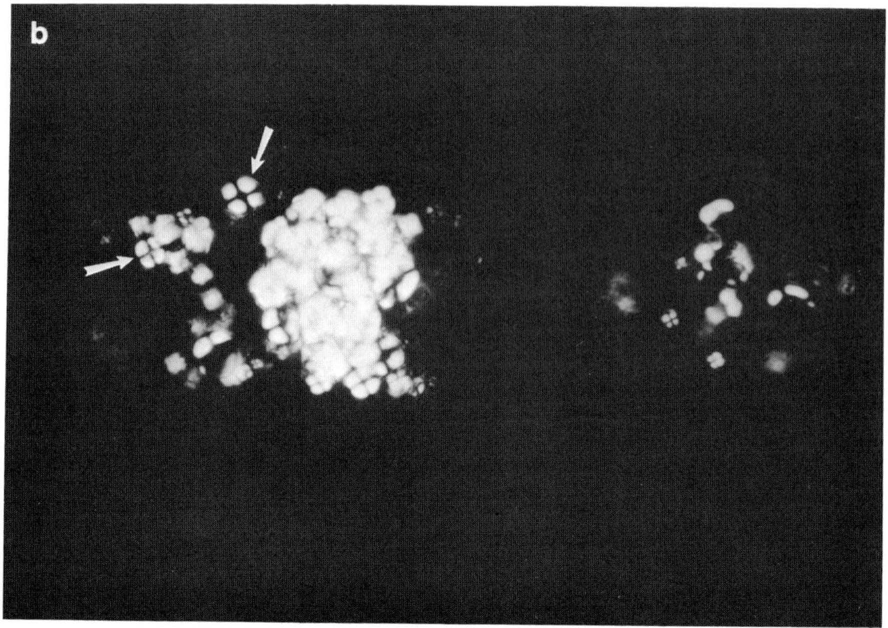

Figure 9-12b. The fatty cast shown in Fig. 9-12a as examined under polarized light. Note the typical Maltese cross appearance (arrows) (×400).

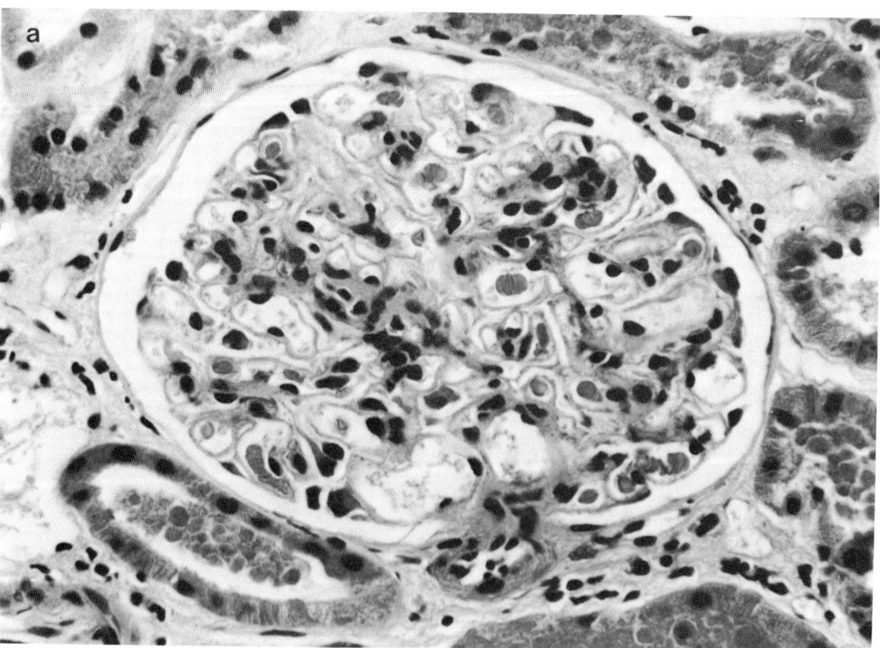

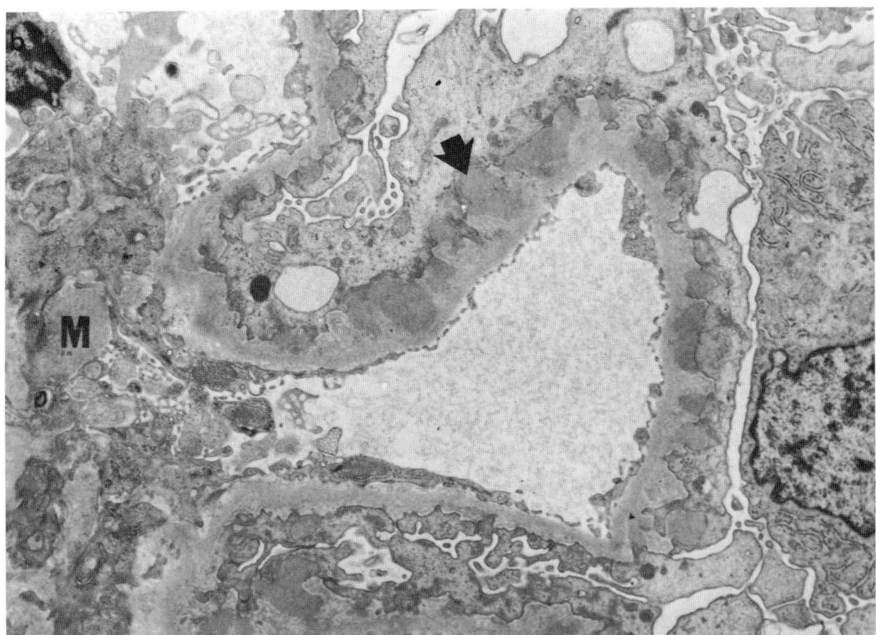

Figure 9-13b.   This transmission electron micrograph of a glomerular capillary loop shows regularly distributed, subepithelial electron-dense deposits (thick arrow) in its upper part. In the lower part, conspicuous spikes give rise to an edentulous jaw appearance. An increase in the mesangial matrix (M) can also be seen (UA + LC, ×4,000).

of hypertension. He was referred here from a community hospital in Millen, Georgia, where he was noted to have blood pressures of 200/150 mm Hg and a 3^+ proteinuria by dipstick. He had a history of facial and lower extremity swelling for one month before admission. The admission physical examination was negative except for a 2^+ pitting edema of the lower extremities and a blood pressure of 164/104 mm Hg.

Admission laboratory studies included a peripheral WBC count of 11,300/mm^3; serum sodium, 142 mEq/liter; serum potassium, 3.3 mEq/liter; serum chloride, 103 mEq/liter; serum bicarbonate, 32 mEq/liter; serum glucose, 90 mg/dl; serum urea nitrogen, 18 mg/dl; and serum creatinine, 2.6 mg/dl. A urinalysis showed 4^+ protein and 3^+ blood. A 24-hr urinary study showed 22.6 g of protein and a creatinine clearance of 72 ml/min. A urine sample was collected for TEM study. A left percutaneous renal biopsy was

Figure 9-13a.   This glomerulus shows a uniform thickening of all peripheral capillary loops, which is consistent with membranous glomerulonephritis. The thickness of the capillaries, with no or a slight increase in the mesangial matrix, suggests stage II membranous glomerulonephritis (H & E, ×400).

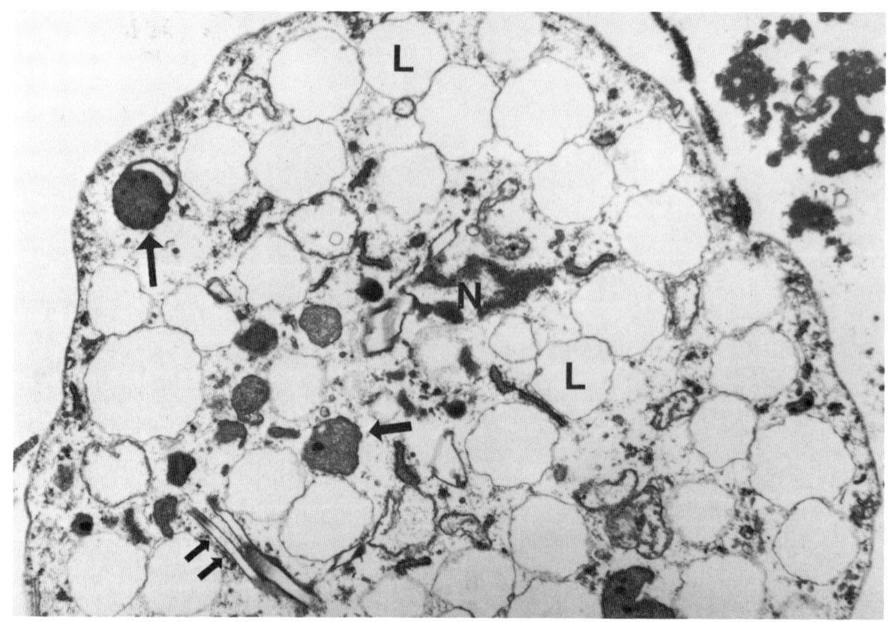

Figure 9-14.   This tubule cell is studded with lipid droplets (L). The nucleus (N), mitochondria (arrows) and cholesterol crystals (double arrows) are also evident (UA + LC, ×5,000).

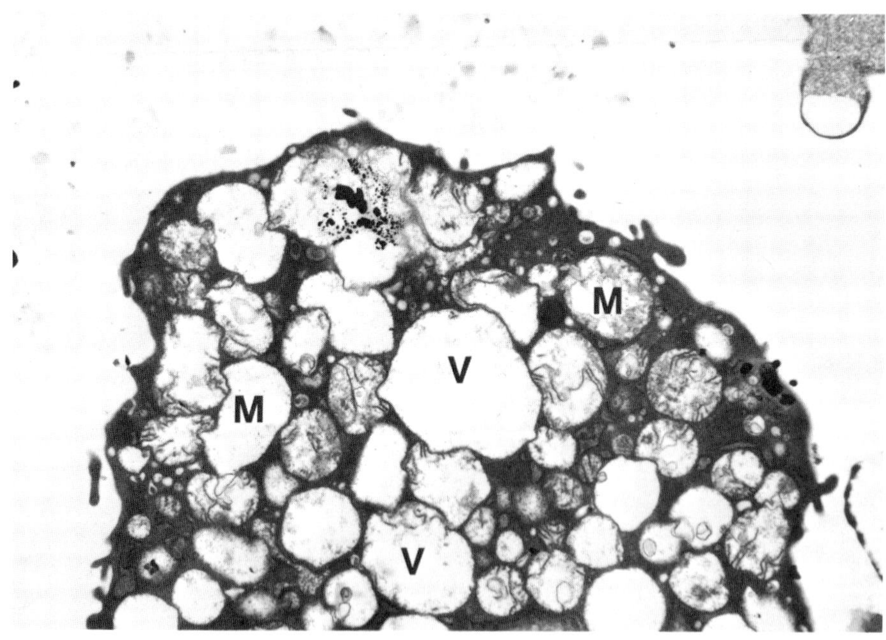

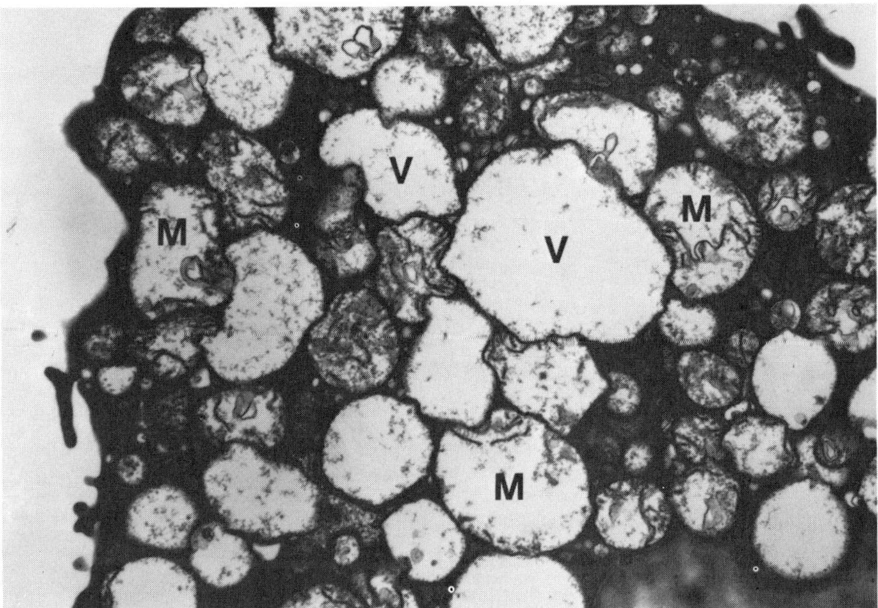

Figure 9-16. Another swollen tubule cell showing numerous vacuoles (V) at a higher magnification. These vacuoles appear to have originated from disintegrated mitochondria (M) (UA + LC, ×10,000).

performed and the tissue was studied using light, immunofluorescence, and transmission electron microscopy.

The urinary sediment TEM showed hyaline casts, lipid-laden cells (Fig. 9-14), vacuolated and swollen tubule cells (Figs. 9-15 and 9-16), free fat droplets (Fig. 9-17), and fatty casts. The hyaline and fatty casts from the urinary sediment of this patient were shown in Chapter 2. An occasional tubule cell was seen (Fig. 9-18). Renal histopathological studies showed some crescent formation in several glomeruli by LM. The immunofluorescence microscopy (IFM) showed a mild to moderate coarse granular fluorescence for IgG, IgM, and C3. The TEM of renal tissue revealed discrete subepithelial electron-dense deposits that appeared more as atypical humps than as typical humps. A diagnosis of a resolving postinfectious (acute) glomerulonephritis was made.

The patient was readmitted on April 7, 1985 for placement of vascular access and hemodialysis. His admission serum urea nitrogen and serum creatinine were 107 mg/dl and 11.6 mg/dl, respectively. Hemodialysis has been three times a week since then.

Figure 9-15. In contrast to Fig. 9-14, the tubule cell shown here is studded with vacuoles (V), which appear to be swollen mitochondria as is evident from the slightly less affected mitochondria (M) (UA + LC, ×7,500).

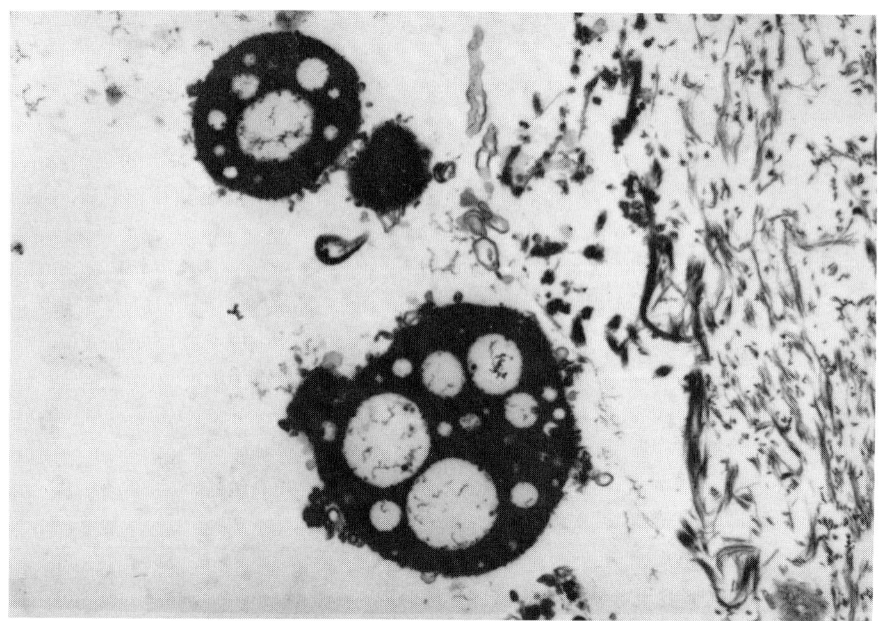

Figure 9-17.   These free lipid droplets have electron-lucent (light) and electron-dense (dark) areas. The electron density varies with the saturation of the fatty acids (UA + LC, ×10,000).

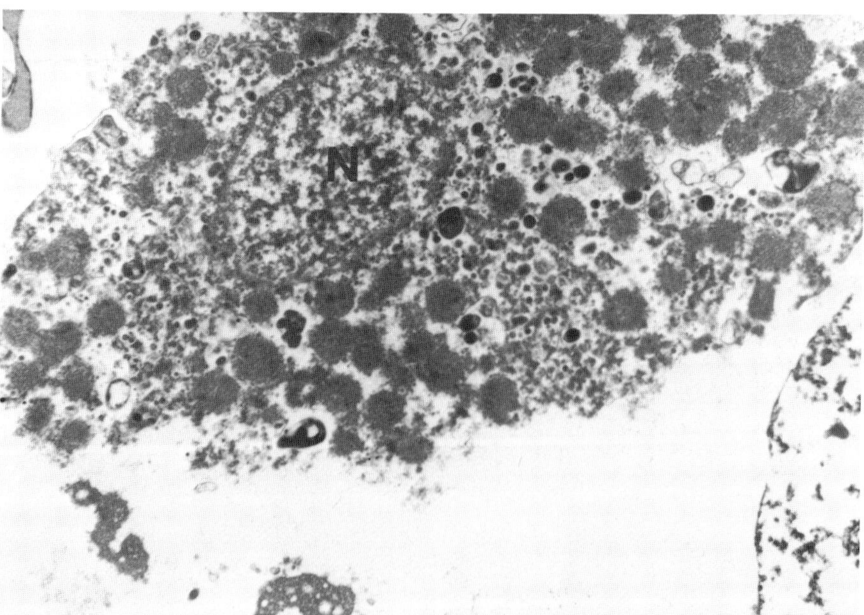

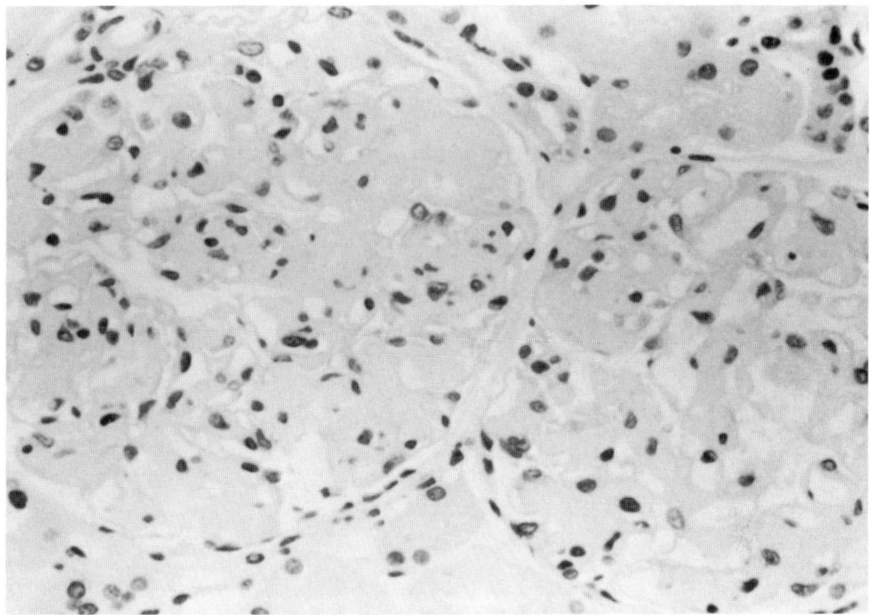

Figure 9-19.   Homogeneous eosinophilic material, seen in all the glomeruli, is consistent with amyloid. Congo red staining of the sections provided green birefringence under polarized light (H & E, ×400).

Patient No. 6, C. B., a 62-year-old white male, was referred to the Medical College of Georgia Hospital, Augusta, Georgia, on March 3, 1986, for follow-up and treatment of a nephrotic syndrome. He had been found to have a primary renal amyloidosis by an open renal biopsy in August, 1984 (Fig. 9-19). A thorough evaluation for potential secondary causes of the amyloidosis, including numerous serum protein electrophreses and a bone marrow examination, disclosed no sign of multiple myeloma or any other disease that might cause secondary amyloidosis.

The patient gave a history of occasional pedal edema, intermittent mild fatigability, and scratch purpura. The physical examination showed a pitting edema around the ankles, a blood pressure of 160/70 mm Hg, without orthostatic changes, and a grade I ejection systolic murmur.

Laboratory studies on this visit showed a serum urea nitrogen of 27 mg/dl; serum creatinine, 2.8 mg/dl; serum total protein, 4.8 g/dl, with an albumin of 2.2 g/dl; serum cholesterol, 396 mg/dl; and serum triglyceride, 265 mg/dl. The patient had a proteinuria of 16.7 g/24 hr. A sample of urine was collected for TEM analysis on March 3, 1986.

Figure 9-18.   The tubule cell seen here appears to be intact, with a well-preserved nucleus (N) and numerous mitochondria (UA + LC, ×3,300).

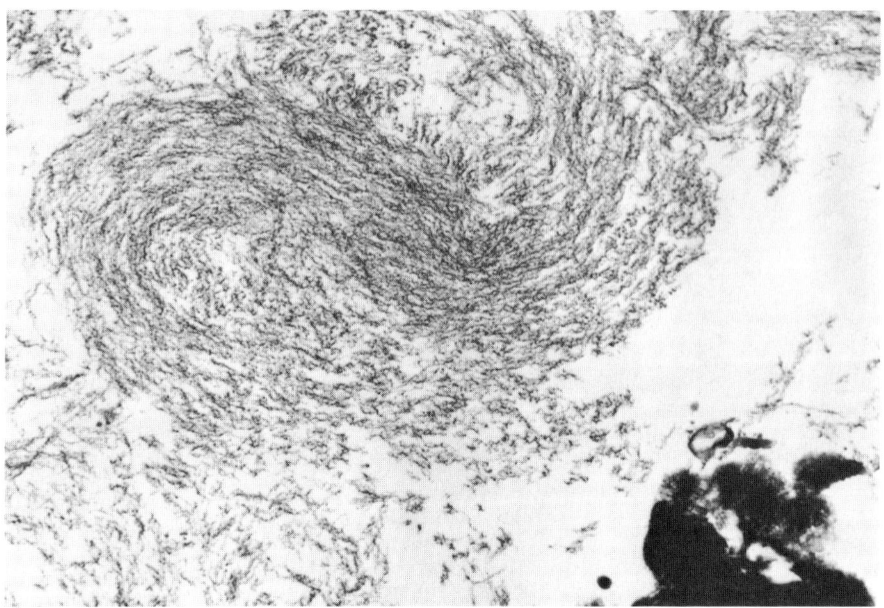

Figure 9-20. These nonstriated, nonbranching fibrils are considered to be amyloid fibrils. A close inspection will reveal dark beaded materials rather than striations (UA + LC, ×7,500).

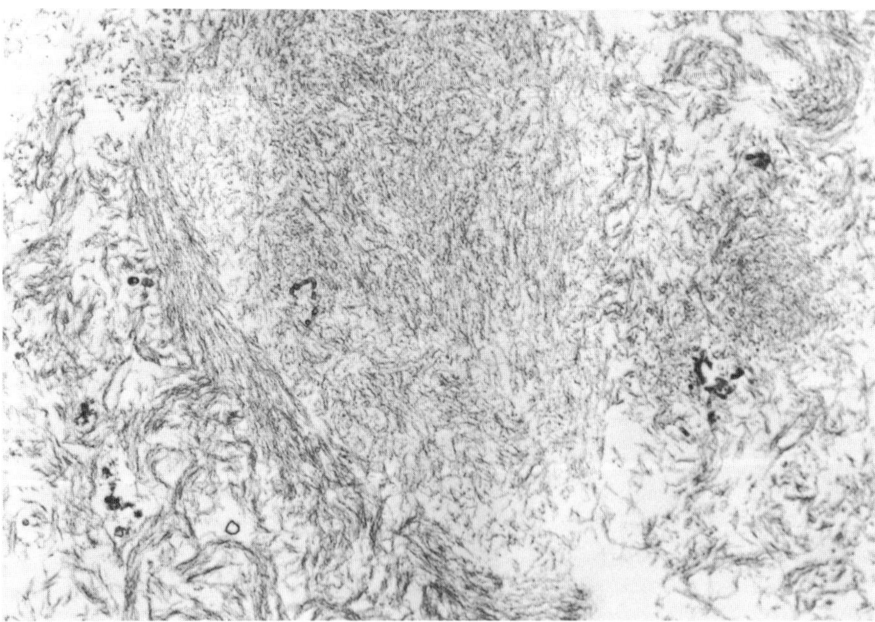

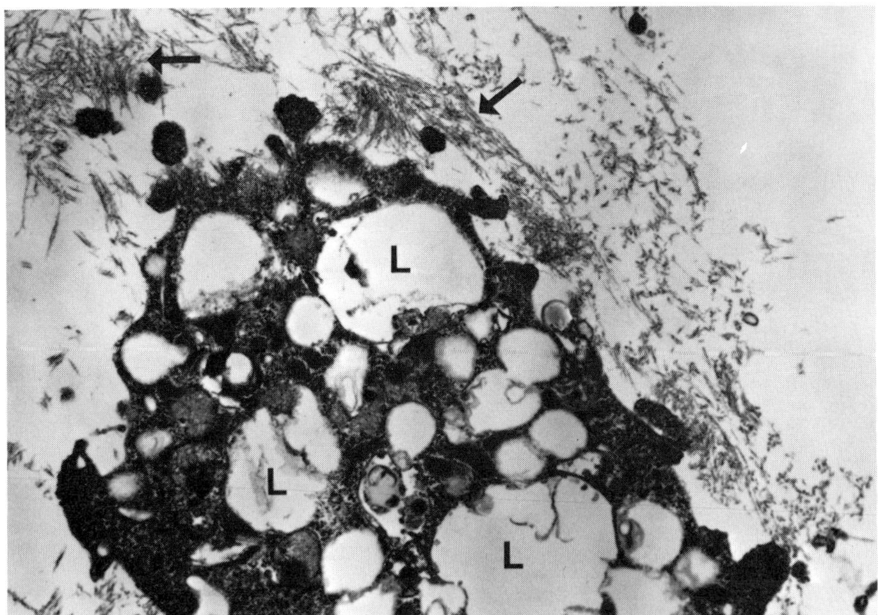

Figure 9-22. This tubule cell is filled with lipid droplets (L) and surrounded by many nonstriated amyloidlike fibrils (arrows) (UA + LC, ×7,500).

The TEM analysis of urine showed several lipid-laden cells, but the conspicuous finding was the presence of collections of long nonbranching and nonstriated fibrils (Figs. 9-20 and 9-21). A close inspection of the fibrils revealed fine dark beadlike structures but no cross striations (Fig. 9-21). These fibrils were from 240 μ to 826.7 μ in length; the average length was 388 μ. The diameter of these fibrils varied from 3.8 to 17.3 μ; the average diameter was 10.9 μ. These dimensions are consistent with those for amyloid fibrils. The fibrils were found around the lipid-laden cells (Fig. 9-22), which suggested amyloid infiltration of the tubules.

Patient No. 7 is the same patient as patient No. 2 (J. B.) in Chapter 8. For the last three months, this patient's disease process has progressed, as shown by an increased proteinuria (8–9 g/24 hr) and a moderate renal insufficiency (serum creatinine, 4.7–6.1 mg/dl). A massive edema of both lower extremities was also seen. The Bence Jones protein was repeatedly positive.

Figure 9-21. At a higher magnification, these individual, nonstriated fibrils (Fig. 9-21) are more easily seen. The beading here is more obvious (UA + LC, ×15,000).

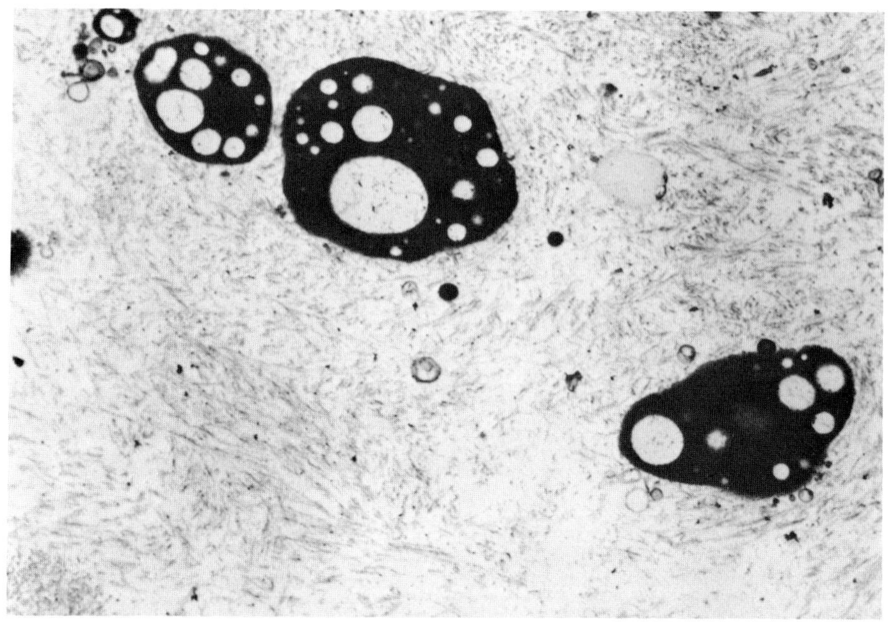

Figure 9-23. These free lipid droplets (cf. Fig. 9-17) consist of electron-lucent (light) and electron-dense (dark) areas (UA + LC, ×7,500).

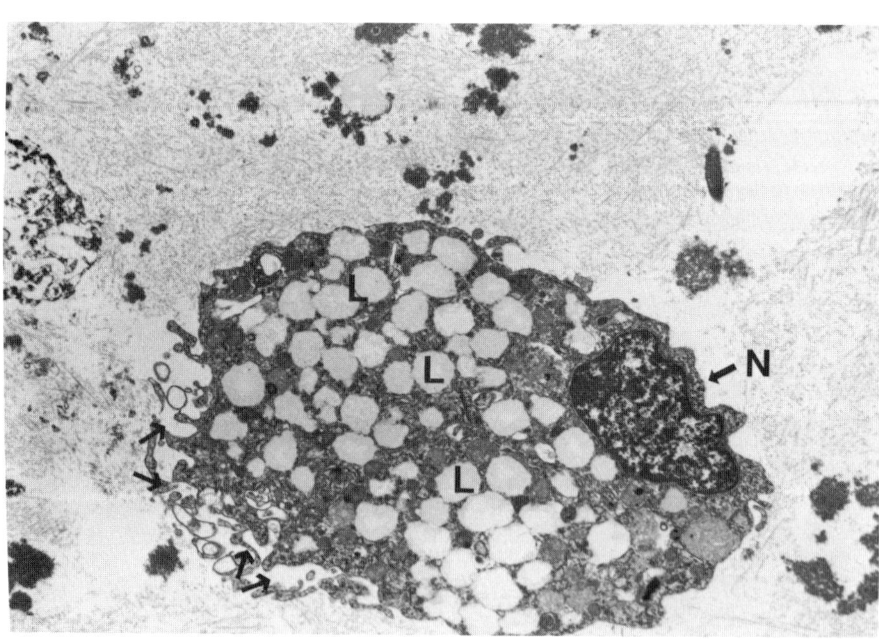

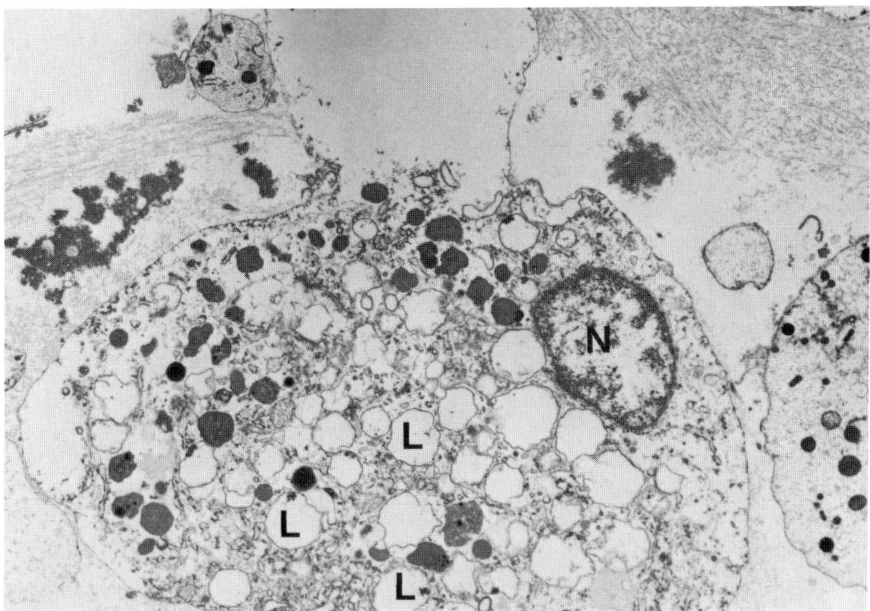

Figure 9-25.   This cell of unknown origin cannot be identified. Note the intact nucleus (N) and the many lipid droplets (L). It can thus be described as an oval fat body. The cells in this figure and in Fig. 9-24 are surrounded by prominent fibrils. More of these fibrils, which appear to be amyloid fibrils, are shown subsequently (UA + LC, ×5,000).

A second sample of urine was collected for TEM analysis on March 21, 1986. A third sample of urine was collected on May 28, 1986, after a few hemodialysis treatments. The TEM study of sediments from these two urinary samples revealed many lipid droplets and lipid-laden cells (Figs. 9-23–9-25). A few tubule cells with ischemic changes in the mitochondria were also found (Fig. 9-26). The most conspicuous finding in the third urinary sample was abundant nonstriated and nonbranching fibrils that resembled amyloid fibrils (Figs. 9-27–9-30). These fibrils were found in large aggregates deposited in the tubules and around the tubule cells. They were from 400 to 1,000 μ in length; the average length was 653.33 μ. The diameter of these fibrils was from 20 to 57.7 μ; the average diameter was 21.5 μ.

Figure 9-24.   An intact, possibly proximal tubule cell, identifiable by its microvilli (arrows pointing), has a well-preserved nucleus (N). The cell, loaded with lipid droplets (L), is called an oval fat body (UA + LC, ×4,000).

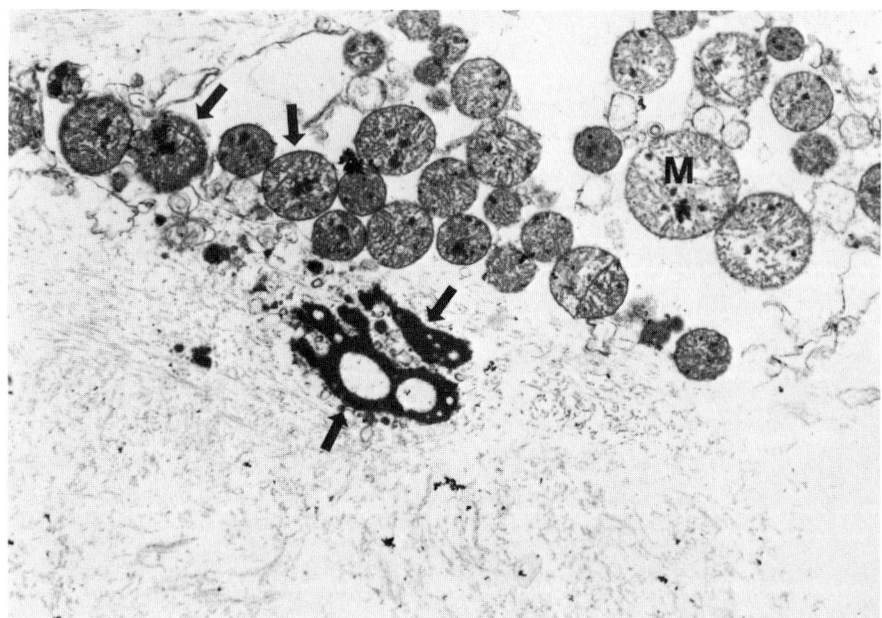

Figure 9-26.   This tubule cell has a nucleus (between arrows) and many mitochondria. Some mitochondria are swollen (M), whereas others contain dark bodies (arrows), considered to be a sign of ischemia (UA + LC, ×7,500).

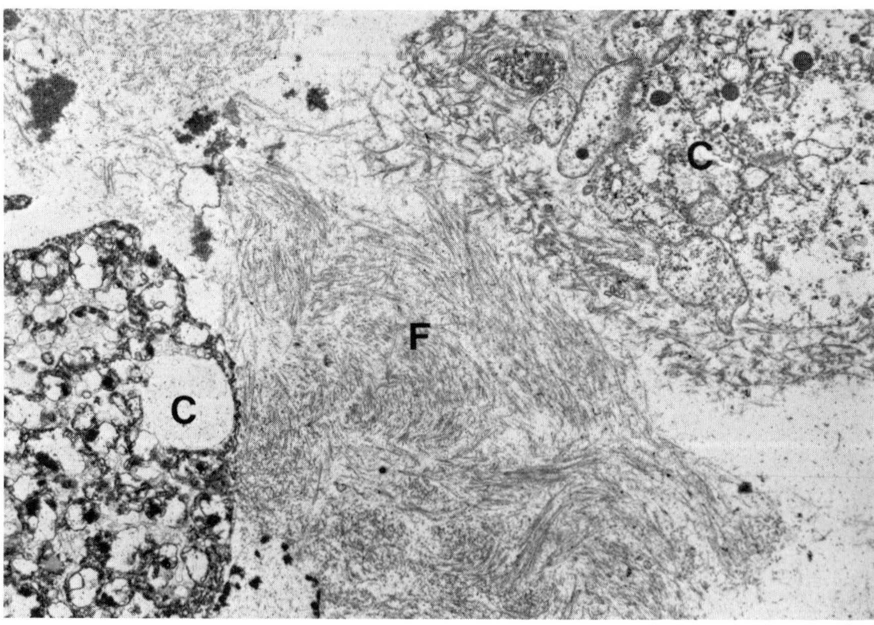

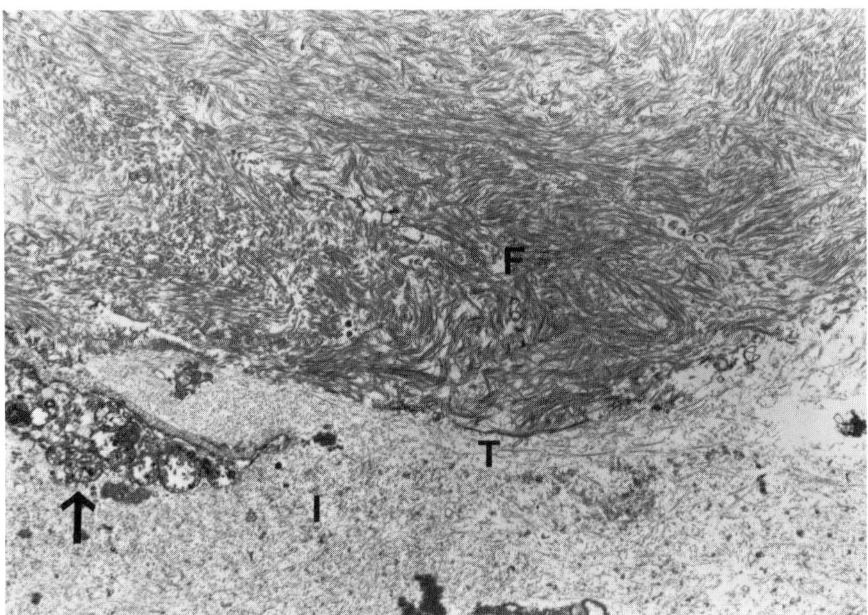

Figure 9-28.   In this transmission electron micrograph, a collection of hairy fibrils (F) is attached to a tubule (T). A fibroblast (arrow) in the interstitium (I) can be seen (UA + LC, ×4,000).

GENERAL COMMENTS

Urinary sediment TEM in nephrotic syndrome has demonstrated a common pattern of abnormalities irrespective of whether the nephrotic syndrome was produced by glomerulonephritis or amyloidosis. These abnormalities include lipid-laden cells (oval fat bodies), lipid-droplets, and fatty casts. Hyaline casts and cellular casts are infrequently found, free tubule cells, occasionally. These structures in the urinary sediment have been described using conventional LM and by using polarized light microscopy. These techniques, however, do not show sediment structures in detail. Study by TEM shows the distinctive sediment structures more clearly and leads to a better understanding of the composition of the structures. For example, the polarizing lens (LM) imparts a Maltese cross appearance to the characteristic oval fat body.

Figure 9-27.   Abundant nonstriated, hairy fibrils (F) are observed between tubule cells (C) (UA + LC, ×5,000).

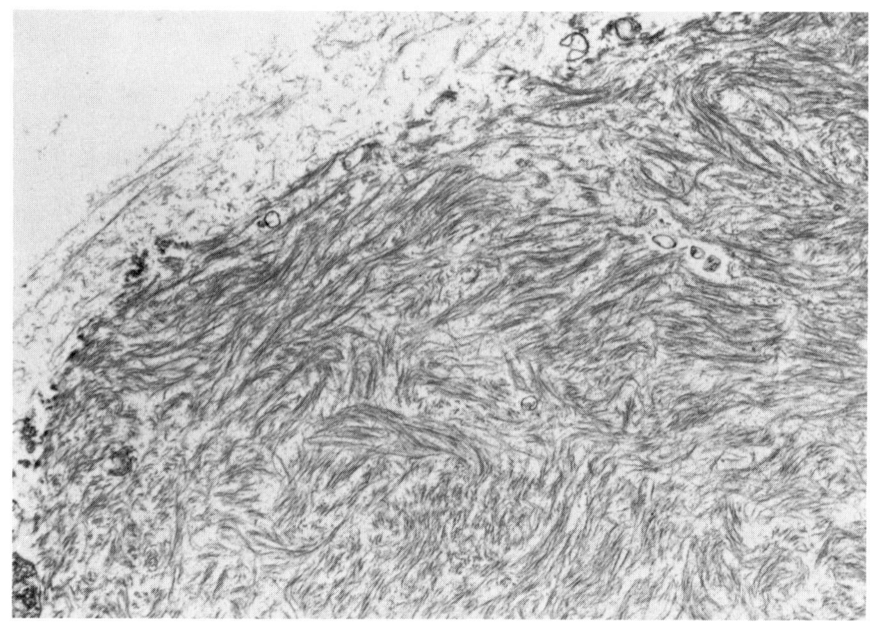

Figure 9-29. These fibrils appear in bundles and are nonstriated (UA + LC, ×3,000).

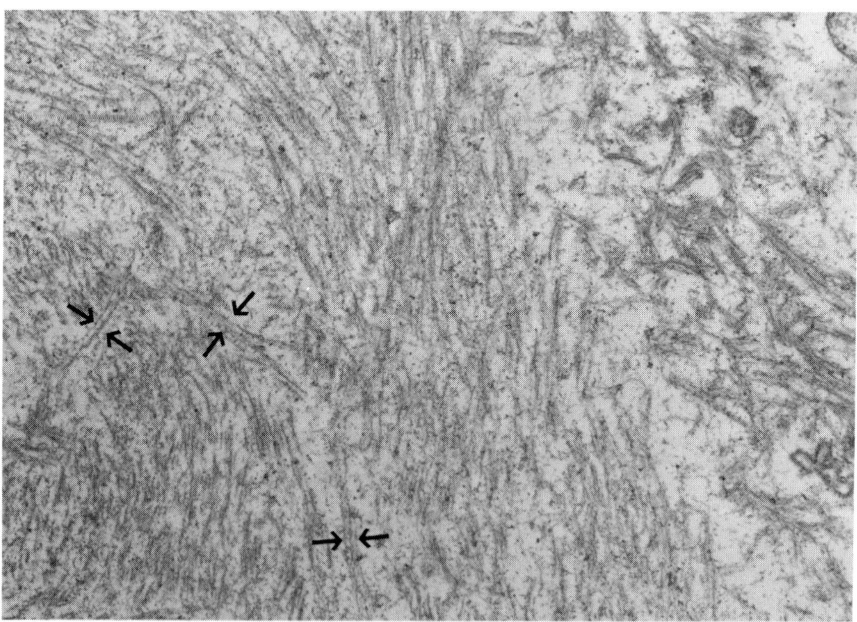

Figure 9-30. At this high magnification, individual fibers (between arrows), which are beaded in appearance, are discernible. No striations are evident (UA + LC, ×13,000).

The TEM study revealed that an oval fat body consists of a tubule cell largely filled with lipid droplets and that these lipid droplets are almost always electron lucent which suggests a higher saturated fatty acid than unsaturated fatty acid content. In another study, it has been shown by the author that saturated fatty acids are not osmiophilic and are electron lucent (gray) in appearance. Furthermore, the concomitant presence of cholesterol crystals (Fig. 9-14), supports the idea of a saturated fatty acid composition of these oval fat body lipid droplets. Unsaturated fatty acids are osmiophilic and, as lipid droplets, are electron dense.[2] It is not known how these lipid-laden cells are formed. Since the nephrotic syndrome is associated with hyperlipidemia, large amounts of fatty acids are filtered and reach the tubule cells. One might speculate that when these lipids overfill tubule cells, the cells detach and are shed in the urine. In most instances, these tubule cells appear to be viable; therefore, their detachment is unlikely to be caused by ischemia or necrosis. In addition, tubular injury, if any, is minimal, since few or no tubule cells appear in the urinary sediment in the nephrotic syndrome.

Identification of the amyloid fibrils in the urinary sediments of patients with amyloidosis was attempted.[3–5] In one study, TEM of urinary sediment showed fibrils that were indistinguishable, by their ultrastructural features, from the amyloid fibrils. These urinary fibrils, however, upon amino acid analysis, were not similar to amyloidosis of amyloid protein (AA) or amyloidosis of light chain protein (AL) protein, nor were they immunoreactive with anti-human AA protein.[3] These large bundles of fibrils found in the urinary sediments of patients No. 6 and No. 7 in this study, however, constitute an important finding. Although occasional fibrils may be found in random urinary sediments of patients with nonamyloid renal disease, collections of hairball-like fibrils as seen by TEM in patients No. 6 and No. 7 have never been observed before by this author, in a study of at least 150 urinary sediments, nor have such large amounts of urinary fibrils been reported by anyone else. Furthermore, patient No. 6 had primary amyloidosis and patient No. 7 had light chain nephropathy, with some signs of amyloidosis as documented by renal biopsy specimens. Therefore, an electron microscopist, in a routine TEM study of urinary sediment, apparently attaches no importance to a few urinary fibrils. But when heavy collections of urinary fibrils are found in the urinary sediments of only two patients with documented amyloidosis, in a series of 150 urinary sediments or more, the TEM studies of patients without renal amyloidosis seem significant.

Finally, the contributions made by TEM of urinary sediment in acute glomerulonephritis were trivial compared to those in acute tubular necrosis, aminoglycoside nephrotoxicity, or transplant rejection.

The bulk of the urinary sediment is made up of tubule cells, inflammatory cells, or such other structures as myeloid bodies. When no or a few tubule cells are seen, this seems to account for the small amount of urinary sediment in glomerular disease. This finding, however, shows that desquamation of tubule cells, and therefore, tubular injury, is minimal in glomerular disease. From this limited study, it can also be stated that glomerular structures are rarely shed into the urine. Therefore, urinary sediment TEM does not appear to be a sensitive procedure in the diagnosis of glomerular disease.

REFERENCES

1. Mandal AK, Mask DR, Nordquist J, Chrysant KS, Lindeman RD: Membraneous glomerulo-nephritis: Virus-like inclusions in glomerular basement membrane. *Annu Intern Med* (Letter) 1974; 80:554–555.
2. Mandal AK, Frohlich ED, Chrysant K, et al: A morphological study of the renal papillary granule: Analysis in the interstitial cell and in the interstitium. *J Lab Clin Med* 1975; 85:120–131.
3. Shirahama T, Skinner M, Cohen, AS, et al: Uncertain value of urinary sediments in the diagnosis of amyloidosis. *N Engl J Med* 1977; 297:821–823.
4. Winer RL, Wuerker RB, Erickson JO: Ultrastructural examination of urinary sediment. *Am J Clin Pathol* 1979; 71:36–39.
5. Shemer J, Messer GY, Pras M, et al: Amyloid in urinary sediments as a diagnostic technique. *Annu Intern Med* 1979; 90:61–62.

10

Acute and Chronic Interstitial Nephritis

HYPERSENSITIVITY ACUTE INTERSTITIAL NEPHRITIS

Historical Background

The appearance of eosinophils in the urine, or eosinophiluria, has been reported in allergic conditions of the urinary tract.[1] Other investigators have reported eosinophiluria in 9 of 14 rejection episodes after kidney transplantation and in 1 case without evidence of rejection; the number of eosinophils, however, never exceeded 5% of the total number of granulocytes in the urine.[2] In one study, urine specimens from 228 patients were examined. Of these 228 patients, 87 had chronic pyelonephritis, 56 had cystourethritis, 75 had other renal diseases, and 10 had bronchial asthma or some other allergic condition. The percentage of eosinophiluria was as follows: 90 patients had less than 1% eosinophils; 40 patients had 1 to 5% eosinophils; and 14 patients had 6 to 33% eosinophils on at least one occasion. In the latter 14 patients, renal histopathological studies did not reveal eosinophils. The authors concluded that eosinophils are excreted from the renal pelvis, though they may originate from the ureters or bladder.[3] In another study, urinary sediments from 65 patients showed eosinophils. In 35 of these 65 patients (54%) with eosinophiluria, the eosinophil count ranged from 1 to over 10% of the total white blood cells (WBC) in the urine; the vast majority, however, had between 1 and 5% eosinophils. The remaining 46% of patients had fewer than 1% of eosinophils.[4] In this study, infections of the upper or lower urinary tract accounted for the largest proportion (45%) of the clinical conditions associated with eosinophiluria. Several individuals had reported eosinophiluria in association with hypersensitivity acute interstitial nephritis.[5]

Diagnosis of Eosinophiluria in Acute Interstitial Nephritis

Normal urine does not contain eosinophils. Therefore, their presence in the urine sediment, or eosinophiluria, appears to be a sign of pathology. Urinary eosinophils have been detected thus far by staining urinary sediment with Wright stain,[4,5] or with May–Grunwald Giemsa stain,[3] in exactly the same way as regular blood films. There is very little information available about the sensitivity and specificity of eosinophiluria as detected by these staining techniques. There are, however, two studies that support the nonspecificity of Wright staining of the urinary sediment in the diagnosis of eosinophiluria. This is shown by the finding that urinary sediments from six patients without clinical evidence of renal or urinary tract disease had eosinophiluria. None of these patients exhibited pyuria or a significant decline in renal function.[4] Also, there is rather firm evidence in that eosinophils are absent in the renal tissue in the face of 6 to 33% urinary eosinophils reported in 14 patients.[3] It is difficult to explain this disparity, and the origin of the urinary eosinophilia.

It can be stated that analysis of the urinary sediment by Wright stain or May–Grunwald Giemsa stain is liable to give false positive or false negative results for eosinophiluria; these staining techniques, however, are fast and economical.

Acute hypersensitivity interstitial nephritis accounts for an unspecified number of acute renal failures (ARF). Because this is a reversible process, especially upon withdrawal of the offending agent, which is often a drug, and upon the institution of corticosteroid therapy, a firm diagnosis of acute interstitial nephritis in the spectrum of ARF is imperative. Eosinophiluria should be considered a hallmark of acute interstitial nephritis, especially when it is accompanied by oliguria and azotemia, though not everyone would agree. Therefore, the presence of eosinophiluria should be precisely established.

In the author's experience, a more definitive method than Wright staining of the urinary sediment to demonstrate eosinophiluria is the analysis of urinary sediment by transmission electron microscopy (TEM). As will be seen, duplicate urinary sediments from two patients were fixed for TEM study on the premise that these urinary sediments were positive for eosinophils when they were stained with Wright stain. The purposes of this study were to determine the reliability of Wright staining of urinary sediment compared to TEM of urinary sediment for eosinophils and to demonstrate the superiority of TEM in assessing urinary sediment for eosinophiluria.

Patient No. 1, H.B., a 53-year-old black male, was admitted to the Medical College of Georgia Hospital, Augusta, Georgia, on August 31, 1985, after open fractures of his right tibia and fibula. The patient underwent surgical repair of the fractures, with debridement of the wounds, and was placed on prophylactic antibiotics (cefazolin and gentamicin) postoperatively for 48 hr.

Subsequently, the patient required multiple debridements and graft procedures and was begun on ticarcillin and tobramycin on September 23, 1985, for suspected infection. On September 26, 1985, his serum urea nitrogen (SUN) and serum creatinine (Scr) were normal (6 mg/dl and 0.7 mg/dl), respectively. On October 14, 1985, antibiotics were discontinued because of a sharp elevation of temperature to 103° F. On October 17, 1985, three days after the antibiotics were discontinued, the patient became oliguric and showed elevations of SUN to 90 mg/dl and Scr to7.2 mg/dl. He also exhibited a 37% peripheral blood eosinophilia (total WBC, 17.4 $\times$ 10^3/mm^3). On October 17 and 24, 1985, light microscopy (LM) of Wright-stained urinary sediment showed many eosinophils; on October 25, 1985, however, a Wright-stained sediment was negative for eosinophils. There was no history of arthralgia, nor was any skin rash found. A diagnosis of acute interstitial nephritis secondary to ticarcillin was made. On October 27, 1985, treatment with prednisone (60 mg orally) was initiated. The patient required temporary hemodialysis for volume overload. In two weeks, his renal function returned to normal. On November 8, 1985, his SUN and Scr were 13 mg/dl and 1.1 mg/dl, respectively, and a blood count showed 7.5 $\times$ 10^3 WBC/mm^3, with 5% eosinophils.

Two separate urinary sediments taken one day apart, October 24 and 25, 1985, were fixed for TEM study in glutaraldehyde–formalin (7:3) in acid medium (pH 5) and with a high osmolality (900 mOsm/kg). Thick or semithin (0.5 μ) sections of the first sediment, when examined by LM, revealed numerous polymorphonuclear leukocytes, some with conspicuous granularity (Fig. 10-1). The prominent granularity suggested that these cells were eosinophils, but the findings were not confirmed by LM. The LM study of the thick sections also revealed many hyaline casts (Fig. 10-2). Thin (300Å) sections were stained with uranyl acetate and lead citrate (UA + LC). The TEM study of the first urinary sediment showed many eosinophils. The eosinophils were confirmed unequivocally by the presence of crystals or crystalloid materials within the granules (Figs. 10-3 and 10-4). No neutrophilic leukocytes were seen, but a few lymphocytes and monocytes were found (Fig. 10-5). As noted earlier, hyaline casts and a few cellular casts (Fig. 10-6) were seen. In the TEM study of the second urinary sediment, there were fewer eosinophils. As in the first sediment, the eosinophilic granules were conspicuously crystalloid (Figs. 10-7–10-9). In one eosinophil, the membrane was disrupted and the granules freed (Fig. 10-9). In the second sediment, however, more lymphocytes and monocytes were found than in the first urinary sediment (Fig. 10-10). As in the first urinary sediment, there were no neutrophilic leukocytes.

Patient No. 2, M.B., a 34-year-old white male, developed multiple infections secondary to quadriplegia following a gunshot wound in the neck on August 24, 1985. He was transferred to the Veterans Administration Medical Center, Augusta, Georgia, from a community hospital in Athens, Georgia, September 23, 1985. He received aminoglycoside antibiotics from January 23 to February 16, 1986. He also received cimetidine, which was initiated on January 23, 1986. His peripheral blood eosinophil count progressively increased, reaching a maximum of 14% on February 21. On the following day, his serum creatinine peaked at 4.9 mg/dl. A Wright-stained urine sediment was reported as showing many eosinophils. Thus a picture of peripheral eosinophilia accompanied by eosinophiluria provided a diagnosis of cimetidine-induced acute interstitial

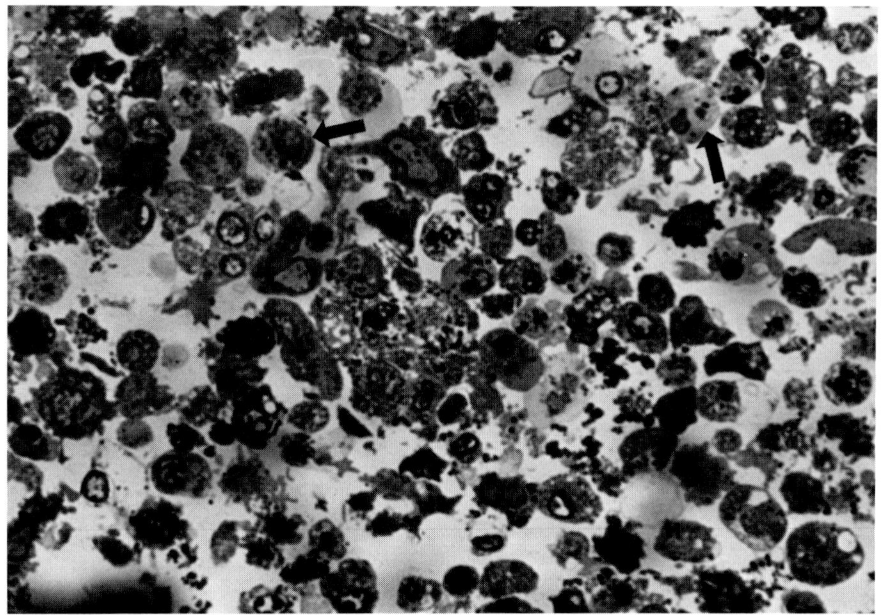

Figure 10-1. Pleocytosis can be seen in this light micrograph, but nucleated cells, with granules, that appear to be eosinophils (arrows) are discernible (toluidine blue and basic fuchsin, ×400).

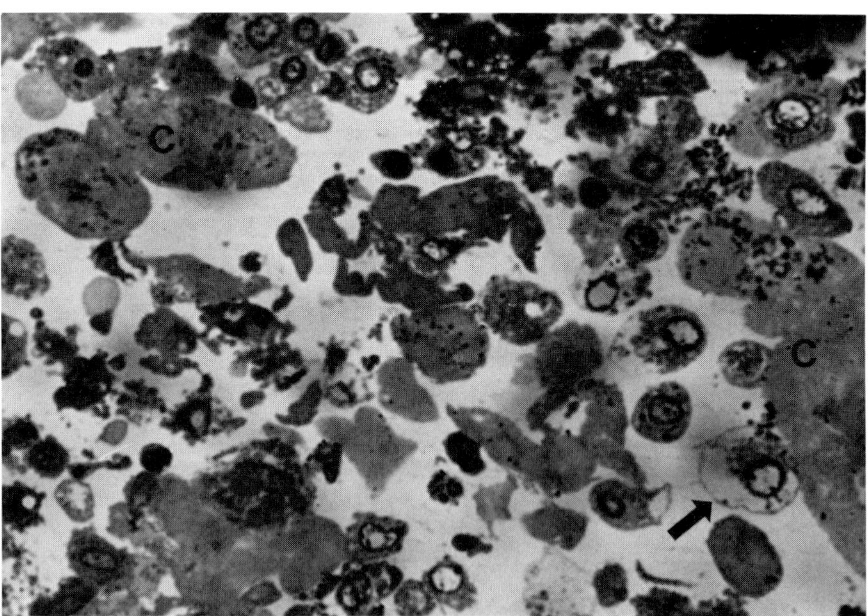

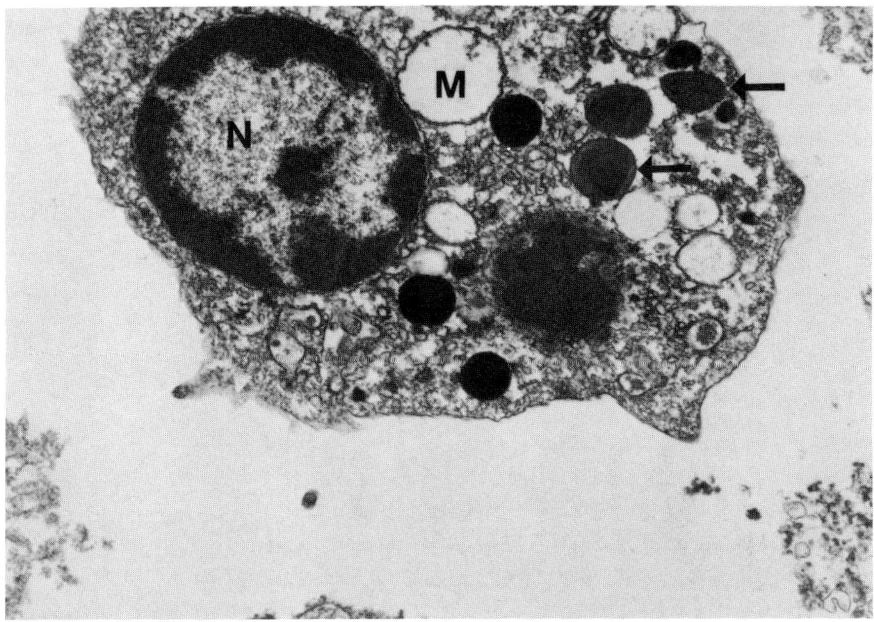

Figure 10-3.   Crystalloid material can be seen within the granules (arrows) of this eosinophil. The cellular membrane and the nucleus (N) appear to be intact, though the mitochondria (M) are swollen (UA + LC, ×10,000).

nephritis. On February 22, cimetidine was discontinued. On February 26, a sample of urine was collected for TEM analysis.

The TEM analysis of the urinary sediment showed tubule epithelial cells and many intracellular and extracellular myeloid bodies. Though numerous inflammatory cells—neutrophils, lymphocytes, and plasma cells—were found (Figs. 10-11 and 10-12), there were no eosinophils.

Patient No. 3, a 63-year-old black male, developed a high fever, accompanied by chills, arthralgia, and a sore throat. He was treated with indomethacin (25 mg) and potassium penicillin (250 mg) each four times daily. Over the following two weeks, the fever, arthralgia, and sore throat improved, but he developed pruritus and an exfoliative dermatitis and his urine output decreased.

Laboratory studies included a peripheral WBC count of 15,000/mm^3, with 36% eosinophils; a serum urea nitrogen level of 116 mg/dl; and a serum creatinine level of

Figure 10-2.   Many hyaline casts (C) and many eosinophils, some releasing granules (arrow), are seen (toluidine blue and basic fuchsin, ×400).

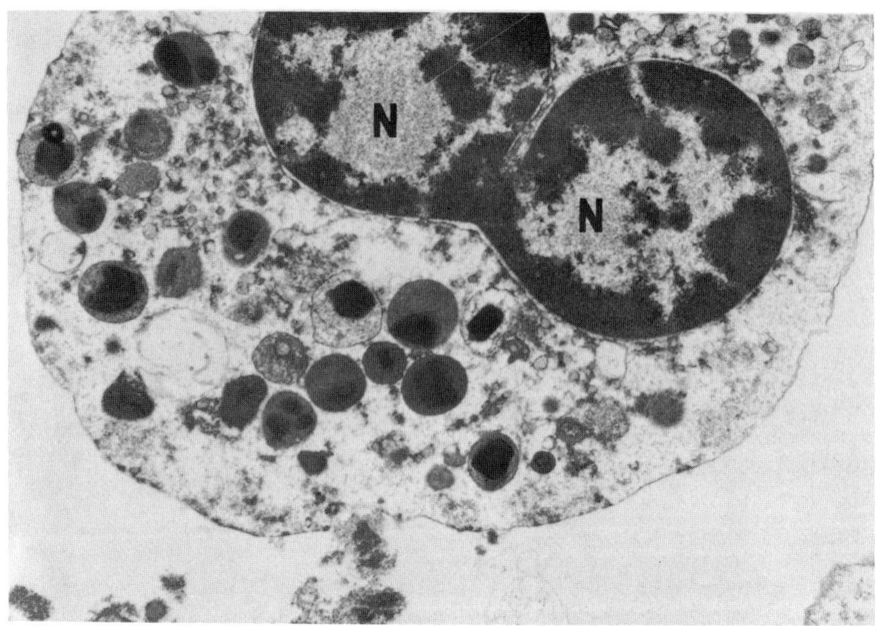

Figure 10-4. In this eosinophil, the intragranular crystalloid material forms conspicuous structures. A bilobed nucleus (N) and an intact cellular membrane can be seen (UA + LC, ×7,500). From *Seminars in Nephrology,* Vol. 6, 1986, with permission.

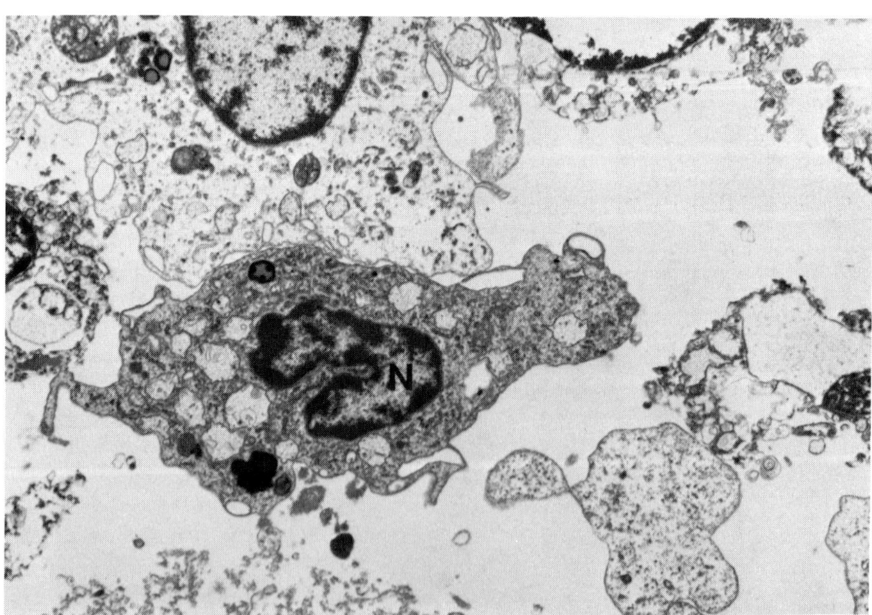

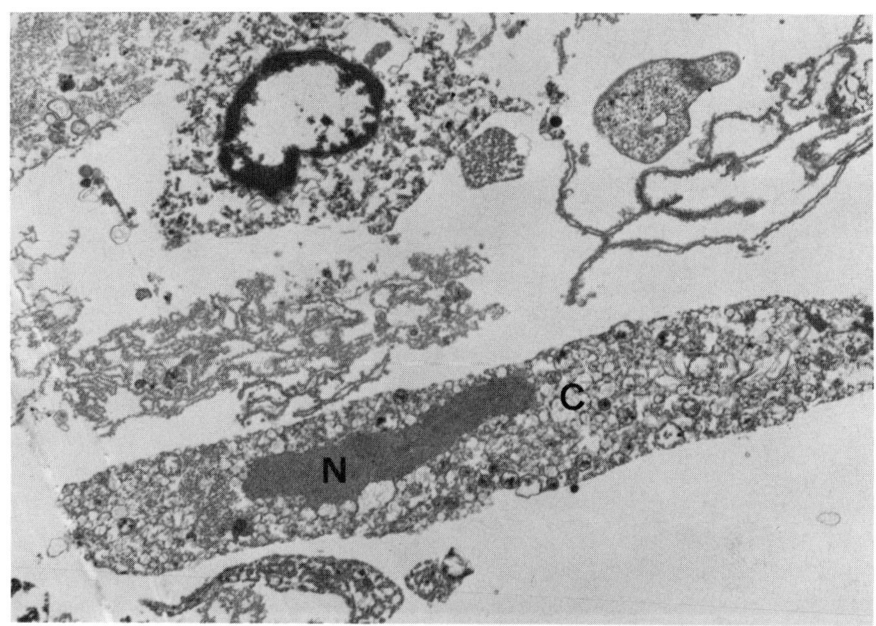

Figure 10-6.   This transmission electron micrograph shows a cellular cast (C) and the nucleus (N) of an epithelial cell (UA + LC, ×4,000).

8.2 mg/dl. There was no proteinuria or hematuria. A percutaneous renal biopsy study revealed a hypersensitivity interstitial nephritis, with numerous eosinophils infiltrating the parenchyma (Fig. 10-13).

Comments: The Wright-stained urinary sediments from patients No. 1 and No. 2 presented here showed eosinophils. Duplicate urinary sediments from these two patients, when fixed simultaneously for TEM analyses, revealed eosinophils only in patient No. 1. The urinary sediment TEM of patient No. 2 revealed many neutrophils but no eosinophils. As mentioned earlier, LM of Wright-stained urinary sediment can be false positive or false negative. Our study exemplifies these problems. In another study, we observed two patients who developed acute interstitial nephritis; one presumably the result of furosemide administration and the other of a nonsteroidal antiinflammatory agent. Urinary sediment, studied by Wright staining, was negative for eosinophils, but renal histopathological studies showed numerous eosinophils for both patients. (See

Figure 10-5.   A monocyte is characterized by a bifid nucleus (N) (UA + LC, ×4,000).

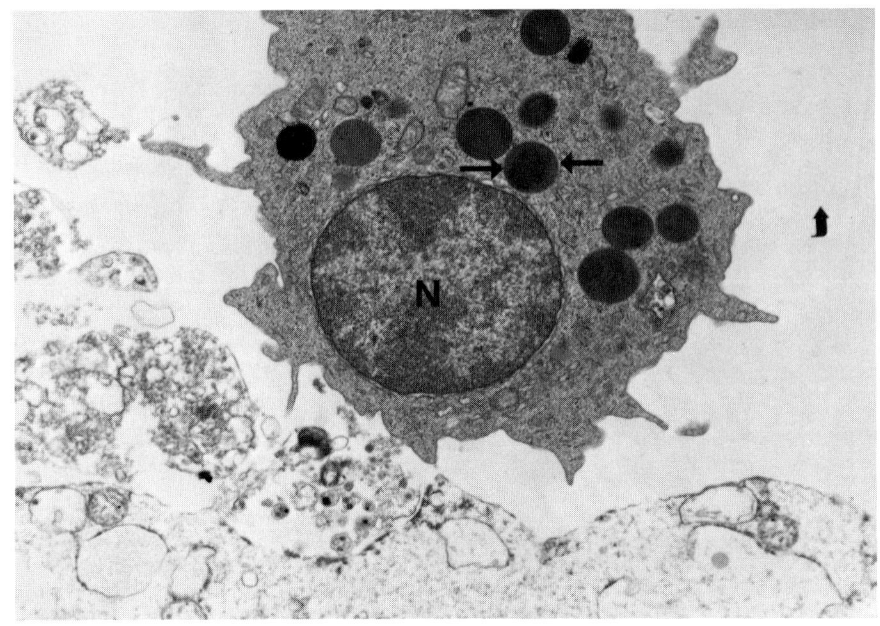

Figure 10-7. This eosinophil shows few granules with intragranular crystalloid material (between arrows) and an intact cytoplasmic structure. The nucleus (N) can also be seen (UA + LC, ×7,500).

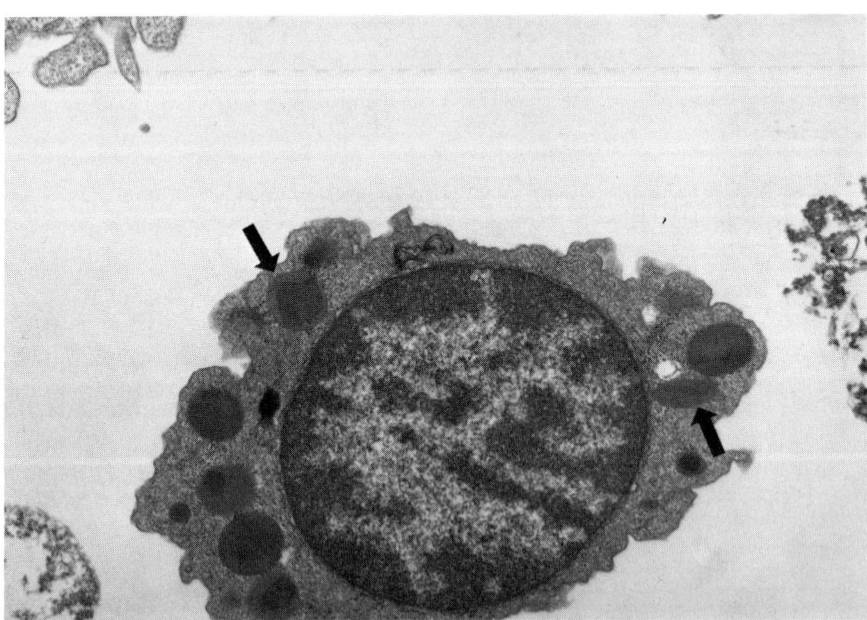

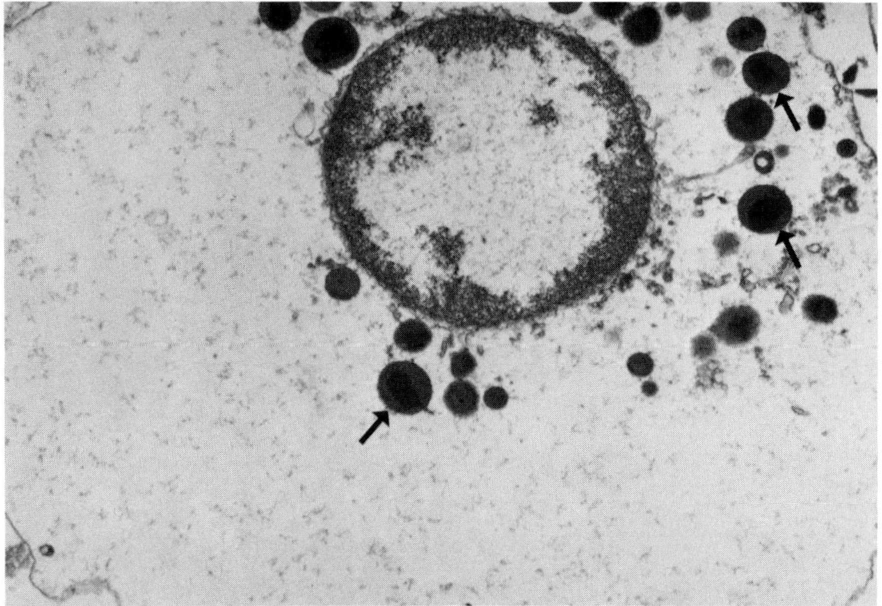

Figure 10-9.   In this eosinophil, the membrane is disrupted, but the intact granules show intragranular crystals (arrows) (UA + LC, ×7,500).

the chapter on drug- and toxin-induced renal disease in the *Diagnosis and Management of Renal Disease and Hypertension*.[6])

It is reasonable to argue that the Wright staining technique is not sensitive enough to detect eosinophiluria, even under the best of circumstances, because of the low optical density of the material under examination and the low resolution of LM. Even though staining increases the optical density of the media to facilitate better visualization of sediment structures, LM cannot delineate the granular crystals or crystalloid material that discriminate between neutrophils and eosinophils. In a Scandinavian study, the dissociation between numerous eosinophils in the urinary sample and the total absence of eosinophils in the renal tissue seemed contradictory. This contradiction raises a serious question about the validity of Wright staining in the examination of urinary sediment for eosinophils. The technique in examining renal tissue, however, is less questionable. If a renal

←

Figure 10-8.   This intact eosinophil contains intragranular crystal and crystalloid material (arrows) (UA + LC, ×10,000). From *Seminars in Nephrology*, Vol. 6, 1986, with permission.

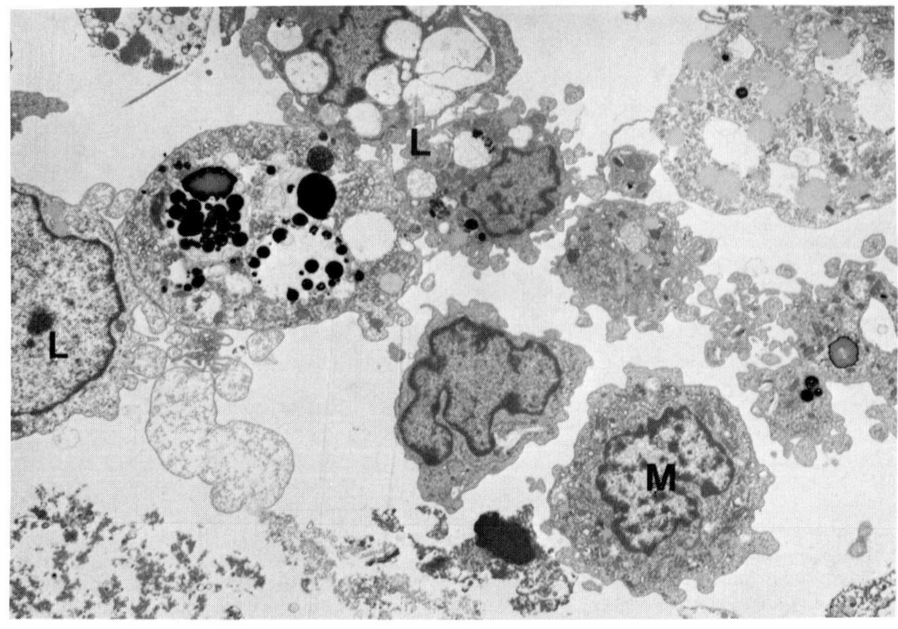

Figure 10-10.   Several lymphocytes (L) and monocytes (M) can be found in this transmission electron micrograph (UA + LC, ×2,500).

biopsy demonstrates eosinophils, as shown in Fig. 10-13, the value of eosinophiluria determined by Wright staining is definitely enhanced.

These pitfalls associated with LM of Wright-stained urinary sediment to determine the presence of urinary eosinophils emphasize the importance of TEM urinary sediment studies. The author's observation underscores the need for TEM analysis of urinary sediment, especially when acute interstitial nephritis is suspected and when the diagnosis depends upon the demonstration of eosinophiluria.[7]

Diagnosis of Hypersensitivity Acute Interstitial Nephritis

Hypersensitivity acute interstitial nephritis is almost always drug induced. The penicillins, most commonly, methicillin; sulfonamides; and diuretics are often incriminated as the cause of acute interstitial nephritis.[8] The exact interval between the administration of the drug and the onset of the pathological process is unknown; overt manifestations, however, are not seen under day 10 or 12 of therapy. The onset of acute interstitial nephritis typically can be from day 12 to

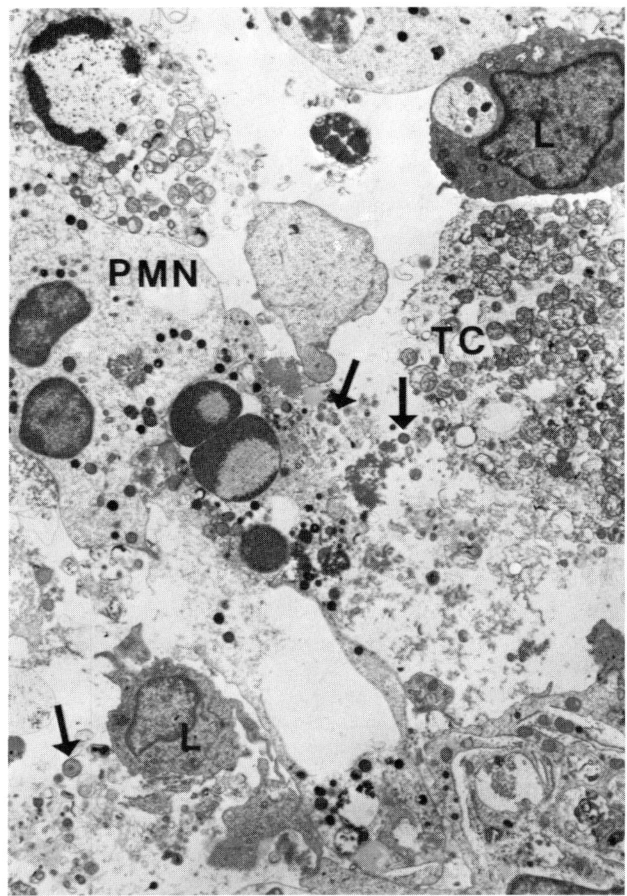

Figure 10-11.   This micrograph shows a tubule cell (TC), neutrophilic leukocytes (PMN), and lymphocytes (L). Many myeloid bodies are seen (arrows) (UA + LC, ×3,000).

21 during the course of therapy. Fever, the most common (100%) presentation, often heralds the onset of acute interstitial nephritis. It may be accompanied by hematuria, pyuria, oliguria, azotemia, or frank ARF, as in patient No. 1. The reported incidence of peripheral blood eosinophilia and eosinophiluria is controversial. Some investigators have reported peripheral blood eosinophilia and eosinophiluria in 100% of their patients[9]; whereas other investigators contend that these two features may be absent in 50% of their patients with histopathologically documented acute interstitial nephritis.[8]

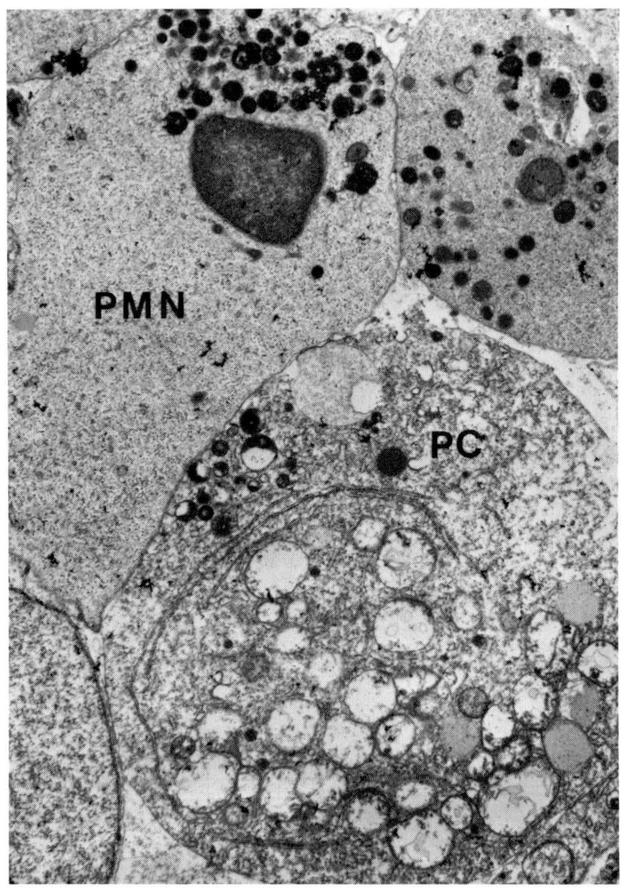

Figure 10-12.   Portions of neutrophilic leukocytes (PMN), and a plasma cell (PC) are visible here (UA + LC, ×5,000).

Short of renal biopsy, there is no definitive diagnostic test that establishes a diagnosis of acute interstitial nephritis. This diagnosis, however, can be established, if urinary sediment TEM reveals eosinophiluria in a patient who develops ARF after receiving allergenic drugs.

Management of Acute Interstitial Nephritis

Management is essentially withdrawal of the drug(s) suspected of causing acute interstitial nephritis and supportive care. Corticosteroid therapy has been shown to enhance recovery of renal function.[8]

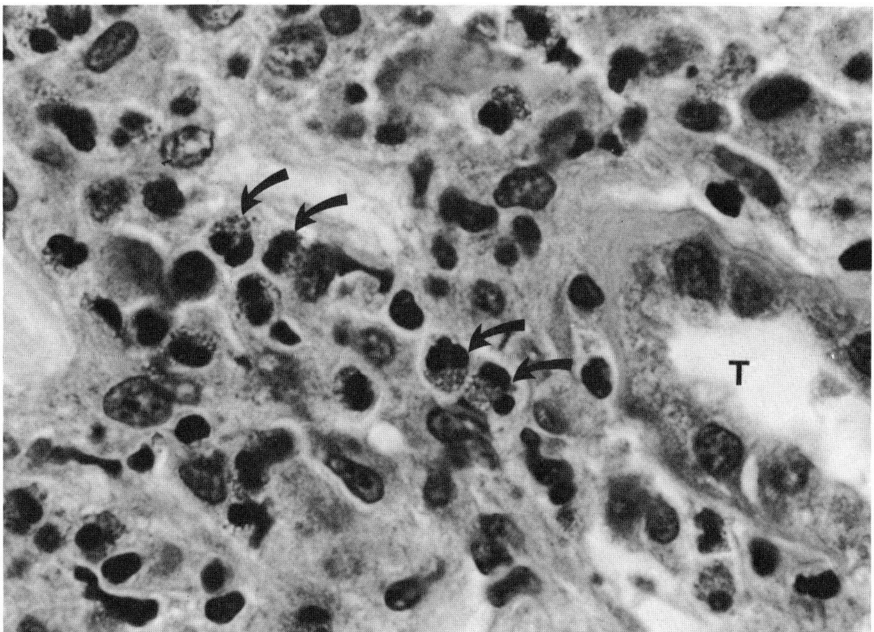

Figure 10-13.   A histopathological study of the renal tissue from patient No. 3 demonstrates the presence of eosinophils (curved arrows) and distal tubule (T) (H & E, ×400).

CHRONIC INTERSTITIAL NEPHRITIS

A 57-year-old while male, E.C., was admitted to the Veterans Administration Medical Center, Augusta, Georgia, on May 17, 1984, for investigation of decreasing appetite, intermittent nausea and vomiting, and elevated serum urea nitrogen and serum creatinine levels. A history of depression with suicide attempts was obtained. He admitted taking six APC (aspirin, phenacetin, and caffeine) tablets daily, as well as Tylenol® and other over-the-counter drugs.

Physical examination was unremarkable. An initial urinalysis showed a few RBC. A repeat urinalysis showed too numerous to count WBC, rare bacteria, rare RBC, and no red blood cell casts. The initial serum chemistry showed urea nitrogen (SUN) 36 mg/dl, and creatinine (Scr) 3.3 mg/dl, but essentially normal electrolytes and CO_2. His urine culture was negative. During his 6-day hospital stay, the patient's SUN and Scr did not change appreciably. A sample of urine was collected for TEM analysis. On the basis of history of heavy consumption of analgesics, sterile pyuria, and renal dysfunction, a diagnosis of analgesic nephropathy was made.

The urinary sediment TEM showed numerous cells that appeared, under low magnification, to be fibroblasts (Fig. 10-14). Under higher magnification, these cells were observed to have long cytoplasmic processes (Fig. 10-15). With still higher magnification,

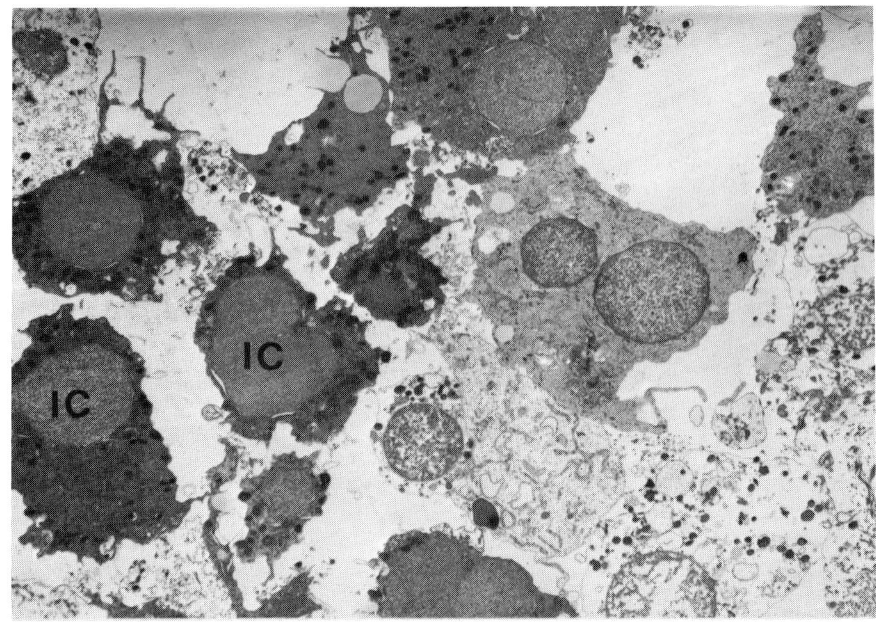

Figure 10-14.   These interstitial cells (IC) have large nuclei and long cytoplasmic processes and contain dark structures that may be granules, which are found in renal papillary interstitial cells (UA + LC, ×1,600).

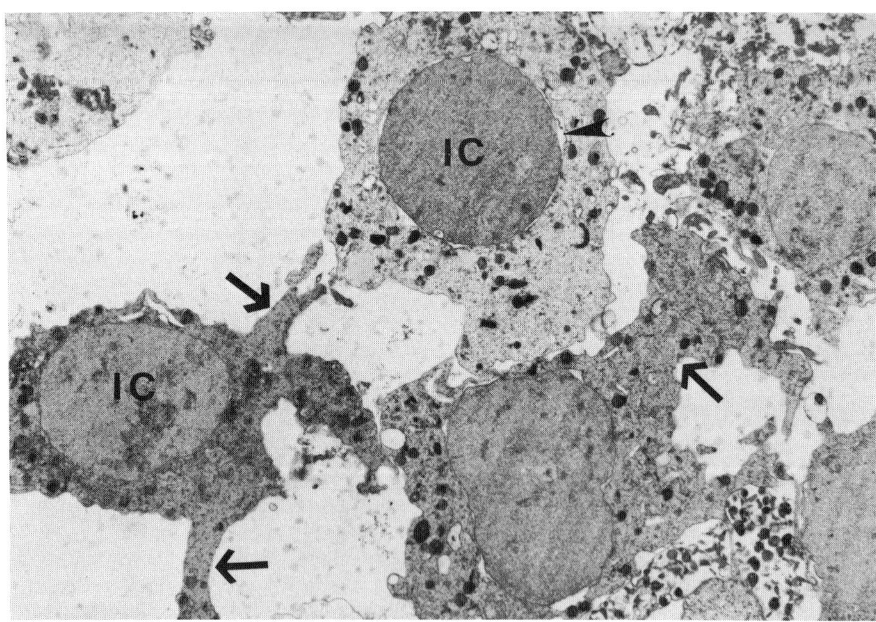

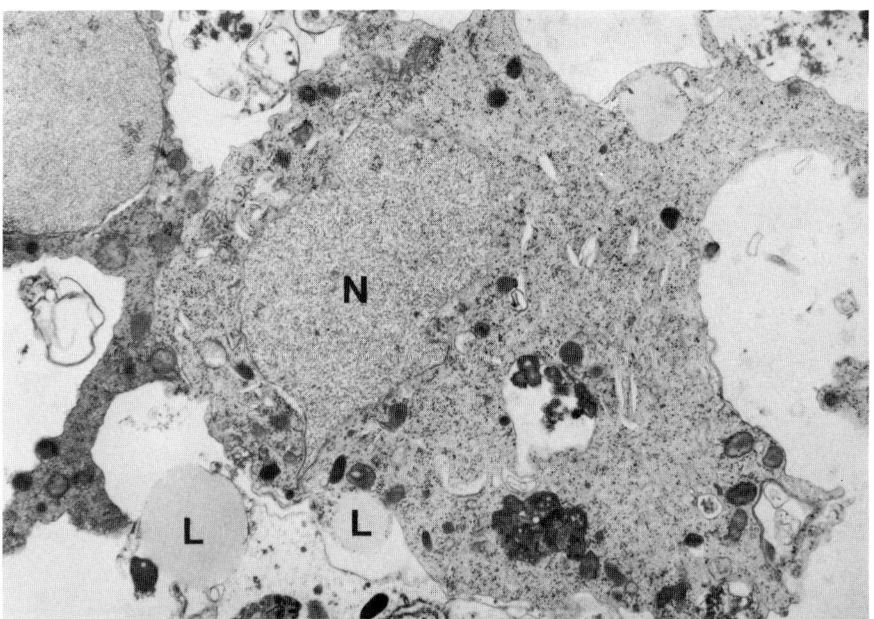

Figure 10-16.   This interstitial cell shows conspicuous lipid droplets (L) and a nucleus (N). The cell is rich in ribosomes (UA + LC, ×5,000).

the cells were found to be rich in ribosomes and to contain many dilated endoplasmic reticula. The striking features of these cells were prominent lipid droplets and occasional calcium deposits (Figs. 10-16 and 10-18).

The patient was advised not to take analgesics or pain medication. A repeat serum chemistry two months later showed an appreciable decrement in serum creatinine (2.2 mg/dl), but his SUN remained essentially unchanged. Subsequently, the patient was lost to follow-up.

The cells found in the urinary sediment were a specialized type of fibroblasts, the interstitial cells. The presence of lipid droplets, abundant ribosomes, and many cytoplasmic processes are typical of type I interstitial cells. These interstitial cells are normally located in the papilla and in the proximal outer medulla.[10] Therefore, the appearance of numerous type I interstitial cells in the urinary sediment in the absence of bacteriuria suggests some type of noninfectious injury involving the renal medulla and/or renal papilla. The sterile pyuria was further evidence. Analgesics and uric acid preferentially affect the

Figure 10-15.   The long cytoplasmic processes (arrows) are clearly evident in these interstitial cells (IC). The perinuclear cisterna (arrowhead) is not dilated, which suggests a well-fixed specimen (UA + LC, ×2,600).

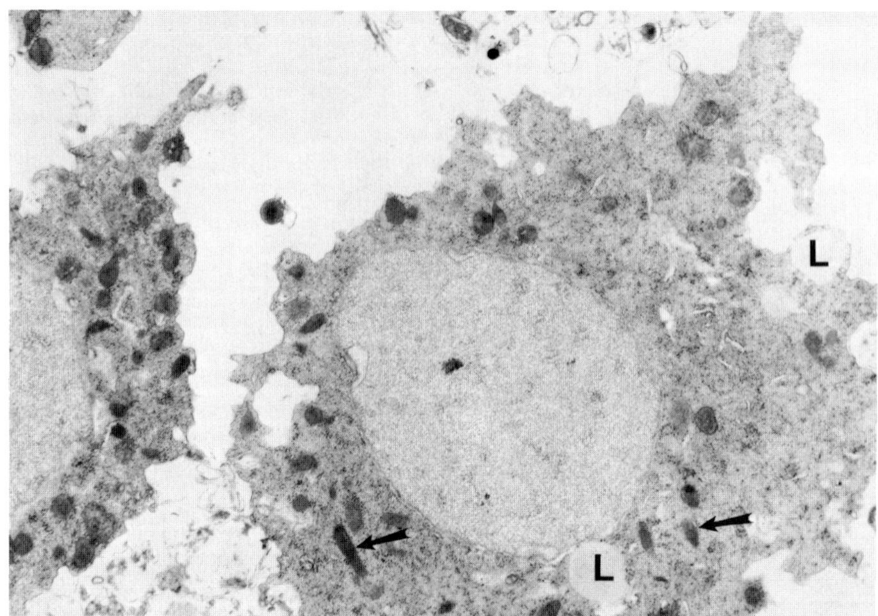

Figure 10-17.   In this interstitial cell, a moderate number of elongated mitochondria (arrows) and prominent lipid droplets (L) can be seen (UA + LC, ×5,000).

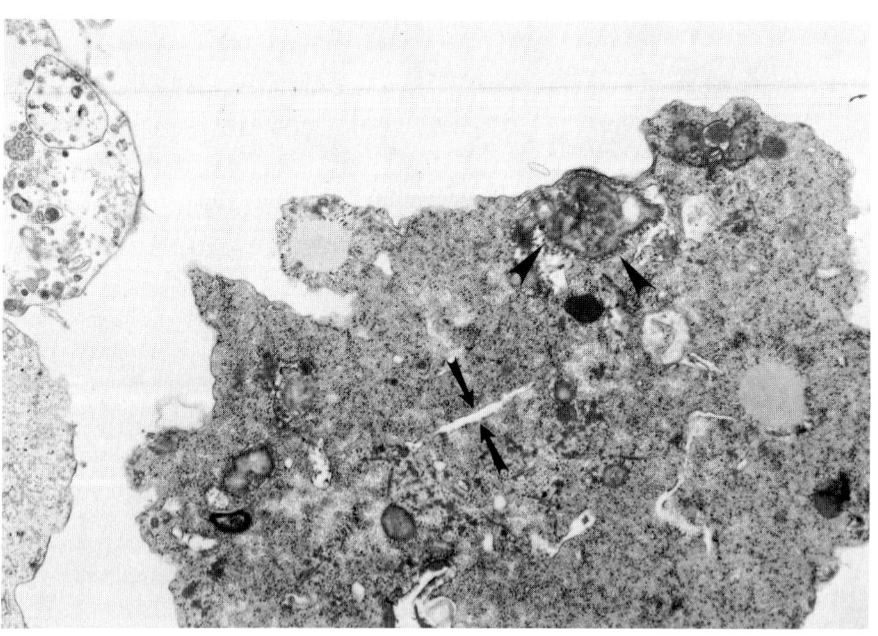

renal medulla. Since this patient had a history of heavy consumption of analgesics and presented with renal insufficiency, analgesic nephropathy was a logical diagnosis.

The pathological lesion of analgesic nephropathy begins in the inner medulla and papilla as focal areas of necrosis, which progress to total papillary necrosis. In the advanced stage of analgesic nephropathy, the necrotic papilla is structureless and often calcified.[11] Calcium deposits were observed in the interstitial cells of the urinary sediment of the patient presented above (Fig. 10-18). For more information on analgesic nephropathy, the reader should consult the chapter on drug- and toxin-induced renal disease in *Diagnosis and Management of Renal Disease and Hypertension.*[6]

Thus far, there is no definitive test, including percutaneous renal biopsy, that establishes a diagnosis of analgesic nephropathy. Furthermore, it is very difficult to biopsy the papilla, in which the most severe lesions are seen. It is equally difficult to confirm a diagnosis of other types of chronic interstitial nephritis. A history of polyuria and nocturia, evidence of impairment in the acidification of urine, anemia, mild proteinuria, an essentially inactive urinary sediment, and irregularly small kidneys by radiological examination are the usual features of chronic interstitial nephritis. None of these features alone is diagnostic. A renal biopsy of a relatively normal area of the kidney can lead to even more confusion in the overall diagnosis.

Since all forms of chronic interstitial nephritis primarily involve the medulla and papilla and are progressive, a technique that delineates the cellular components in the urinary sediment should be useful. Therefore, urinary sediment TEM may provide valuable aid in the diagnosis by showing interstitial cells that distinguish diseases involving the renal papilla from those involving renal cortex and in showing the disease process by serial studies. Numerous urinary interstitial cells may indicate an active process; few urinary interstitial cells may indicate that the disease has run its course. Urinary sediment TEM is particularly important in the diagnosis of analgesic nephropathy, especially when the history of analgesic intake is equivocal.

Management

Management consists first of removal of the cause (for example, analgesic or lead). In the case of analgesic nephropathy, discontinuation of the drug results in renal function improvement. Similarly, treatment of lead nephropathy with

Figure 10-18.   In this interstitial cell, dilated endoplasmic reticula (between arrows) and a calcium deposit (arrowheads) are shown. Note the large number of ribosomes (UA + LC, × 6,600).

edetate calcium disodium (calcium EDTA, a chelating agent) leads to an improvement in renal function. Second, supportive care, and third follow-up of patients. Some patients despite withdrawal of the analgesic or chelation of the heavy metal, progress to develop a chronic renal failure that requires dialysis.

REFERENCES

1. Eisenstaedt JS: Allergy and drug hypersensitivity of the urinary tract. *J Urol* 1951; 65:154–162.
2. Spencer ES, Peterson VP: The urinary sediment after renal transplantation: Quantitative changes as an index of the activity of the renal allograft reaction. *Acta Med Scand* 1967; 182:73–82.
3. Helgason S, Lindqvist B: Eosinophiluria. *Scand J Urol Nephrol* 1972; 6:257–259.
4. Corwin HL, Korbet SM, Schwartz MM: Clinical correlates of eosinophiluria. *Arch Intern Med* 1985; 145:1097–1099.
5. Linton AL, Clark WF, Driedger AA, et al: Acute interstitial nephritis due to drugs. *Annu Intern Med* 1980; 93:735–741.
6. Jennette JC, Mandal AK: Drug and toxin-induced renal disease, in Mandal AK, Jennette JC (eds): *Diagnosis and Management of Renal Disease and Hypertension*. Philadelphia, Lea & Febiger, 1987.
7. Mandal AK: Transmission electron microscopy of urinary sediment in renal disease. *Sem Nephrol* 1986; 6:346–370.
8. Linton AL, Lindsay RM: Drug-induced acute interstitial nephritis. *The Kidney* 1982; 15:1–4.
9. Galpin JE, Shinaberger JH, Stanley TM, et al: Acute interstitial nephritis due to methicillin. *Am J Med* 1978; 65:756–765.
10. Bohman, SO: Ultrastructure of the renal medulla and the interstitial cells, in Mandal AK, Bohman SO (eds): *The Renal Papilla and Hypertension*. New York, Plenum Medical Book Co, 1980, pp 7–28.
11. Heptinstall RH: Renal complications of therapeutic and diagnostic agents, analgesic abuse, and addiction to narcotics. In *Pathology of The Kidney*, Boston, Little, Brown, 1983, pp 1195–1255.

Index